Queering Nutrition and Dietetics

This book presents the experiences of LGBTQ+ people relating to food, bodies, nutrition, health, wellbeing, and being queer through critical writing and creative art.

The chapters bring LGBTQ+ voices into the spotlight through arts-based scholarship and contribute to experiential learning, allowing for more understanding of the lives of LGBTQ+ people within the dietetic profession. Divided into three parts, the first explores eating, food, and bodies; the second discusses communities, connections, and celebrations; and the final part covers care in practice. Topics include body image, eating disorders, weight stigma, cooking and culinary journeys, queer food culture, queer practices in nutrition counselling, and gendered understandings of nutrition. Exploring not only experiences of marginalization, homophobia, transphobia, and cisheteronormativity within dietetics and nutritional healthcare, this collection also dives into the positive connections and supportive communities that food can create. Special attention is paid to the intersections of oppression, colonialism, social justice, and politics.

This book will be beneficial to all health professionals, educators, and students creating and fostering safer, more inclusive, and more accepting environments for their LGBTQ+ clients.

Phillip Joy is an assistant professor at Mount Saint Vincent University. His research focuses on queer nutrition and health. He is the co-editor for *Rainbow Reflections: Body Image Comics for Queer Men.*

Megan Aston is a professor and the associate director of Research and International Affairs at Dalhousie University in the School of Nursing. She teaches and researches in the areas of social justice, community, family, and perinatal health.

Queering Nutrition and Dietetics

LGBTQ+ Reflections on Food Through Art

Edited by Phillip Joy and Megan Aston

Routledge
Taylor & Francis Group

NEW YORK AND LONDON

Cover image created by Phillip Joy and Maritza Miari

First published 2023
by Routledge
605 Third Avenue, New York, NY 10158

and by Routledge
4 Park Square, Milton Park, Abingdon, Oxon, OX14 4RN

Routledge is an imprint of the Taylor & Francis Group, an informa business

ISBN: 978-1-032-10795-0 (hbk)
ISBN: 978-1-032-10794-3 (pbk)
ISBN: 978-1-003-21712-1 (ebk)

DOI: 10.4324/9781003217121

Typeset in Baskerville
by Deanta Global Publishing Services, Chennai, India

Contents

PART 2
Communities, Connections, and Celebrations 107

Figures

About the Editors

Aston, Megan, PhD, RN

Dr Aston (she/her) is a registered nurse and professor at the School of Nursing, Dalhousie University, Canada. She uses feminist poststructuralism informed by discourse analysis to examine issues of social justice and how healthcare professionals and clients negotiate beliefs, values, and practices regarding healthcare that have been socially and institutionally constructed through relations of power. Her research primarily focuses on community, family, and perinatal and newborn health, as well as children with intellectual disabilities, their families, and healthcare professionals who care for them. She teaches Qualitative Health Research and Family and Community Health Nursing. She can be contacted at megan.aston@dal.ca

Joy, Phillip, PhD, RD

Dr Joy (he/him) is a registered dietitian with the Nova Scotia Dietetic Association (NSDA) and an Assistant Professor at Mount Saint Vincent Univeristy, Halifax, Nova Scotia, Canada. His research interests are driven by his own experiences as part of the LGBTQ+ community. His research perspective is through the lens of poststructuralism and queer theory and provides both a personal and political perspective on the topic of nutrition, gender, sexuality, nutrition pedagogy, and health. His research often uses arts-based methodologies, such as photography and comics, that can disrupt the foundations of nutrition and health research. He was co-editor of *Rainbow Reflections: Body Image Comics for Queer Men*. He can be contacted at phillip.joy@msvu.ca

Contributors

Aden, Andronicus Andronicus Aden completed his MPhil in English from Jadavpur University, Kolkata, India. He received his MA in English from Jadavpur University and his BA in English from Scottish Church College (University of Calcutta), Kolkata, India. His areas of interest include postcolonial Shakespearean studies, Lepcha folklore, and Nepali literature. He has contributed a chapter in the edited volume titled *Asian Interventions in Global Shakespeare: "All the World's His Stage"* (Routledge, 2021). He is an amateur cook who is interested in the ethnic food cultures of North Bengal.

Alexander, Marissa Marissa Alexander (she/her or they/them), RD, works as a regional dietitian on the traditional territory of the Lheidli T'enneh. In her role she has the opportunity to work with all 55 First Nations communities in the Northern Region of BC, Canada. She is passionate about advocacy, social justice, and the intersection of food and aims to bring this passion into her work as much as possible. As a dietitian of colour, she prioritizes anti-racism in her work and life, and this journey has led her to pursue a Masters in Interdisciplinary Studies with a focus on equity.

Anderson, Mikey Mikey Anderson, MAAT, LPC (they/them & he/him), is a queer artist–art therapist who graduated from the School of the Art Institute of Chicago, USA, with a BFA in fine art and an MA in art therapy and counselling. Their art practice is informed by a community-driven art therapy practice, which incorporates fibre crafts, illustrations, queer theory, and activism. Their artworks range from embroideries and quilts to comics and a handmade plush toy line they call "Yarnies." Their artworks are soft, bubbly, cuddly, and invite participation. These artworks entice people to come closer, where the underlying message about queer advocacy becomes evident. They strive to broaden queer representation by way of both their art and art therapy practices. Through the sessions they run, the community-based art projects they facilitate, and the Yarnies they create, they are committed to queer advocacy.

Aphramor, Lucy Lucy Aphramor is a radical dietitian and spoken word poet based in England. They wrote the popular HAES book *Body Respect* with Lindo Bacon. Lucy recognizes *Body Respect* as a manifesto for coloniality and, with apologies, encourages anyone (else) who missed this to revisit the text holding space for new awareness. Lucy is also an associate professor of Gender, Power, and the Right to Food at Coventry University, England. Contact Lucy at: aa0059@coventry.ac.uk

Armstrong, Emerson "Kai" Emerson "Kai" Armstrong (MA, Saint Louis University) is a doctoral student in the Department of Communication & Journalism at the University of New Mexico, USA.

Baeza Scagliusi, Fernanda She has a degree in Nutrition from the University of São Paulo, São Paulo, Brazil, a PhD in Physical Education, also from the University of São Paulo, and a post-doctorate in Public Health Nutrition from the School of Public Health at the University of São Paulo. She is a professor at the University of São Paulo, School of Public Health, Department of Nutrition. She has experience in Nutrition, emphasizing Food and Culture in interface with Gender, Food Consumption and Food Vulnerabilities, Stigma, and other subjects. fernanda.scagliusi@gmail.com

Bockus-Thorne, Laura Laura Bockus-Thorne is a Registered Dietitian (RD), Master's graduate, researcher, and mixed-media artist, currently residing in Dartmouth, Nova Scotia, Canada. She enjoys combining her passion for nutrition and art to create interactive educational tools and therapeutic art pieces. Her distinctive personal style as an artist aims to tell a story, whether it is a journey through healthy eating for different chronic disease states, advocating for healthy fruit and vegetable intakes, or delving into critical dietetics. Laura hopes to further explore options for combining her love of research, dietetics, and artistry.

Brennan, David J. Dr David J. Brennan, MSW, RSW, PhD, Professor and Associate Dean, Research, serves as an OHTN HIV Endgame Leadership Chair in Gay and Bisexual Men's Health (Social Work) and the founding director of the CRUISElab, an interdisciplinary social work research lab that is centred on community-based research that investigates issues related to HIV/STBBIs, as well as broader issues of the health and wellbeing among gay, bisexual, Two-spirit, and other men who have sex with men (GB2M). His work focuses on online apps and tools for sociosexual connections, health education, and service access among GB2M. Professor Brennan serves as the lead for the Investigaytors Toronto team, a community-based research training programme for young GB2M. Professor Brennan's work is focused on community-based research methods that include quantitative, qualitative, and mixed-methods designs.

Brisco, Anna Anna Brisco (they/them or she/her), RD, MEd, is passionate about relational pedagogies that honour narratives, embrace embodiment(s), and imagine equitable futures. They hold a Bachelor of Science in Food, Nutrition, and Health (2016) from the University of British Columbia, Canada, and work in the field of education. Their masters (2022) focused on transformative, justice-oriented, and decolonizing approaches to dietetic education and K-12 health science curricula. Anna, a settler of European ancestry, lives in unceded, traditional, and shared Sḵwx̱wú7mesh (Squamish), xʷməθkʷəy̓əm (Musqueam), and səĺílwətaʔɬ (Tseil-Watuth) territories (Vancouver, BC) with their partner Shila, and their fluffy cat.

Castle, Maxie Maxie is a white community organizer, prison abolitionist, and writer living in unceded Wurundjeri Country in so-called Australia.

Chamberlain, Edward Dr Edward Chamberlain is an Associate Professor of Cultural Studies at the University of Washington Tacoma, USA. His research interests include the study of food, gender, and migration across the Americas. Dr Chamberlain's recent monograph is titled *Imagining Latinx Intimacies: Connecting Queer Stories, Spaces, Sexualities* (2020). He also has published research in such journals as *Lateral, Pacific Coast Philology,* and *The CEA Critic.* He is currently working on a new monograph that examines the sociopolitical connections of queer food experiences and consumption in several cultural contexts.

Coffey, Melik D.H. Melik D.H. Coffey, MSW, LCSW, (he/him/his) is a licensed mental health clinician with over a decade of experience in clinical services such as individual, family, and group therapy, crisis intervention, and case management. As a graduate of the Brown School of Social Work at Washington University, Saint Louis, USA, Melik has chosen to base his area of clinical focus on Child and Adolescent Mental Health, Youth Violence Prevention, Human Trafficking and Sexual Exploitation, and Criminogenic Risk and Behavioural Health Needs. Melik has furthered his education and learning at the Saint Louis Psychoanalytic Institute, where he was trained in psychodynamic practice to better treat individuals and families who have experienced compound and complex trauma.

Collins, Mikhail Mikhail Collins is a recent graduate of Arizona State University, USA, with a bachelor's degree in Queer and Sexuality Studies and minor in Sociocultural Anthropology. They live in sunny Phoenix, Arizona, and spend most of their time writing. They hope to continue their education with graduate school within the field of women and gender studies and queer theory in the coming years.

Crack, Shelly Shelly Crack is a Scottish, Irish, English, Canadian settler who was born and raised on 100 acres of land on Robinson-Superior Treaty territory, which is the traditional territory of the Anishnaabeg. Shelly trained as a dietitian at UBC and moved to the northern region of BC, Canada, where she is raising her two children, Freya and Huxley, with her wife Traci. Shelly enjoys yoga, swimming, dancing, and cooking. Shelly has a passion for unlearning current colonial systems and supporting social justice through local food system work. She has gratitude for the unceded land of the Haida Nation where she lives, works, and plays.

Davies, Adam W.J. Dr Adam Davies, PhD, OCT, RECE, is an Assistant Professor of Family Relations and Human Development at the University of Guelph, Canada, and an Ontario Registered Teacher and Ontario Registered Early Childhood Educator. Adam's research interests are in gay masculinities, anti-oppressive approaches to education and social work, sexuality education, queer theory, and critical disability studies. Adam's current project investigates psychosocial determinants of supplement usage and gendered ideologies amongst gay, bisexual, queer, and non-binary communities. Adam has a PhD in Education and Sexual Diversity Studies and Women and Gender Studies from the Ontario Institute for Studies in Education, University of Toronto.

Dimitrov Ulian, Mariana Mariana Dimitrov Ulian is a nutritionist who graduated from the Federal University of São Paulo, São Paulo, Brazil, and holds a Master of Science from the same institution. She also holds a PhD from the University of São Paulo – School of Public Health – and participates in the Food and Culture Research Group of the University of São Paulo. She works mainly on the themes of obesity, food choices, culture, and the body. She has experience in applying care proposals based on expanded clinical nutrition and nutritional counselling for people with obesity. Currently, she is a post-doctoral fellow at the School of Public Health at the University of São Paulo. mari_dimi @hotmail.com

Doll, Kaitrin aka Big Poppa Kaitrin Doll (they/them) is a second-year doctoral student at the Factor-Inwentash Faculty of Social Work, University of Toronto, Canada. Through queer, anti-oppressive, and intersectional frameworks, Kaitrin is committed to research that will support more affirmative, representative, and inclusive policies and practices to support queer, trans, and gender-diverse people. Kaitrin's doctoral research will focus on the experiences of queer, trans, and gender-diverse people who play roller derby and any connection with resilience and mental wellness. They have research experience with sexual gender minority youth and information communication technologies, social work and mental health, LGBTQIA+ populations, people experiencing homelessness, and youth social enterprise. When not working Kaitrin can be found cycling, park skating, exploring with their partner and their dog (Doc), and not so patiently waiting for the return of roller derby. Kaitrin.doll @mail.utoronto.ca

Eguchi, Shinsuke Shinsuke Eguchi (PhD, Howard University) is an Associate Professor in the Department of Communication and Journalism at the University of New Mexico, USA.

El-Khoury, Dalia Dr Dalia El-Khoury is an Assistant Professor of Applied Human Nutrition in the Department of Family Relations and Applied Nutrition at the University of Guelph, Canada. Dalia received a BSc in Nutrition and Dietetics (2002) and an MSc in Nutrition (2005) at the American University of Beirut, Lebanon. Dalia completed a PhD in Physiology and Physiopathology at the University of Pierre et Marie Curie, France (2008).

Dalia served as a lecturer at the American University of Beirut (2009–2010), and as a postdoctoral fellow and lecturer at the University of Toronto (2010–2014). Dalia is a Licensed Dietitian in Lebanon and has recently obtained the status of Registered Dietitian in Canada. Dalia's research interests have primarily focused on the role of functional ingredients/foods in the regulation of appetite, food intake, glycemia, and metabolism in healthy individuals and individuals with nutrition-related disorders including overweight/obesity, hyperinsulinemia, and metabolic syndrome.

Fernandez Unsain, Ramiro Ramiro Fernandez Unsain holds a degree in Anthropology and a Masters in Anthropological Sciences both from the University of Buenos Aires, Argentina, and a PhD in Health Sciences from the Federal University of São Paulo, Brazil. He is a post-doctoral fellow at the University of São Paulo, School of Public Health, and has experience in anthropology, with emphasis on Anthropology and Sociology of Health and Food, working on public health, food, and food choices/practices, obesity, intersectionality, sexuality, gender, identity, ethnicity, and research methodology. He is a researcher at the Research Group on Food and Culture, University of São Paulo, a guest researcher at the University of Buenos Aires, and a professor in the Universidad San Francisco Xavier, Bolivia. ramirofunsain@yahoo.co.uk

Forrest, Michelle Michelle Forrest is Professor of Philosophy of Education, Mount Saint Vincent University, Kjipuktuk (Halifax), Mi'kma'ki (Nova Scotia), Canada. Having trained as an actor and classical singer and taught secondary-school English and Drama, she writes and teaches pre- and in-service teachers about the ethics of teaching, collaborative inquiry, feminist pedagogy, and the value of art and philosophy in challenging bias and closed-mindedness. Her recent publications include "Valuing a Feminist Ethics of Care in Pandemic Times," *Global Feminist Autoethnographies During COVID-19*, Routledge, 2022; "Out of the Closet and into Quarantine: Stories of Isolation and Teaching" with Phillip Joy, Atlantis: Critical Studies in *Gender, Culture, and Social Justice* 42.1, 2021; and *Scripting Feminist Ethics in Teacher Education*, with Linda Wheeldon, University of Ottawa Press, 2019. Michelle actively supports her faculty union, having served in several executive positions, and cherishes her career-long involvement in the Canadian Association of Foundations of Education. She has been managing and general editor of *Philosophical Inquiry in Education* and sits on the advisory board of *The Canadian Journal of Education*. She and her wife live in coastal Nova Scotia, where she has worked with a community organization to save the local lighthouse as a federal heritage site.

Fraser, Kathryn Kathryn, MScAHN PDt (they/them, she/her), is a queer, non-binary dietitian originally from a small town in South Shore, Nova Scotia, Canada. They have a passion for helping people expand their worlds by recognizing and healing challenging relationships with food and bodies by drawing upon a trauma-informed, anti-diet, inclusive, and body-liberating lens of recovery from disordered eating and eating disorders. In their spare time they enjoy fermenting, pickling, attempting to make jam, and knitting. Occasionally they can be found dabbling in academia on the side.

Gingras, Jacqui Jacqui Gingras, PhD, is an Associate Professor in the Department of Sociology at X University in T'karonto, Ontario, Canada. Her research explores social health movements, fat studies, radical democratic pedagogies, and decolonization of health professions within the entanglements of colonial neoliberal economics and intersectional feminisms. She has published in the *Fat Studies Journal*, *Journal of Sociology*, and *Critical Public Health*. She is an Associate Member of the Communication and Culture graduate programme, a joint programme between X and York Universities. She is the founding editor of the *Journal of Critical Dietetics*, an open-access, peer-reviewed journal at https://journals.library.ryerson.ca/index.php/criticaldietetics/index

Greening, Alo Alo Greening (they/them) is a queer-identifying psychology student who spends their time working on school, attending therapy, watching anime, and reading. Their interests lie in gender and sexuality, social media, and mental illness.

Gupta, Gunita Gunita is a high school English and Foods teacher in Langley, BC, Canada. She is currently pursuing doctoral studies in education at the University of British Columbia. Her research interests include exploring the ways in which local/personal knowledge might function as a counternarrative to normative discursive constructions of food and nutrition. Despite living in a temperate rainforest all her life, Gunita has lately come to realize that she is a solar-powered individual. In no particular order, she loves dogs, bikes, cooking, eating, reading, and being outside.

Hanson, Treena Treena Hanson is a retired Dietitian and Certified Diabetes Educator. She worked the majority of her career at the Diabetes Centre at St Paul's Hospital in Vancouver, Canada, and was actively involved with Diabetes Canada, volunteering her time at Diabetes Days and participating in activities such as "Ask the Dietitian." Treena was a member of Team Diabetes and participated in running events around the world and a mountain biking event in Iceland. She finished her career as a Coordinator of a Diabetes Education programme in Tillsonburg, Ontario. She is very proud of her accomplishments and all the wonderful people she met over the years.

Hoffelmeyer, Michaela Michaela Hoffelmeyer is a PhD candidate in Rural Sociology and Women's, Gender, and Sexuality Studies at Pennsylvania State University, USA. Michaela's research interests include gender and sexuality in agriculture, sustainability, and food justice. Michaela has conducted research related to LGBTQ farmers, rural and urban women farmers, and sustainability initiatives. They are working on a dissertation about the experiences of meatpacking plant workers in Iowa across different scales of meat production. Michaela's research works to understand how social location and power in the agrifood system affect rural livelihoods and community vitality. Email: mkh40 @psu.edu. Twitter handle: M_Hoffelmeyer

Kaner, Esther Esther Kaner is a postgraduate student in Biosocial Medical Anthropology at UCL, UK, with interests in the anthropology of food and nutrition, community health activism, chronic illness, and the emergence collective care and mutual aid under neoliberalism. She has been a member of the Public and Patient Involvement Group for Integrating Care for Trans Adults, a large-scale research project exploring barriers to integrating transgender-related healthcare in the UK, for over two years. She can be found on Twitter: @EstherKaner.

Kasten, Gerry Gerry Kasten (any pronoun) loves food! He was born to a farming family and still helps their brother bring in the harvest each year. She has an Honours Diploma in Commercial Cooking and both Bachelors and Masters degrees in Nutrition. His Masters research was on food choices amongst gay men. They worked in Public Health in British Columbia, Canada for 30 years. She has a chequered past which led him to a critical analysis of the constructions of gender, particularly as they are enacted through food. He lives and plays on the traditional, unceded land of the Sḵwx̱wú7mesh, Səlílwəta?, and xʷməθkʷəy̓əm peoples.

Ketchum, Alex Dr Alex Ketchum (alexketchum.ca) has been the Faculty Lecturer of the Institute for Gender, Sexuality, and Feminist Studies of McGill University, Canada, since 2018. Alex is the author of the forthcoming book, *Ingredients for Revolution* (2022), a history of lesbian feminist restaurants, cafes, and coffeehouses in the United States from the 1972 to the present. She is the founder of The Feminist Restaurant Project (www.thefeministrestaurantproject.com) and the co-founder and editor of The Historical Cooking Project (historicalcookingproject.com), a website dedicated to food history scholarship. Twitter: @aketchum22 and Instagram: @dr.alexketchum

Klassen, Ben Ben Klassen is a white queer settler living and working on the unceded and ancestral territories of the Musqueam, Squamish, and Tsleil-Waututh peoples. He is a Research Manager at Community-Based Research Centre Society (CBRC), Canada, where he oversees several LGBTQ+ research studies. Ben holds an MA in History from Simon Fraser University, Canada, where he studied queer narratives of the HIV/AIDS epidemic in Vancouver, with a primary focus on oral history. He has extensive experience in community-based research, qualitative methods, and applied ethics and has co-authored papers on a range of queer health topics, including blood donation policy and HIV treatment and prevention.

Lachowsky, Nathan Dr Nathan Lachowsky (he, him, his) is a settler researcher and uninvited guest on the traditional territory of the Lekwungen peoples. He is an Associate Professor in the School of Public Health and Social Policy at the University of Victoria, Canada, and Research Director for the national

Community-Based Research Centre Society (www.cbrc.net). Championing interdisciplinary and community-based approaches, he has conducted population health research with sexual and gender minoritized communities across Canada and Aotearoa New Zealand. Nathan's research focuses on social and behavioural epidemiology and the importance of developing and analyzing mixed-methods data to inform public health practice, health service provision, interventions, and policy. He conducts interdisciplinary research within a social justice framework in order to achieve health equity for marginalized communities.

Lam, Peter Peter Lam was brought up in a typical Asian family where they hoped that he would become a doctor, lawyer, or engineer. However, Peter eventually became a dietitian because of his ultimate love of food. He grew up in an environment where he was taught to appreciate the many aspects of food and about food. He truly believes that food is good medicine, not just for the body but also for the soul. This is why he has focussed his area of dietetic practice in supporting people with eating and drinking difficulties for the past many years.

Lawn, Fran Fran brings over 25 years of programme development, management, and non-profit leadership within the environmental and sustainability field. His work has been recognized in the field of ecology and environmental education, as well as national recognition for building a horticulture re-entry to workforce programme and partnership for returning citizens in Philadelphia. Fran is currently pursuing a masters degree in Nutritional Sciences. His goal is to combine nutrition coaching and education to help GBTQ men improve their health through better nutrition. As a lifelong environmental advocate with a passion for nature, nutrition, and health, he enjoys helping people make a stronger connection to their environment by building a healthy, active lifestyle through nutrition.

Lee, Deonté Deonté Lee was born in Adelanto, CA, in 1997, receiving his BFA from the University of California, Riverside, in 2021. Deonté's work is rooted in portraiture, queer visual culture, and eccentricity. His subjects are translated through the inverted colours depicting individuals of strength as a homage to religious iconography. His deeply alluring and otherworldly portraits craft a sense of otherness within the viewer because the images are meant to be seen as striking, evocative, and unmundane. The photographs were taken during Lee's research project surrounding underground queer nightlife culture in Rio, LA, London, and NYC. His Instagram is @eclectic.nomad.

Leung, Enoch Enoch Leung is a PhD Candidate in the Department of Educational and Counselling Psychology at McGill University, Canada. His primary areas of interest lie in working with (1) students with disabilities and (2) the LGBTQ+ student population. Being educated and learning under various cultures, Enoch grounds his work primarily through an intersectional approach to better understand the environments students are situated in. Additionally, in an educational setting, Enoch abides by the philosophy of Universal Design for Learning to understand the barriers and obstacles marginalized students will experience in their environment and ensure equity in schools. With over nine years of experience working in educational institutions across daycare, elementary, high school, CÉGÉP (*College d'enseignement general et professionnel*), and at the university level, Enoch's primary passion lies in actively listening to those students who feel disempowered or encounter barriers at their institution and problem-solve collaboratively to remove those obstacles.

Leung, Jon Jon Leung, RD, is a second-generation Asian Canadian living in Vancouver, Canada. He graduated from the University of British Columbia with a Bachelor of Science in Food, Nutrition, and Health. Jon is a Certified Nutrition Support Clinician and currently works as an ICU dietitian at an acute care hospital. He holds an appointment with the university as a Clinical Instructor and supports dietetics students as a preceptor. In his free time, Jon likes to binge-watch cartoons, play video games, or explore the Vancouver restaurant scene with his partner, Lucas.

Linsenmeyer, Whitney Whitney Linsenmeyer, PhD, RD, LD (she/her) is an assistant professor of nutrition at Saint Louis University, USA, and a spokesperson for the Academy of Nutrition and Dietetics. Her research and clinical practice centre on nutrition care for the transgender community. She is passionate about the powerful role that nutrition and physical activity can play in the lives of transgender individuals. Whitney lives in Saint Louis, Missouri, with her partner (Justin), kids (Charlie, Marea), and dog (Tater Tot).

Lutz-Barabé, Fabien Fabien is an artist/cartoonist living in Tantallon, Nova Scotia, Canada. Originally from Montreal, in 1997 he moved here with his partner and husband. Last of 11 children he is from a large family and entertained his nieces and nephews with his hand-drawn original comics and superhero stories. In 1985 he moved from the Eastern Townships to Montreal and had his first cartoon The Spice of Life published in two weekly newspapers. Inspired by the beauty of Nova Scotia, he developed his painting skills. The majesty of the province is often used as the muse for his works. He joined the Peggy's Cove Area Festival of the Arts in 2010 and has participated in the annual Paint Peggy's Cove, the Studio Tour, and other various art exhibitions.

Ng, David David is the Co-Artistic Director of Love Intersections. His work has also recently included collaborations with Primary Colours/Couleurs primaires, which is an initiative to decolonize the Canadian art system by putting Indigenous arts practices at the centre, through the leadership of Indigenous artists, supported by artists of colour. David has been a filmmaker for 22 years, and more recently through Love Intersections, he has produced over 15 short films, which have screened internationally at over 60 film festivals. His last film, *Yellow Peril: Queer Destiny*, screened at the Academy Award Qualifying festivals: The Leeds International Film Festival and the Aesthetica Film Festival. He is currently a PhD candidate at the Social Justice Institute at the University of British Columbia, Canada. He holds a Master of Social Sciences from the African Gender Institute at the University of Cape Town, South Africa, a BSoSc (hons) from the University of Cape Town, and a BSoSc in gender studies from Simon Fraser University, Canada.

Ly, Gordon Gordon Ly (he/him), RD, is a racialized settler on the traditional territory of the Tsleil-Waututh and Qayqayt Nations. He is grateful his family was able to flee war-stricken Southeast Asia and seek refuge in the lands he currently occupies. He holds a Bachelor of Science in Food, Nutrition, and Health (2014) from the University of British Columbia, Canada, and a Certified Diabetes Educator designation (2018). His interests lie in the many intersections between race, gender, paediatrics, chronic disease, and nutrition. Seeking out a diversity of professional experiences, he has joyfully found himself working in education and advocacy. Outside of his work, you can find him on the mountain, in the forest, or by the river – undoubtedly accompanied by delicious food.

Moran, Kelsey Kelsey Moran (she/they) is a licensed psychologist currently working in the Counseling Center at the College of the Holy Cross, USA, as the Coordinator of LGBTQIA+ (lesbian, gay, bisexual, trans, queer/questioning, intersex, asexual/aromantic, and all other people who exist under the rainbow) Counseling Services and Programming. The work that they are lucky enough to do there with students is profoundly meaningful to them, both professionally and personally. Kelsey is, at least as far as she currently understands herself, a white, bisexual, non-binary, and fat person who is happily in recovery from an eating disorder. They live in Rhode Island with their absolutely incredible fiancée, a ridiculous cat, way too many plants, and a fully stocked cheese drawer.

Morris, Bonnie Bonnie J. Morris is a women's history lecturer at the University of California-Berkeley, USA, a finalist for the 2020 Excellence in Teaching Prize, and a nationally recognized expert on the role of women's music and culture. The author of 19 books, she has devoted more than 30 years to documenting the women's music movement, first publishing *Eden Built by Eves*, a finalist for the Lambda Literary Award, and more recently *The Disappearing L* and *The Feminist Revolution*. Her research on women's music, Olivia Records, and American lesbian culture will one day be housed at the Radcliffe Institute's Schlesinger Library. In recent years Dr Morris won a D.C. Arts and Humanities grant and a writing residency in Wales; organized the first-ever exhibit on the women's music movement at the Library of Congress; arranged for Olivia albums to be part of the Smithsonian; received the Ruth Rowan Believer Award from the National Women's Music Festival; and accepted the exciting role as Olivia Records' official historian and archivist. Dr Morris has been a featured speaker at conferences and museums throughout the country and continues to profile women's music history for the Smithsonian. As a fiction writer, she also published the time travel novel *Sappho's Bar and Grill*, a finalist for the Foreword national award in LGBT fiction and winner of the Devil's Kitchen award from Southern Illinois University. Coming soon: a history of women's sports, entitled *What's the Score?* www.bonniejmorris.com

Ó Baoill, Fergal Fergal Ó Baoill (MPhil) is a graduate of Gender Studies at Trinity College, University of Dublin, Ireland. His Masters thesis explored femininity in relation to neoliberalism and the impact of cisgender gay men's choice of sexual partner on the wider Irish queer community. He intends to pursue a doctorate study in the field of queer subjectivity and the creation of communities in opposition to neoliberal economics.

Peters, Lynette Lynette A. Peters is a Doctoral Candidate in Health at Dalhousie University, Nova Scotia, Canada. She is the artist and founder of Cerberus Pottery. While her research interests include pottery and CAF Veterans who transition from service, her artistic innovations continue to place clay in novel spaces in order to challenge others to uncover meaning.

Pradhan, Anil Anil Pradhan is a PhD candidate and UGC Senior Research Fellow at the Department of English, Jadavpur University, Kolkata, India. He received his MPhil and MA in English from Jadavpur University and his BA in English from Presidency University, Kolkata. His areas of interest include queer cultural studies and queer literature and films about India and its diaspora. His research articles have been published in *Jadavpur University Essays and Studies, Journal of Media & Communication, Café Dissensus, Rupkatha, In Plainspeak, Studies in Canadian Literature, Interdisciplinary Studies in Literature and Environment, Journal of Comparative Literature and Aesthetics,* etc.

Quathamer, Nat As a young LGBTQIA+ professional in the health education field, Nat (PDt, they/them, he/him, she/her) has found a passion for empowering their community to become food, health, and science literate. He works to bring the fields of health equity and food justice together – while applying an environmentally ethical lens – to give all people unconditional access to what they need to maintain or improve any aspect of their health they wish to pursue.

Robinson, Margaret Margaret Robinson is a Mi'kmaw scholar and a member of Lennox Island First Nation who grew up in Sheet Harbour, in the Eskikewa'kik district of Mi'kma'ki, Canada. She is Two-spirit, bisexual, and queer, and passionate about food justice, Indigenous self-government, and vegan cooking. Margaret works as an Assistant Professor at Dalhousie University, where she holds the Tier 2 Canada Research Chair in Reconciliation, Gender, and Identity.

Russell, Julia Julia is a doctoral candidate at the University of Waterloo, Canada. Her research focus is on veganism and wellbeing. Julia has a Master of Science degree in community health science from the University of Northern British Columbia and an honours Bachelor of Science from the University of Toronto, where she completed a specialist programme in international development studies and a major in environmental science. Julia's past research experiences have largely been in the areas of Indigenous health and wellbeing and food-related topics.

Simpson-Theobald, Jason Jason is the HIV specialist dietitian at Nottingham University Hospitals NHS Trust (Nottingham, UK); he has worked in HIV for over ten years. He completed his Masters in Advanced Dietetic Practice with his research project relating to nutrition and chemsex. He is passionate about inclusive, holistic dietetic care and is a member of the HIV Care Specialist Interest Group of the British Dietetic Association. He is a proud member of the LGBTQIA+ community and promotes diversity within the profession, and more widely, whenever he can. He can be contacted via Jason.simpson -theobald@nuh.nhs.uk

Sotto, Jeffrey Jeffrey Sotto lives and works full time in Toronto, Canada. He is an advocate for eating disorder awareness and recovery through his role as a peer mentor at Eating Disorders Nova Scotia (EDNS) and having shared his journey on various platforms including CBC Radio and Global News. In 2019, he published a novel called *Cloud Cover* based on his experience with mental health issues, specifically eating disorders. His second novel, *The Moonballers: A Novel about The Invasion of a LGBTQ+ Tennis League by … Straight People (GAY GASP!)*, was published in April 2022. Jeffrey can be found on his website, jeffreyasotto.com, Facebook, and Instagram at jeffreyasotto.

Sungshine, Jen Jen Sungshine is a queer Taiwanese Canadian interdisciplinary artist/activist, community facilitator, and cultural producer based in Vancouver, Canada. She is the Co-Artistic Director and Co-founder of Love Intersections, a media arts collective producing intergenerational and intersectional Queer, Trans, Black, Indigenous People of Color (QTBIPOC) stories through documentary film. Her most recent works include *Yellow Peril: Queer Destiny* (2019), winner of the Gerry Brunet Memorial Award for best BC Short and visual arts exhibit, *Yellow Peril; Celestial Elements* (2020) at the SUM Gallery. She is a co-producer of CURRENT: Feminist Electronic Art Symposium and currently serves on the board of Vancouver Artists Labour Union Cooperative (VALU CO-OP). www.jensungshine.com

Thill, Lee Ann Lee Ann Thill, PhD, ATR-BC, LPC, is a visual artist, art therapist, and lecturer at Lesley University, USA. Her doctoral research was an art-based inquiry of vegan women with food and body image issues. Her research interests are human/animal relationality, gender/sexuality, disability/madness, food/body, ecofeminism, and art-based methodology. She has been an Intersectional Justice Conference co-organizer, Institute for Critical Animal Studies presenter, and founder-organizer of online art-based patient advocacy initiatives. Lee Ann lives with her husband and rescued animal family in New Jersey, USA. Social Media Website: www.leeannthill.com Twitter @adrartlady Instagram: @drartlady

Whebby, Marin Marin (she/her, they/them, ve/ver) brings a trans voice to the world of food and nutrition. Her research interests focus on feminist food studies, trans-inclusive nutrition practice, the ways we relate to bodies, and socially just approaches to wellness. Beyond school, Marin likes to cook, garden, gush about food and movies, read, and cuddle with their dogs.

Wilson, Megan L. Megan Wilson is a PhD candidate in English and American Studies at the University of Manchester, UK. She holds a BA in Film Studies from King's College, London, and a MA in Gender, Sexuality, and Culture from the University of Manchester. Her research interests encompass queer cinema and history, with a particular focus on contemporary lesbian films and audiences.

Zoller, L.M. L.M. Zoller is a white non-binary writer, zinester, and artist living on the unceded Coast Salish land known as Seattle, WA, USA. Their work focuses on the intersection of food, gender, and queerness. They are the co-author of *The Queer Language of Flowers* and *The Corners of Their Mouth: A Queer Food Zine* and the author of *Midwestern Transplant Presents* zine series. Their work has been featured in *Compound Butter*, *Dinner Bell Mag*, *GRLSQUASH*, and *Comestible*. Find them on social media @illmakeitmyself (Instagram, Twitter, Facebook, Patreon) or online at illmakeitmyself.net or thecornersoftheirmouthpress.com.

A Rainbow of Acronyms: Language Notes

Phillip Joy and Megan Aston

The way we talk about and the way we talk within our communities is extremely important. Within our rainbow groups are many identities and experiences that we need to acknowledge, honour, and create inclusive spaces in which people feel seen and known. Within this book, we use the acronym LGBTQ+ (lesbian, gay, bi, trans, queer, and other sexual- or gender-minority identities), but we acknowledge that this acronym sometimes does not include all of our experiences or identities. There are many other acronyms that we could have used including:

- 2SLGBTQ+ which is an acronym that acknowledges Two-spirit (2S) Indigenous people who were the first sexual- and gender-minority people in North America. At the time of writing, this acronym is not often used outside North America.
- LGBTQIA which includes intersex and asexual identities.
- LGBTQQIP2SAA which includes lesbian, gay, bisexual, transgender, questioning, queer, intersex, pansexual, Two-spirit, androgynous, and asexual identities.
- LGBTIQAPD which includes lesbian, gay, bisexual, transgender, queer, intersex, asexual, pansexual, and demisexual identities.

We have chosen the shorter acronym simply for readability and not to exclude any voices. In fact, we have consciously tried to include as many voices from our communities in this book as possible. We, therefore, made the decision to have many shorter chapters (which we think is a little queer in the academic world itself) to support our aims of giving voice. But we also acknowledge that many voices may still be underrepresented. We hope you enjoy exploring and reflecting upon the contributions in this collection.

Phillip and Megan

Preface: Queering Dietetics through Arts-Based Methodologies

Phillip Joy and Megan Aston

Queer is a word with many meanings. The *Cambridge Dictionary* (2022) defines it as an old-fashioned adjective to describe something or someone that is strange, unusual, or not expected. The boys who chased me through my school halls screaming queer at me obviously found me strange, unusual, and unexpected. I was not a boy like them, and they could sense it. Queer turned to fag and their hatred was a daily experience for me. Years later I recognize that I was not alone in these experiences. Many of us who did not fit within the cisheteronormative ideas, or the universal assumptions of cisness and straightness, shared the hurt of such words. Some of us, however, were able to reclaim the word queer. Through activism and social transformation, queer is now an adjective of pride.

The *Cambridge Dictionary* (2022) also defines queer as a verb. To queer something is to change something so that it no longer fits cisheteronormative ideas. In the 1990s, queer theory emerged as a critical theory to challenge the notion that straight desire was the only acceptable form of desire. Halperin (1995) suggested that "queer is by definition whatever is at odds with the normal, the legitimate, the dominant. There is nothing in particular to which it necessarily refers" (p. 62) and, over the years, scholars from other disciplines began using queer theory to explore and to queer other topics. But it is important not to forget the historical and painful meanings of what queer and queering meant to gender and sexually diverse people. In this book we use queer in both of these ways as a way to bring queer voices to the field of nutrition and dietetics and to critically challenge many ideas about food, eating, and bodies within the profession and our wider society. We feel the stories of queer lives are central to the challenging, resisting, and dismantling of cisheteronormative constructs. We cannot have one without the other.

Ways for individuals to resist, subvert, and reveal new possibilities of knowing and living is through creativity and art. Queer art in the 20th century has been shaped by both the need to remain hidden and the desire to be visible (Burk, 2015). As liberation movements began to grow, activists, social commentators, and others working within social and activist movements used art in various forms to critique, challenge, and disrupt notions of gender and sexuality within political, social, and healthcare systems. For example, photographers like the American Nan Goldin were queering gender and sexuality through their art decades before Teresa de Lauretis (1991) first used the term queer theory. Goldin's work explored many queer issues, including the post-Stonewall gay era, queer bodies, the AIDS crisis of the 1980s, and gender politics. The photographs in The Other Side destabilized binary concepts of gender as by documenting the lives of drag queens and trans people living in New York City in the 1970s (Skodbo, 2007).

In Leavy's (2018) *Handbook of Arts-Based Research* one can find a multitude of arts-based methodologies from various disciplines, ranging from education, sociology, natural sciences, and health sciences like the field of nutrition and dietetics. Leavy (2018) provides a starting point for understanding the breadth and diversity of arts-based research and inquiries, describing arts-based research as an umbrella term to include all artistic approaches to research and inquiry that draw connections between art, artmaking, and scholarship. These methodologies are grounded in a philosophy that recognizes multiple ways of knowing: knowing through sensory, kinaesthetic, and imaginary ways. Art-based research and scholarship can represent emotions, bodies, and identities and the process of creating art can allow people time for reflection and to express themselves in thoughtful and purposeful ways (Finley, 2008). Finely (2008) suggested that "to claim art and aesthetic ways of knowing as research is an act of rebellion against the monolithic 'truth' that science is supposed to entail" (p.73). Arts-based methodologies can, therefore, disrupt the foundations of research that propose knowledge is found only in rigid number sets or knowledge that is supposedly removed from human experiences and becomes critical in knowing the self and others (Leavy, 2018).

Arts-based research and scholarship is as diverse as art itself and may take literary forms. Essays, experimental writing, poetry and parables, personal narratives, reflections, and autoethnographies are literary forms. While music, songs, dance, and theatre are performative forms (Leavy, 2018). Research and scholarship may also be expressed visually through collage, photography, sculpture, comics, paintings, needlework, and quilts or combined with audio in the forms of film and video (Leavy, 2018). Within this collection, you will find many of these forms that are disruptive to normative views of sexuality, gender, bodies, food and nutrition, and dietetic knowledge and practices while contributing to social transformation through the expression of new perspectives and new ways of being. From the many arts-based forms of scholarship within this collection, we include autoethnographies and reflective essays, prose, parables, photography, comic art, sculpture, collages, quilt work, and analysis of films divided into three main parts. Within the first part, we explore experiences of eating, food, and bodies for queer folx. In the second part are chapters that explore issues of communities, connections, and celebrations of queer experiences. In the third part, we provide contributions that explore issues of queer care within nutritional and dietetic professions.

In this collection, we have brought together a diverse range of queer voices, sharing their beliefs, values, and experiences of food, eating, care, health, and queerness. We feel there is no better way to queering the sciences of nutrition and dietetics than through art and art-based methodologies. As Lucy Aphramor proclaims inside this collection,

> Queering is an orientation to the world not a marker of who or how we desire or fuck. Queering and Creativity are vital in allowing us to think, feel and dream dietetics differently by animating and re-indigenizing our faculties of analysis, perception, and communication.

References

Burk, T. (2015, November 4). *Queer Art: 1960s to the Present*. Art History Teaching Resources. http://arthistoryteachingresources.org/lessons/queer-art-1960s-to-the-present/

Cambridge Dictionary. (2022). *Queer*. Retrieved February 26, 2022, from https://dictionary.cambridge.org/dictionary/english/queer

De Lauretis, T. (1991). *Queer theory: Lesbian and gay sexualities* (Vol. 3, No. 2). Indiana University Press.

Finley, S. (2008). Arts-based research. In *Handbook of the arts in qualitative research* (J. G. Knowles and A. L. Cole Eds). (pp. 71–81). SAGE Publications.

Halperin, D. (1995). *Saint Foucault: Towards a gay hagiography*. Oxford University Press.

Leavy, P. (Ed.). (2018). *Handbook of arts-based research*. Guilford Publications.

Skodbo, T. N. (2007). *Nan Goldin: The other side: Photography and gender identity* [Master's Thesis]. University of Oslo.

About the Cover Art: The Other Half

Phillip Joy

The Other Half

Broken in two;
Can our halves ever be mended?
Are we destined;
To remain one and one ended?

Phillip Joy

The Faeries are everywhere. As magical creatures of light, colour, and love, they play in the realm of man with unbounded delight. All a human needs to do is look, listen, and open themselves up to the queer possibilities of the universe to catch a glimpse of these enchanting beings.

The sensual nature of the Faerie is explored in a collection of work, entitled *Playgrounds of the Faerie*. This collection by Phillip Joy and Maritza Miari contains over 20 pieces of art that capture the endless ways Faeries amuse themselves. The collection is a unique collaboration between these artists using different media to create cohesive and integrated pieces of art. The artists traverse the boundaries between photography and illustrations, as well as blur the realms of man and Faerie.

The word "fairy," like the word "queer," has been historically used as an othering and derogative term for gay men. Brontsema (2004) traces the context of these words, noting both gender and class differences between the men identified by these terms. Both fairy and queer were used to describe men who were attracted to and loved other men, but fairy was used to describe effeminate and flamboyant men, whereas the word queer referred to more traditionally masculine men whose class often put them at professional risk if any signs of femininity were displayed (Brontsema, 2004).

The image on the cover, *The Other Half*, finds a solitary Faerie, sitting in the broken ends of an egg. He holds the *Symposium* by Plato. In his reading of Aristophanes's speech found within the pages, the Faerie learns about the origins of humans. He discovers that humans were once rounded, doubled creatures with two heads, four arms, and four legs (Dover, 1966; Plato & Gill, 1999). The Faerie reads how, at this time, humans had three sexes. One sex was descended from the sun and were all male. Another sex was descended from the Earth and were all female. The third sex was descended from the moon and were "androgynous" or half male and half female (Plato & Gill, 1999). The humans were ambitious and tried to reach the Gods of Olympus, and in his anger, Zeus split the humans in half. Humans became what we know of today, with one head, two arms, two legs, and a constant, never-ending desire to reunite with their other half. The Faerie learns that humans may only find their other half if they are devout enough to the Gods (Dover, 1966; Plato & Gill, 1999).

This myth was retold in the song, *The Origin of Love*, featured in the award win-ning 2001 American musical film, *Hedwig and the Angry Inch* (Mitchell, 2001). The film follows the life of a genderqueer rocker after botched gender reassignment surgery. These stories and songs were the inspiration for the cover art.

References

Brontsema, R. (2004). A queer revolution: Reconceptualizing the debate over linguistic reclamation. *Colorado Research in Linguistics, 17.* https://doi.org/10.25810/dky3-zq57

Dover, K. J. (1966). Aristophanes' speech in Plato's symposium. *The Journal of Hellenic Studies, 86,* 41–50.

Mitchell, J. C. (2001). *Hedwig and the angry inch* [Motion picture]. Killer Films.

Plato, & Gill, C. (1999). *The symposium*. Penguin Books.

Acknowledgements

Our book is a product of the love, support, passion, and compassion from many individuals. We would like to start by thanking those who supported our vision and first steps to creating the book. Thank you to Kathleen Chan for helping us with social media and recruitment of contributors as we began the project. Thank you to those at Routledge Press for guiding us through the process of submitting our proposal for the book with much enthusiasm and support. We would especially like to acknowledge the brilliant and compassionate authors and artists who have shared their knowledge and personal stories in the pages of this book. It was such a pleasure to receive each submission for the first time and engage in their powerful experiences that they so generously shared through the written word and visual art.

Part 1
Eating, Food, and Bodies

1 Double Visioning

A Two-Spirit Reflection on Food

Margaret Robinson

As a health researcher, food is part of my work. Food is embedded with cultural and personal meaning and evokes memories through taste and smell. Due to food's central role in our lives, it shapes our whole selves, including our physical, mental, emotional, and spiritual wellbeing. My identity as a Two-spirit person helps me examine these connections. Two-spirit is a term some Indigenous people use to describe our gender or sexual difference, but the identity can also connect us to a history of similar people who held valued roles in our nations. Two-spirit theory is particularly useful for examining food issues because it combines queer theory's analysis of how power creates categories of gender and sexuality with an analysis of colonialism rooted in first-hand experience.

For most of our nations' histories, Indigenous people maintained thriving economies of hunting, fishing, and cultivation that kept us intimately connected to the lifeways, cycles, and specificities of our territories and the beings that live there. Our languages and cultures describe and encapsulate our knowledge about our specific territory. Indigenous food can support wellness for Two-spirit people by connecting us to others through feasting, food preparation and sharing, and the rediscovery of food knowledge that connects us to our territories. This ability to connect us to our culture is something food has in common with the Two-spirit identity. Indigenous culture is so central to Two-spirit identity that Two-spirit scholar Alex Wilson (2008) describes embracing the identity as "coming in" (to community), rather than "coming out."

Colonialism severs our connection to lands, disrupting the transmission of our languages and of our territorial knowledge and practices of relation. One of the ways Indigenous people are separated from our territories and cultures is by settlers usurping control over our food economies – what and how people eat, where our food originates, and how much it costs. Intentional starvation was a tactic used to "pacify" Indigenous nations in the plains, with settler governments intentionally killing off sources of food, such as the buffalo (Isenberg, 1992, p. 227), and withholding contracted rations to force Indigenous people to leave their territories (TRC, 2015).

In Canada today, as in other settler states, food is a commodity sold for profit. Within a for-profit food system, colonialism is normalized. Like many Canadians, I grew up buying food from "Dominion," a national grocery chain named in 1919 to

DOI: 10.4324/9781003217121-2

reflect Canada's position at that time as a self-governing nation of the British Empire. Yet even when colonial processes are unacknowledged, they continue to shape how we eat. Like many others, Indigenous people eat what we can afford and what is available where we live, so food indicates our places in hierarchies of power. The places we can afford to live may lack access to fresh nutrient-rich food, creating "food deserts" (USDA, 2009). In my own territory, the settler government forced Mi'kmaw people to live in isolated areas to preserve farmable land for settlers. As a result, Mi'kmaw diets reflect the availability of cheap processed food over fresh nutritious produce (Travers, 1995). Racism, classism, sexism, and other dominations are expressed and reinforced through food. The absence of familiar foods – on university cafeteria menus, for example – can signal that we are unwelcome in that space.

One factor shaping contemporary Indigenous food practices are settler-run residential and boarding schools, which three quarters of First Nations youth were forced to attend between 1884 and 1996. The residential school system in Canada attempted to assimilate Indigenous children into settler society as a servant class (Fournier & Crey, 2006). Boys were trained to farm (a feminine activity in some Indigenous nations) and girls were trained to cook and clean. Two-spirit children were forcibly re-gendered and food traditions (such as participating in both sides of a gendered food economy; Callender et al., 1983) and other roles involving them were nearly exterminated (Robinson, 2019a).

Children were forced to perform most of the work required to keep residential schools running, with students at one Ontario facility performing 7.5 hours of heavy labour every day (Maclean, 2005, pp. 114–115). Despite their long work hours, inmates at residential schools reported that hunger was constant. Ian Mosby and Tracey Galloway calculate the average daily caloric intake for children held in residential schools to have ranged from 1,000 to 1,450 calories per day (2017, p. E1044). The Ministry of Health for the Province of Ontario (2016) reports that youth aged 13 and older require an average of 2,000 calories per day, and children between the ages of 4 and 12 need 1,500 daily calories. Survivors detail how some hungry students resorted to eating compost (Mosby & Galloway, 2017). The Truth and Reconciliation Commission of Canada reports that the Federal Government

> knowingly chose not to provide schools with enough money to ensure that kitchens and dining rooms were properly equipped, that cooks were properly trained, and, most significantly, that food was purchased in sufficient quantity and quality for growing children.
>
> (2015, p. 92)

The impact of residential schools on food practices was rarely acknowledged prior to Mosby's (2013) study revealing that nearly 1,000 Indigenous children had been unknowingly subjected to experiments that relied upon their malnutrition. Follow-up work has found that malnourishment stunted the growth of residential school inmates and increased their insulin resistance, leading to type 2 diabetes and immune system problems (Mosby & Galloway, 2017). Colonial starvation policies also affect those whose parents and grandparents are residential school survivors, causing similar health issues in the second and third generations (Mosby & Galloway, 2017).

Indigenous Health

Research in Canada tends to frame Indigenous malnutrition as a failure of Indigenous people to make good food choices. In a review of 76 studies funded between 2018 and 2021, 73% aimed to change how Indigenous people eat or exercise, and 8% implied a genetic cause for weight gain (Robinson, 2019b). Health interventions often targeted Indigenous women and children with messages about body size from the settler diet industry. Only 16% of the funded studies planned to consider policy solutions, and only 3% named colonialism as a factor shaping health. The tendency of health researchers to focus on changing how Indigenous people eat ignores the role of government policy in food economies and fails to connect factors shaping food choices, particularly land dispossession and the destruction of natural ecologies for economic gain.

Indigenous nations are aware of how ongoing colonization damages the health of their citizens. Some Indigenous people have urged a return to traditional diets, sharing stories of physical, cultural, and spiritual benefits to be gained. One such story focuses on Bossy Ducharme, a Métis man from Duck Bay, Manitoba, who resolved "not … to put anything in my body that was not here before the Europeans arrived" (National Post, 2012). Ducharme stopped consuming processed foods and animals imported by settlers, such as chickens, cattle, or pigs, and began eating buffalo, elk, wild rice, seeds, berries, and regional vegetables (National Post, 2012). Ducharme connects Indigenous malnutrition to colonialism and poverty, explaining that those of us raised in poverty "eat what you can afford. You spend the money on bigger portions — the pastas, the sugars" (National Post, 2012).

Ducharme reports that thanks to his dietary changes he has "more energy and both a clearer complexion and mind," and now feels "so present in my daily life" (National Post, 2012). Efforts to take up a traditional diet may be a form of what Anishinaabe scholar Gerald Vizenor (2008) calls "survivance" – Indigenous resistance to domination, paired with our physical and cultural survival as a people. Taking up practices such as harvesting, preparing, serving, and eating traditional foods may support immersive embodied experiences that contribute to survivance by sensually affirming our resistance in daily life.

However, stories about life improvements after dietary changes may also uncritically mimic success stories from the settler diet industry, reducing the problem of malnutrition to size and the benefits of traditional eating to numbers on a scale. The article about Ducharme, for example, sounds remarkably like an advertisement when it reports that he "was 223 pounds, and managed to drop to 145 pounds, without exercising." A similar article, about a dietary experiment in Alert Bay (this one informed and voluntary), reports that within a year "some 1,200 pounds had been collectively shed by the 80 or so residents of the fishing village," with one man reporting he "not only lost 40 pounds, but no longer requires drugs to treat his diabetes" (Sin, 2008). Indigenous people must consider how to reclaim our food economies without replicating the diet industry's gendered body shame. Focusing on individual eating habits fails to consider factors such as the theft of Indigenous lands for commercial agriculture, the objectification of animals used for food, and the ongoing destruction of the Indigenous food economies by the colonial governments occupying their territories.

Solidarity Art

The paper sculpture collection, *Take it With a Grain of Salt*, by Toronto-based artist Meegan Lim (2020a), presents a challenge to colonial narratives that deny Indigenous food knowledge. Lim is an artist of Chinese-Malaysian descent whose work "engages people with stories about food, culture & social change" (Lim, 2021). Lim revisions the packaging of "pantry staples" common in Canada – flour, sugar, salt, and lard – contextualizing them historically (Figure 1.1). These items are produced on stolen land, were forced on Indigenous people in the form of government rations, and came to form a bready filler food many people call "bannock," with a nutritional value similar to a sugar loop doughnut (Tim Hortons, 2021). Lim reveals these items as staples of settler colonialism.

The scale, text, and images on Lim's works are small, inviting close examination. The side panel of "White Sugar," for example, includes images of the

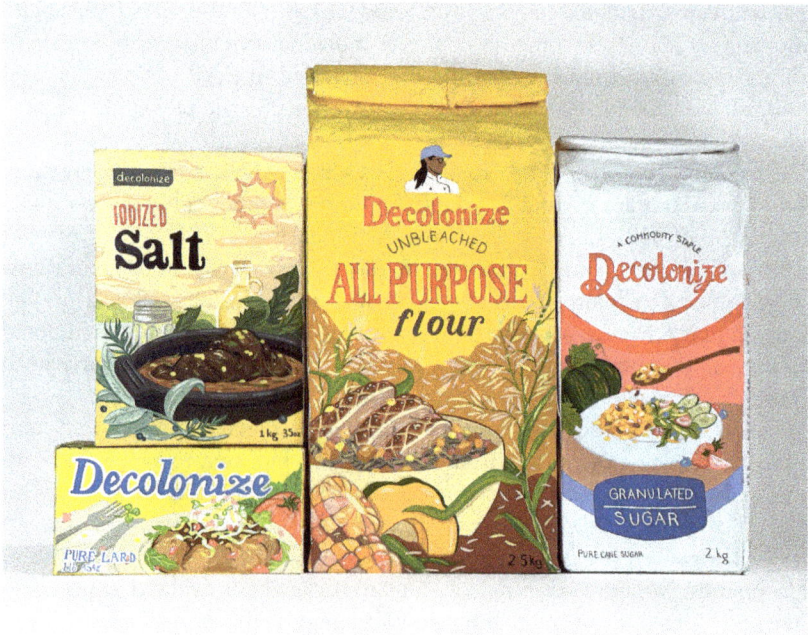

Figure 1.1 Take it With a Grain of Salt. Meegan Lim.

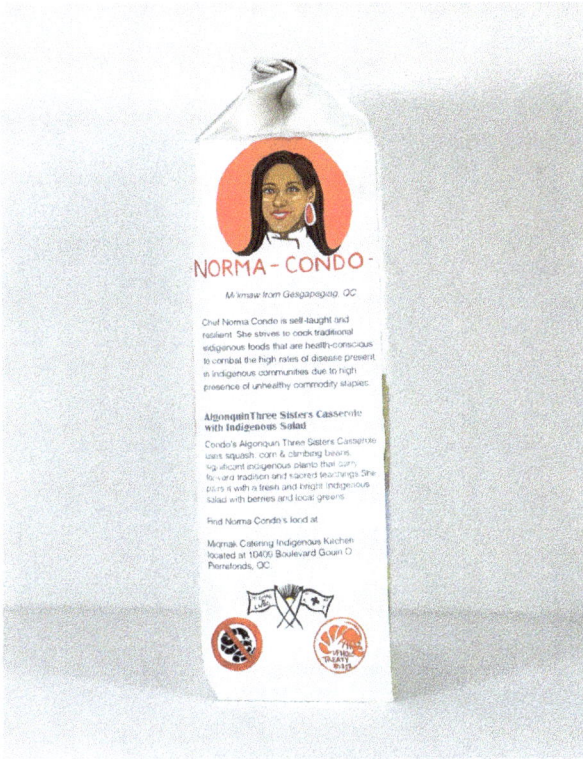

Figure 1.2 White Sugar. Meegan Lim.

Mi'kmaw National Flag, an anti-pipeline snake, and a lobster with "uphold treaty #1752" (Figure 1.2) This image refers to a Peace and Friendship treaty signed by Peregrine Thomas Hopson, who claimed Governorship of Nova Scotia, and Jean-Baptiste Cope, the saqamaw of Sipekne'katik. The lobster refers to Provision 4 in that treaty, that the Mi'kmaq "shall not be hindered from but have free liberty of Hunting and Fishing as usual" (Daugherty & Savage, 1983, p. 58). In a video showing the creation process, Lim (2020b) effaces colonial packaging with gouache before adding content that centres Indigenous foods and Indigenous food experts. The result feels like a restoration.

The piece "All Purpose Flour" revises the familiar yellow Robin Hood flour bag to read "Decolonize Unbleached All Purpose Flour" above images of wild rice, squash, corn, and duck meat (Lim 2020a). On a side panel (Figure 1.3), where nutritional information would be, Lim adds facts about wild rice, including settler attempts to eradicate the plant. Each work in the series showcases an Indigenous chef, undermining assumptions that Indigenous people lack food knowledge. On "All Purpose Flour," the chef is Brian Yazzie (Dené), whose approach is described

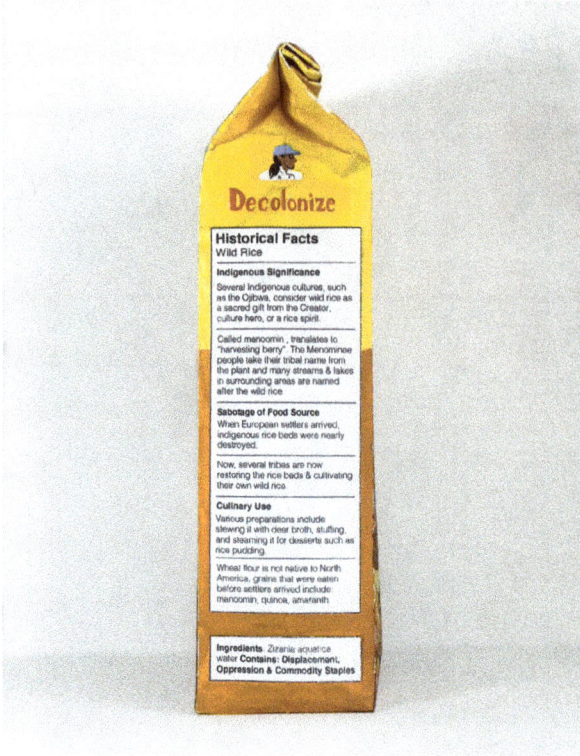

Figure 1.3 All Purpose Flour. Meegan Lim.

as "bringing together hyper-local Indigenous ingredients" and combining "ancestral knowledge with modern techniques" (Lim, 2021).

Given its re-membering of history, I classify Lim's *Take it With a Grain of Salt* collection as solidarity art. By revising settler pantry staples Lim envisions a decolonized present in which Indigenous foods hold a central place and Indigenous food expertise is acknowledged and celebrated. By posting the series on social media Lim disrupts colonial practices of amnesia – the suppressing and "forgetting" of negative history in order to feel innocent. Lim's critical stance may be possible in part because settler privileges are not accessible to, nor claimed by, every non-Indigenous person (Lawrence & Dua, 2005; Phung, 2011).

Decolonized Staples

Reclaiming control over our food economies is a daunting task, as food is intertwined with commercial colonialism through settler agriculture's use of stolen land and stolen labour to produce marketable food. Residential schools disrupted the teaching of Indigenous food terms, philosophies, spiritualities, and practices (especially around animal death), skills of leadership and diplomacy that maintained our trade networks, and the land-based knowledge required to run our food economies. Colonial regulations pushed Indigenous women and Two-spirit people out of positions of power and residential schools subordinated them further. Some of this damage can be undone by restoring roles of respect and responsibility to women and Two-spirit people and acknowledging the key role they play in protecting the land on which we all depend. Decolonizing food further requires us to question commercialization, which makes food something to buy, not something to earn through knowledge of the land and its inhabitants. Health research will remain inadequate until it extends its vision to encompass communitarian, rather than individualistic approaches to eating. Two-spirit scholarship is essential to this work, and to decolonizing food economies, because of its "critique of heteronormativity as a colonial project" (Driskill, Finley, Gilley, & Morgensen, 2011, p. 3). Such analysis helps oppose colonial body management practices that focus on women's appearance and reproduction (Robinson, 2019b).

Those who challenge colonial food systems risk being targeted by state violence. Examples can be seen in attacks against Indigenous land protectors as well as in how Canada's Federal Government maintains ongoing legal opposition to environmental protections and Indigenous land claims. Practices such as the copyrighting of seed by multinational corporations extends food issues beyond the border of any given settler nation. To decolonize our food economies may therefore be an international, even global, undertaking.

References

Callender, C., Kochems, L. M., Bleibtreu-Ehrenberg, G., Broch, H. B., Brown, J. K., Datan, N., & Strathern, A. (1983). The North American berdache [and comments and reply]. *Current Anthropology*, *24*(4), 443–470. https://www.jstor.org/stable/2742448

Daugherty, W., & Savage, E. (1983). *Maritime Indian treaties in historical perspective*. Treaties and Historical Research Centre. https://www.sac-isc.gc.ca/DAM/dam-cirnac-rcaanc/dam-tag/workarea/dam/texte-text/tremar_1100100028967_eng.pdf

Driskill, Q. L., Finley, C., Gilley, B., & Morgensen, S. (2011). The revolution is for everyone: Imagining an emancipatory future through Queer Indigenous critical theories. In Q. L. Driskill (Ed.), *Queer Indigenous studies: Critical interventions in theory, politics and literature* (pp. 211–221). University of Arizona Press.

Fournier, S., & Crey, E. (2006). Killing the Indian in the child: Four centuries of church-run schools. In Maaka, R., & Andersen, C. (Eds). *The Indigenous experience: Global perspectives* (pp. 47–80). Scholars Press.

Isenberg, A. C. (1992). Toward a policy of destruction: Buffaloes, law, and the market, 1803–83. *Great Plains Quarterly*, 227–241. https://www.jstor.org/stable/23531659

Lawrence, B., & Dua, E. (2005). Decolonizing antiracism. *Social Justice*, *32*(4), 120–143. https://www.jstor.org/stable/29768340

Lim, M. (2020a, December 12). Take it with a grain of salt [Paper and gouache sculpture]. https://m.facebook.com/MeeganLimIllu/videos/299821878057125/?locale2=ne_NP

Lim, M. (2020b, December 11). A closer look of "take it with a grain of salt" [Video.1:13 mins]. https://www.facebook.com/MeeganLimIllu/videos/299821878057125/?__so__=channel_tab&__rv__=all_videos_card

Lim, M. (2021). *Welcome, I'm Meegan!* https://www.meeganlim.com

MacLean, H. (2005). Ojibwa participation in methodist residential schools in upper Canada. *The Canadian Journal of Native Studies, 25*(1), 93–137. https://vdocument.in/ojibwa-participation-in-methodist-residential-schools-main-aboriginal-nation-living.html

Mosby, I. (2013). Administering colonial science: Nutrition research and human biomedical experimentation in Aboriginal communities and residential schools, 1942–1952. In *Histoire sociale/social history* (Vol. 46, No. 1, pp. 145–172). https://muse.jhu.edu/article/512043

Mosby, I., & Galloway, T. (2017). "Hunger was never absent": How residential school diets shaped current patterns of diabetes among Indigenous peoples in Canada. *Canadian Medical Association Journal, 189*(32), E1043–E1045. https://www.cmaj.ca/content/189/32/E1043

National Post Staff. (2012, May 18). Yes to berries, no to salt: Aboriginal man goes back to his dietary roots in order to lose weight, live healthier. *National Post.* https://nationalpost.com/news/yes-to-berries-no-to-salt-aboriginal-man-goes-back-to-his-dietary-roots-in-order-to-lose-weight-live-healthier

Ontario Ministry of Health. (2016, December 29). Calories on menus. https://www.ontario.ca/page/calories-menus

Phung, M. (2011). Are people of colour settlers too? In A. Mathur, J. Dewar, & M. DeGagné (Eds.), *Cultivating Canada: Reconciliation through the lens of cultural diversity* (pp. 289–298). Aboriginal Healing Foundation.

Robinson, M. (2019a). Two-spirit identity in a time of gender fluidity. *Journal of homosexuality, 67*(12), 1675–1690. https://doi.org/10.1080/00918369.2019.1613853

Robinson, M. (2019b). The big colonial bones of Indigenous North America's "obesity epidemic". In M. Friedman, C. Rice, & J. Rinaldi (Eds.), *Thickening fat: Fat bodies, intersectionality, and social justice* (pp. 15–28). Routledge.

Sin, L. (2008, March 16). The slimming of alert bay: MD returns first nations village to a traditional diet and sees success. *Times Colonist.* https://www.pressreader.com/canada/times-colonist/20080316/281621006042629

Tim Hortons. (2021). Tim Hortons nutritional information. https://cdn.sanity.io/files/czqk28jt/staging_th_ca/00b2310348e26d6b8071e12d29dbf478ffc33772.pdf

Travers, K. D. (1995). Using qualitative research to understand the sociocultural origins of diabetes among Cape Breton Mi'kmaq. *Chronic Diseases in Canada, 16*(4), 140–143. https://epe.lac-bac.gc.ca/100/202/301/chronic_diseases_canada/html/1995/v16n04/www.phac-aspc.gc.ca/publicat/cdic-mcc/16-4/b_e.html

Truth and Reconciliation Commission of Canada. (2015). Final report of the truth and reconciliation commission of Canada. Volume one: Summary "honouring the truth, reconciling for the future". https://irsi.ubc.ca/sites/default/files/inline-files/Executive_Summary_English_Web.pdf

U.S. Department of Agriculture. (2009). *Access to affordable and nutritious food—Measuring and understanding food deserts and their consequences: Report to congress.* U.S. Government Printing Office. https://www.ers.usda.gov/webdocs/publications/42711/12716_ap036_1_.pdf

Vizenor, G. (Ed.). (2008). *Survivance: Narratives of native presence.* University of Nebraska Press.

Wilson, A. (2008). N'tacinowin inna nah': Our coming in stories. *Canadian Woman Studies, 26*(3). https://cws.journals.yorku.ca/index.php/cws/article/view/22131

2 The Unbearable Straightness of Intuitive Eating

Maxie Castle and Lucy Aphramor

And so, we ask you to imagine that you are among a group of people talking about wellbeing and eating. Maybe it's a conference and you're there as a scholar or practitioner. Maybe you're among peers navigating troubled eating. It could be an eating disorder (ED) recovery group. You wanted food with social justice and landed here.

And yet, once again, well-meaning specialists advise you to trust your body signals. You listen for nuance that isn't forthcoming. It is bad enough when the mainstream food conversation erases you; it is its own brand of heartsink when you are not caught in the safety net cast by more socially aware food talk. Yet again, you are reminded that you are an aberration, an outlier, a complex case. The experts who developed the theory behind intuitive eating clearly did not have you in mind.

Lucy (L)

It is a profoundly alienating experience.

The "trust body signals" stance of intuitive eating assumes a safe world, a safely inhabitable body, sanity, and privilege. A world without trauma. I will not be the only person listening who knows what it feels like to be flooded with the clear, compelling, urge to self-harm. There will often, I guess, be other people at the conference wondering how this blanking is possible. If it excludes me, as an adult with so many privileges from thinness, whiteness, class, then it excludes and harms many more marginalized folk.

Maxie (M)

Our bodies hold immense wisdom, no doubt about it. I fully support "trusting your gut," literally and metaphorically. But our "intuitive" body signals are not innate or pure or neutral; they are learnt, shaped, and contoured over time, including by our experiences of harm, violence, and oppression. Working towards being more "attuned" to your body is simply not safe or possible for everyone, and a few intuitive eating worksheets certainly won't get us there.

DOI: 10.4324/9781003217121-3

What's more, we are actively dissuaded from noticing and honouring body signals so much of the time that it can feel confusing, if not hypocritical, for intuitive eating to insist this is the pathway out of our misery. For example, capitalism does not care if your body is telling you that you need to rest, to move more slowly, that you don't feel safe under your current work conditions. In order to function "well enough" under this neoliberal matrix, we are forced to ignore and dismiss the messages our bodies send us. These too are "natural" body signals from which we are systematically alienated, day in and day out.

As queer and trans people, the dominant message we receive from society is that our bodies and our desires are wrong, obscene, laughable, dangerous. It is a particularly insidious form of gaslighting to be told that the solution to your troubled eating lies in simply trusting your body, when that same body, and representations of bodies like yours, has been consistently distrusted and denigrated, ignored and excluded, humiliated and hurt.

L

So, there's this mismatch where intuitive eating is celebrated as anti-oppressive yet embeds the ideologies it denounces. Like healthism: presuming a standard, non-traumatized, non-disabled self ignores the fact that many people will be unwell much of the time, discards people who will never be healthy, and disconnects body-making from power and histories.

It can't account for the body as co-constituted and embedded. Queering would foreground the way that we are fashioned through relational exchange. It could help us make sense of internalized fat stigma, gender rigidity, ableism, and more. Remind us that what we feel is not always a reliable indicator of what's true for us – in keeping with our values – which encourages us to interrogate our feelings. It also challenges the colonial notion of timeless, placeless, fixed truths. Queering rips up the cultural script where we are at the mercy of feelings we have no conscious role in creating, and react to without agency.

Intuitive eating's individualism buries the workings of white supremacist thinking. Our body signals are also contoured by immersion in white supremacy, plus any experiences of privilege. As white people we are coached to expect comfort and primed to develop body signals where we experience Black people as menacing and dangerous. This conditioning stops us from knowing we feel fear because we are co-regulated with systemic racism. Instead, our fear feels "natural" and justified, a logic that sanctions racist emotional reactions as an "acceptable" explanation for harm. So when a white police officer shoots a Black adult or child, "I did it because of my body signals" is normalized as legitimating Black murder.

A liberatory public health narrative would dethrone white comfort and announce that how we develop feelings is strongly shaped by who we are in relation to power.

M

I can't count the number of times I have heard intuitive eating dietitians uncritically state "all babies know when they are hungry." I hate it. Firstly, some babies quickly learn that it is *not* safe to proclaim their hunger, that they will not be fed or held or soothed when they cry. And beneath this is the foundational appeal to innocence, purity, naturalness, normalcy. The infant is held up as an exemplar of the "natural" body, not yet corrupted by outside influences of diet culture or fat stigma or body shame, incontestable proof that we all were once in touch with our bodies and their signals. As though this should give us hope that it is possible, desirable, indeed imperative, for us troubled eaters to one day return to this "natural" state of affairs.

Trans people know that any appeal to the "natural" generally leaves us in the gutter. As babies, our bodies are coercively gendered. As we grow, the world tells us incessantly that our bodies and our desires are *not* natural. I remain wary of origin stories, the promise of a return to a more natural way of being. The "natural" offers us no safe harbour.

In pointing out how the reification of the "natural" body can be decidedly anti-trans, I'm not saying that trans people are simply left behind by intuitive eating. For sure, our personal experiences may be occluded. But what I think we're really getting at in this conversation is how the hegemony of intuitive eating unwittingly reinforces the very things it claims to be against.

L

Absolutely. Intuitive eating uses binary thinking to impose the individualism and power-blankness it rails against. Where "exceptions" like disability and poverty are mentioned, they're tagged on with caveats. That's not a liberatory logic; that's a logic that shoehorns everyone into a flawed framing. It confuses the will to inclusion through assimilation with the will for transformation. As if the central task of scholarship is to construct infallible theory. What happened to praxis?

Defending the intuitive eating critique by saying "it worked for me" implies that personal healing always extrapolates to mutuality and collective benefit. That's wrong of course: a thin person can drop fat shame without dropping thin privilege or other investments in whiteness. Again, yes, everyone deserves healing; some people have benefitted from intuitive eating. But served up through the self-other binary and stripped of context and consequence like this, deservingness morphs into a sense of entitlement where one person's healing doesn't require serious consideration of anyone else. What works for you or me is an important contribution to knowledge but never the last word. There are plenty of things that benefit an individual and lead to other human and non-human people suffering and land desecration.

Intuitive eating doesn't encourage us to understand this. Personal healing gets sold as a right without fostering awareness of mutuality, accountability, or privilege. You can "heal" without any consciousness of intersectionality. I'm not recommending guilt-tripping someone in the grips of an eating disorder, or any time, to "think of others less fortunate." Or burdening someone in crisis with inappropriate emotional, intellectual, or spiritual labour. I'm saying intuitive eating is formed around norms it rejects.

It implicitly casts the undoing of whiteness as outside the immediate relevant sphere of (clinical) concern, something to be named, for sure, but compartmentalized for addressing another time. It misses the ways that its current discourse is already serving whiteness and busy stabilizing the binary.

M

It's such a relief to hear you say that. I've been on the receiving end of a lot of eating disorder treatment over the years, and I've been bombarded by countless dietitians implicitly and explicitly upholding intuitive eating as the pinnacle of recovery, the goal that we should all be working towards. It would be funny if it wasn't so harmful, the way that intuitive eating reinforces the classic body/mind split and the disconnect between the individual and the world "out there." I have always struggled with this myth of self-sufficiency, as though both the problem and the solution to my troubled eating lie entirely within me as an individual. As though our personal pain and healing are not intimately bound up in shared struggles and collective liberation.

In a recent eating disorder inpatient admission, it was striking how any time we "patients" tried to collectivize our approaches to healing, to take on challenges together, to express solidarity with one other, we were shut down by dietitians and psychiatrists alike. We were instructed to "stay in our own lanes," to focus on our own recovery. This says a lot about the fragility of healthcare practitioners and their theories and how easily they are threatened by visions of healing, eating, and caring for one another outside the narrow individualist frame of intuitive eating.

L

Professional socialization guards against deep knowing and transformation. As registered dietitians we graduate with certain of our competence as scientists and healers. Non-diet dietitians treat intuitive eating as a no-brainer, so even feeling concern, never mind voicing it, is going to feel weird. Just acknowledging scholarly critique can feel like a betrayal when your leaders aim to suffocate it with silence. Because the culture is one of orthodoxy, not praxis, members don't develop skills in criticality. Yet in the non-diet community we can feel exceptionally astute, smarter than our diet colleagues and so believe we have good critical skills. Now there's a conundrum. Non-diet dietitians may struggle to grasp what's been said in critiques like this and end up bemused, frustrated, indignant, and hurt. They are trapped by the logic of orthodoxy promulgated by leaders. Not the bit that says intuitive eating or health at every size (HAES) is right. But the belief it is right and cannot be wrong.

The binary logic of intuitive eating creates the world with intuitive eating and the world without. A world without intuitive eating means dieting, so intuitive eating must be good, right? Queering allows for a different world, plurality, a third and fourth theory of eating, rejuvenates ancient food ways.

Naming this good/bad dichotomy is my opportunity to make clear that in confronting the failings of intuitive eating (bad) I'm not claiming to be innocent (good). I've been very wrong about foundational beliefs in the past. I've done all the things. I'm totally capable of being wrong again.

If intuitive eating saves you from peril you'll feel protective. Still, stonewalling dissent is a trauma-forged response – that needs addressing as such – because ultimately it protects the status quo.

M

And the status quo loves to put it all back on us, as the problem, so that we're so busy trying to fix ourselves that we won't have time or energy to fight back. Like how intuitive eating insists that the main obstacles to achieving interoceptive awareness originate from our own minds – it's easy to feel like it's our fault, that we're wedded to the eating disorder and haven't tried hard enough at recovery. For example, I feel shame for still needing a meal plan. Surely I should be done with this by now? Surely I should know what and when and how much to eat? When intuitive eating is positioned as the ultimate goal, the meal plan is cast as a short-term crutch to outgrow as soon as possible. But I'm tired of being made to feel like I'm broken. I'm tired of carrying the burden of shame. And I'm tired of the linear (straight!) teleology of recovery offered by intuitive eating.

So, what would it mean to queer our visions of healing troubled eating? I suspect that in a world without interpersonal and systemic violence, we would *all* be more able to feel safe and present in our bodies, to listen to and respect body knowledge at any given moment. Not only hunger and fullness, but also regarding our safety, our desires and attractions and yearnings, our need for care and rest, our energy levels, our capacity to feel joy and connection, and so on. And so the queer world we are working towards must be the overturning of the capitalist and white supremacist structures of oppression and exclusion that hurt us all.

Along the way, I want to reconfigure the meal plan as queer technology, another queer prosthesis alongside our packers and bras and hormones and binders and fake eyelashes. A means of showing up for ourselves, nourishing and resourcing ourselves, doing what we can to ensure our safety and vitality under the current conditions, as we organize towards a world where we can all thrive. Recognizing that we are no more or less queer, trans, or "recovered," by virtue of the supports, interventions, or technologies that we choose or choose not to engage, to pick up and put down and different times, for a multitude of reasons. Recognizing that our pain and our healing is always in coalition, a matter of solidarity, which is to say, life or death.

L

Queering is a call to understand binary thinking as a logic of domination and disconnect and replace it. Queering nutrition, making it queer- and trans-safe, includes troubling the social contract that presents the gender binary as "normal" and therefore desirable and incontestable. Of course, we need to respect pronouns and kinship arrangements and make sure everyone can use the loo safely. But that's not liberation. Liberation needs a deeper queering, where we are not in thrall to toxic-but-naturalized whiteness. As Black scholars such as Harrison (2021) have been telling us, this means building praxis that centres Black fat trans lives.

That serves the collective, that strengthens the commons. It is a praxis that uplifts disability justice too. Even if we can all feel safer and more present in our bodies, not everyone gets to access embodied knowledge, or feel recovered or healed. Fanon (1961) captures this: "And the day when our human race has fully matured, it will not define itself as the sum of the inhabitants of the globe, but as the infinite unity of their reciprocities."

Plus, who says the "right" way for someone to flourish is minus a meal plan? We can't know that, and we can't know it is possible. Sure, someone might really want this outcome. Queering holds this desire and hope and potential in a narrative that remains open to other possibilities.

Queering embroils us in flux, indeterminacy.

Another queer thing is sharing that dietetics might not be someone's best medicine. As well as changing what we offer as dietitians, we need to use our privileged place in the nutrition tree to undo whiteness and share non-dietetic knowhow that might be useful – the creative arts, plant medicine, ancestral healing, and much more.

So we left the conferences, the recovery groups, and the HAES forums, to write this chapter about our experiences, to break a silence manufactured by power. We have said that intuitive eating presumes personal healing is hermetic; that it fashions "instinct" devoid of embeddedness; that it reifies the non-relational, non-traumatized and "natural" body, is aligned with straightness and whiteness. These harms matter even while we acknowledge and are glad for the fact that advocates of intuitive eating seek to – and may – interrupt personal suffering, fat stigma, and build queer-safe(r) places. This constellation, while important, isn't in itself liberatory. Learning to live well enough in a toxic system is necessary for our survival, but it does not need or compel us to change the system. Any theory or practice that lets us believe our personal positive experience is sufficient to prove universal benefit is entwined with anti-queer individualism and hinders transformation.

We hope for queered responses, for engagements that seek to further our ideas generatively, offering amendments and exploring extensions. As part of this we hope that the story we share registers with intuitive eating advocates in ways that spur them to interrogate their certainties and identify and change the norms in community knowledge-creation that continue to write people out.

References

Da'Shaun, L. H. (2021) *Belly of the Beast: The Politics of Anti-Fatness as Anti-Blackness.* North Atlantic Books.

Frantz Fanon, The wretched of the earth. (1961). Retrieved November 4, 2021, from https://onlinereadfreenovel.com/frantz-fanon/page,6,59498-the_wretched_of_the_earth.html

3 Invisibility – In Visibility

Art-Based Autoethnography of a Bisexual Vegan Woman with Type 1 Diabetes

Lee Ann Thill

I wanted to be invisible from an early age. Diagnosed with type 1 diabetes (T1D) at age five, I grew weary of questions, comments, and teasing, and by second grade, was invested in keeping my diabetes a secret. From there, keeping secrets and going unseen was my default. I struggled with food and body image for years, hiding my eating behaviours and diabetes mis/management, trying to "disappear" through weight loss. For an "invisible illness," hiding T1D required effort to sneak, lie, and be vigilant, which I maintained through my early adult years.

Invisible disability designates a disability that is not apparent. There can be clues that a person has T1D – insulin pump, beeping devices, blood sugar checks – but as a chronic disease, it is largely considered invisible, and diabetic people can conceal T1D (Sanders et al., 2019; Syma, 2019).

At 19, my boyfriend asked if I had sexual thoughts about women. I trusted him and said yes; he erupted in anger and disgust. He was the first person I told. I would eventually share my same-sex desires with other boyfriends and made an uncertain effort to meet women in my late 20s, but I identified as heterosexual into my 30s.

Bisexual invisibility is a consequence of bisexual erasure (Yoshino, 2000). There are three explanations for erasure: ontic, "truth" that the world is comprised of binaries because some binaries exist (i.e., night/day); cognitive, a tendency to assign binaries to complex phenomena; and political, "agonistic politics have bifurcated the continuum," forcing interested parties to choose sides to serve their respective interests (Yoshino, 2000, p. 391).

Non-human animals are similarly metaphorically invisiblized through social exclusion, characterized by "moral disrespect … and absence of gestures of recognition" (Honneth & Margalit, 2001, p. 123). Animals are also literally invisibilized, hidden by the animal agriculture industry, by being renamed as "meat" and by being aggregated (i.e., "livestock") (Rowe, 2011). Animal invisibilization is undergirded by anthropocentrism, which "pervades human–animal relations at the deepest levels and informs hierarchies of the differently seen and cared-for" (Arcari et al., 2021, p. 944).

Queer autoethnography is a relational, political, and scholarly intervention for disrupting business-as-usual violence and the invisibilizing of minoritized others (Holman Jones & Harris, 2019). Art-based inquiry promotes non-linear thinking and allows for the juxtaposition of disparate ideas (McNiff, 2011). Collage and assemblage, specifically, have historically been the purview of women (Schapiro & Meyer, 2015).

DOI: 10.4324/9781003217121-4

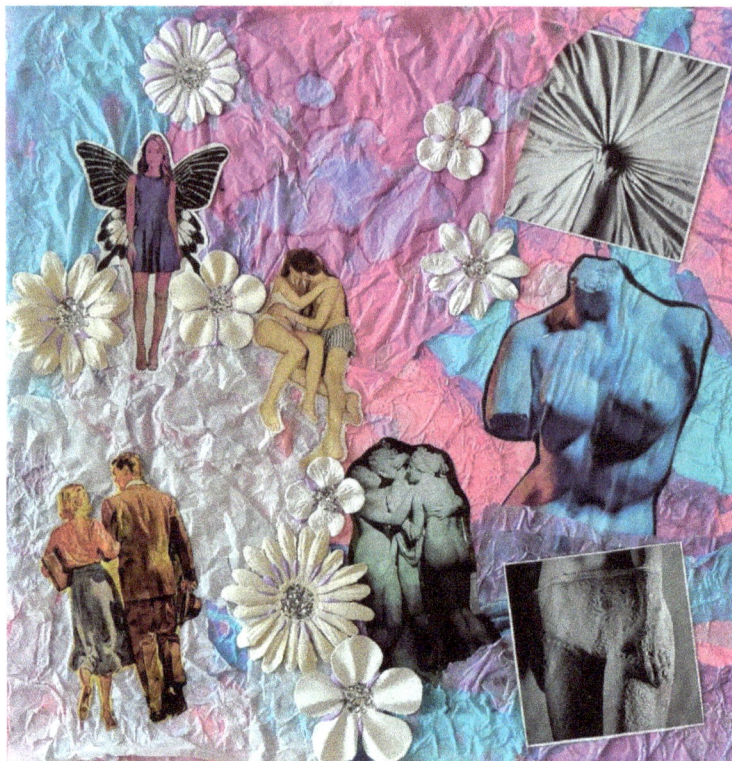

Figure 3.1 Bisexual Invisibility. Lee Ann Thill.

For this inquiry, I completed five mixed-media collages: *Bisexual Invisibility* (Figure 3.1), *That Ham Had Friends* (Figure 3.2), *Bleeding* (Figure 3.3), *Carb Counting* (Figure 3.4), and *Valentine to My Loves* (Figure 3.5). I wrote reflections for each collage about my creative process and the artwork's meaning. Once the art and reflections were complete, I did content analysis, extracting meaning modules, which I grouped by emergent themes.

My experiences – T1D, bisexuality, and veganism – seem disparate, but as strands of a narrative they have a flow and logic. Four underlying themes from the written reflections that have propelled the narrative are explored: presentation and visibility, identity and psychological experience, relationality, body, and physicality.

Presentation and Visibility

The piece, *Bisexual Invisibility* (Figure 3.1), reflects my experience as a bisexual woman in a monogamous marriage with a cis het man. The "public" experience, represented by the white section, is juxtaposed with the "private" experience, the

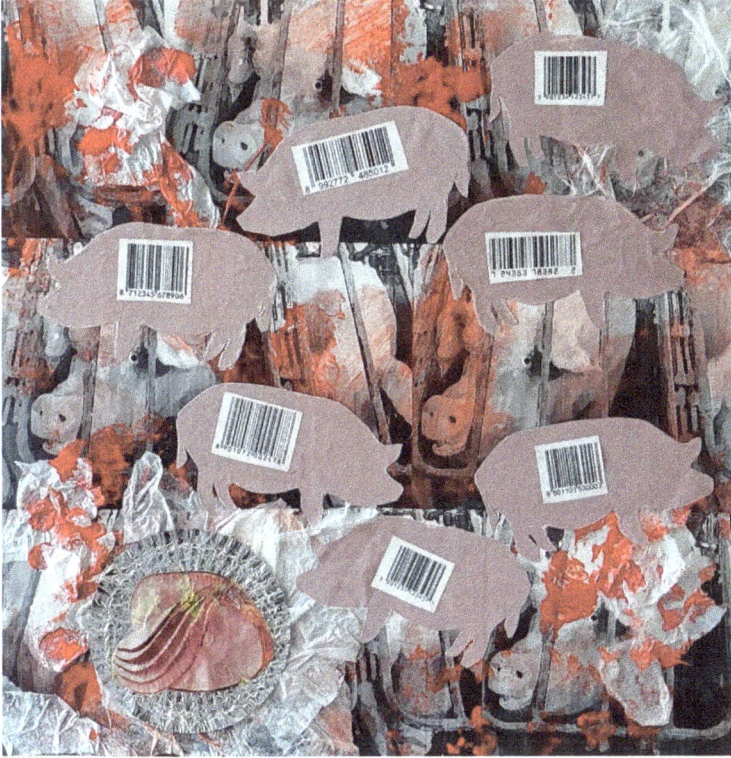

Figure 3.2 That Ham Had Friends. Lee Ann Thill.

blue and pink section. Attention was given to the tension between these spaces representing the visible and invisible.

> *In order to BE bisexual, as in, present as bi, when I am straight-passing in a monogamous relationship with a man, I have to talk about my sexuality. It's not like I look or act bisexual, or present in some kind of way.*

Bisexual people employ strategies for visibility. Direct communication is associated with higher identity centrality and affirmation, and lower internalized bi-negativity and bi-illegitimacy (Feinstein et al., 2021). Using pride symbols, such as the pink, purple, and blue bi flag, also improves visibility and validity (Hayfield, 2021).

> *I liked the effect of dripping water on the tissue. That started as an accident, but then I started playing with it more. The blending and bleeding of colours symbolizing bisexuality seem to represent something about the lived experience … who do I appear to be in this moment.*

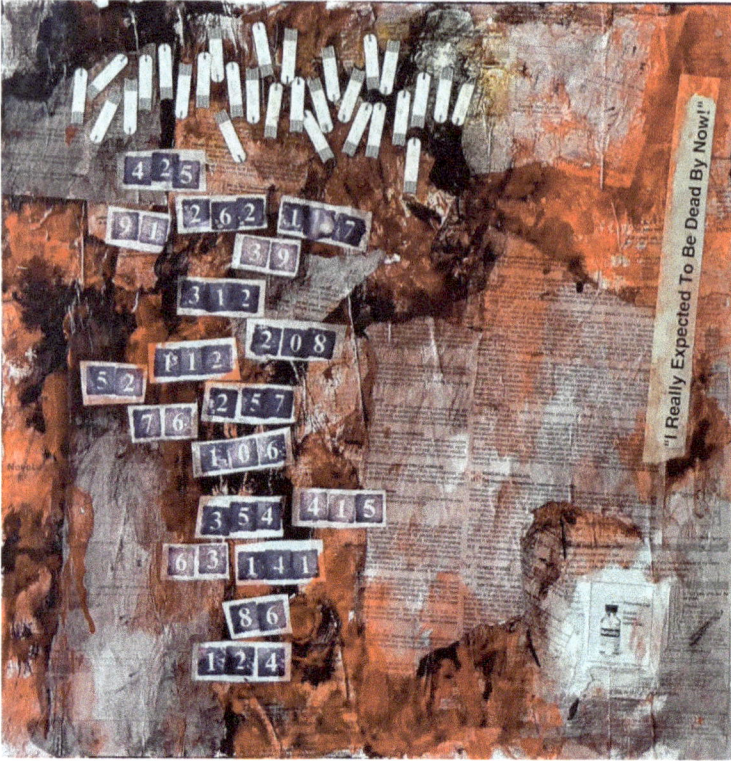

Figure 3.3 Bleeding. Lee Ann Thill.

Notably, visual displays of bisexuality, like flags, were associated with higher anticipated bi-negativity and discrimination from heterosexual people (Feinstein et al., 2021). That risk elicited feelings of vulnerability I have about "coming out" with this collage, when "coming out" is understood as a series of contextual disclosures (Hayfield, 2021; Maliepaard, 2018).

I felt uncertain about the collage representing animals and veganism as a strategy for animal rights. *That Ham Had Friends* (Figure 3.2) was inspired by Adams and Gruen (2014), who asked: "Can negative images that reinscribe oppressive attitudes be contained, by being … dislocated from their original context?" (p. 27). Rowe (2011) answered explicitly: "The visual … puts a struggling, squealing face with the bloody, dead piece of body on my plate" (p. 16).

> *I had the intention of drawing the line from tortured animal to the dinner plate, but I'm anxious about how to represent this violence … "I'm sorry that I'm representing the violent part of your dinner, I'm sorry you have to see the scared animals and the blood," as if it's some big secret.*

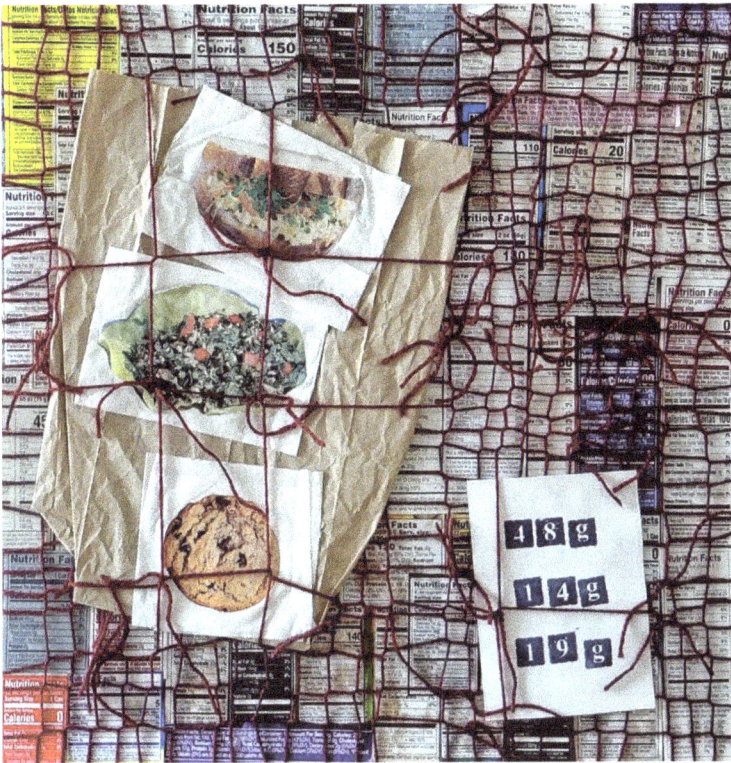

Figure 3.4 Carb Counting. Lee Ann Thill.

Veganism and my regard for animals are implicit in *Carb Counting* (Figure 3.4), which reflects my relationship with food and T1D dietary management. I was conscious of the frameworks I use to select food.

> *I felt pressure to show that a vegan diet can be varied, including treats, like, I'm not eating grass and sticks, as people like to joke. So there's that … I wanted to show a beautiful vegan diet – and I was careful to only use images from vegan recipes.*

Identity and Psychological Experience

The dynamic relationship between visibility, and identity and psychological experiences, was an essential theme of *Bisexual Invisibility* (Figure 3.1). I explored the interaction between the "private" and "public" spheres and their associated impact on my understanding of self.

> *The figure with the wings is like a fairy bi girl, who is probably my conscious effort to present as bi. She represents intention.*

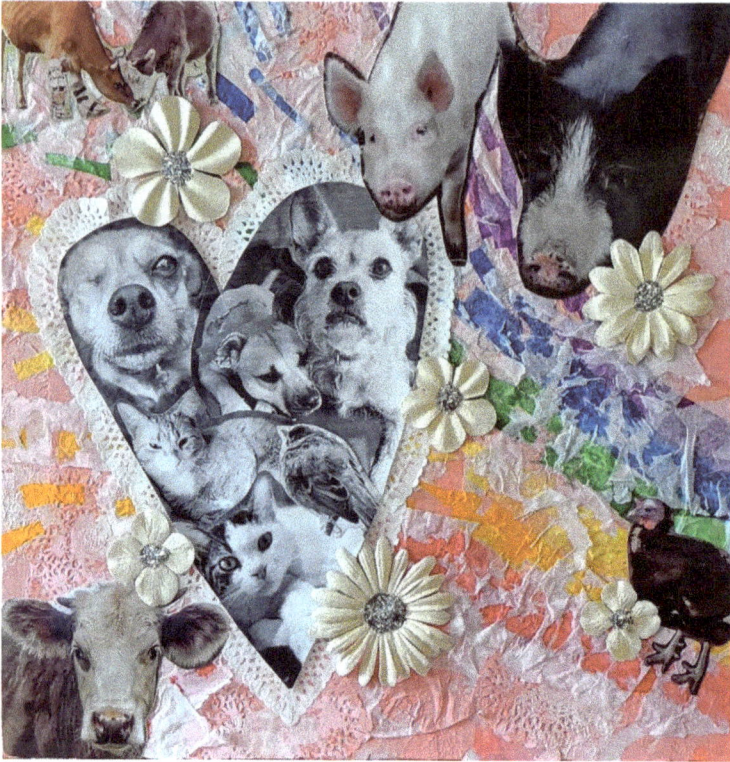

Figure 3.5 Valentine to My Loves. Lee Ann Thill.

The "private" sphere is dominated by images of sculptures of female figures, each of which signifies facets of my identity and psychological experience.

> *A figure without a head or arms, a body, a fantasy without an identity. The figure of the hips with the bound arms, also a reference to not acting on this part of my sexuality, the outcome of which is invisibility. The three female figures also represent the imaginative dimension of my sexuality. And of course, all of these figures are immobilized – no feet, no legs. My bi-ness isn't going anywhere, but my bi-ness is, well, not going anywhere.*

In other words, my bisexuality is intrinsic and stable, but I am in a monogamous heterosexual relationship, so my bisexuality is not fully expressed. The emphasis on female figures is consistent with research that showed bisexual women in different-sex relationships desired intimacy with women, but this did not mean they were dissatisfied with their current relationships (Daly, 2018).

I also alluded to the relationship between presentation and psychological experience of T1D in *Bleeding* (Figure 3.3).

Aside from seeing someone checking their blood sugar, blood sugar management is mental, intellectual, emotional, and not visible. It can engender feelings of frustration and powerlessness when things don't go "right."

Coincidentally, the evening I wrote this, "things did not go right." My blood glucose (BG) was steadily climbing and not responding to my efforts to bring it back into range. I discovered my insulin infusion set had detached from my body, so I was not getting insulin. I related the experience to the artwork, noting my application and visual effect of the paint.

This particular instance also illustrates how trying to identify underlying causes of blood sugar can be inherently opaque.

The infusion set incident was anomalous but exemplifies having the tools and the data – insulin, BG strips, BG readings – but continuously having to account for myriad variables.

Ups and downs ... occur even when someone with T1D is making a "best effort," not because they did something [wrong], but because their pancreas doesn't make insulin.

Naming the underlying physiological mechanism of blood sugar variability is a means of fostering grace towards myself, as opposed to getting entrenched in guilt, shame, and punitive self-talk.

Since food is a primary determinant of blood sugar, these same cognitive and emotional processes are relevant to *Carb Counting* (Figure 3.4). Notably, the initial collage was dissatisfying – lack of clarity about intention resulted in visual disorganization – so I tore it from the surface, and created this collage over the remnants, perhaps a metaphor for transforming my relationship with food over time, including recovery from an eating disorder.

It's not like I have the option to be fully at peace with food though, although I think this is as close as it gets. Type 1 diabetes will forever include intellectual and emotional labour.

The finished piece represents efforts to eat "normally" that conflict with inescapable complexities of T1D dietary management. It also elicited memories of eating challenges I had as a child with T1D.

There are automatic thoughts about how indulgent a meal appears to others – will I be judged for eating too many carbs, or having a sweet treat? It's funny because I had a lot of self-conscious feelings as I chose the images for this meal, feelings that are not unfamiliar to me when actually choosing a meal. As a kid, I was watched when I was eating, and those thoughts have become like muscle memory. In this particular case, the weight of that is more apparent because this isn't even a real meal – these are images depicting a meal – and yet, the thought processes and emotional reflexes are the same – shame, doubt, fear of judgment.

Even when T1D is invisible, the person with diabetes understands that observers who know could be interpreting and judging seemingly innocuous actions like what the person with T1D eats. This ongoing experience of feeling surveilled has been associated with self-consciousness and shame (Lucherini, 2016).

Relationality

My relationship with my partner is a central element of *Bisexual Invisibility* (Figure 3.1).

> *It's good that I could be more open and expressive about my sexuality, like I've felt safe with my husband ... The image of the couple kissing represents het affection and physical intimacy, but it's positioned between the spaces. It's the conventional assumption about a straight-presenting marriage, so it's partially in that space, but it's also in the private space that is both within my marriage, and my internal experience.*

Conversely, relating to people in the "public" sphere about bisexuality is not consistently affirming.

> *I think people should have some basic level of awareness that other people's sexuality might not be how it looks on the surface.*

Similarly, interacting with people about T1D requires mutuality, as noted in my response to *Bleeding* (Figure 3.3).

> *If one were to interact with the art in person, they would need to lean in to make out the images, analogous to the way T1D is visible – one needs to lean in, so to speak, by being observant, engaged, and patient.*

There are limits to learning though, even for the most loving and curious people who are committed to understanding, like caregivers and partners.

> *Conveying the lived experience to others always seems shallow and incomplete, which is deeply unsatisfying emotionally and relationally. That's isolating because the never-ending-ness of it is invisible.*

The unsettling nature of *That Ham Had Friends* (Figure 3.2) compelled me to create *Valentine to My Loves* (Figure 3.5), an alternative narrative about animal relationships that embraces queerness.

> *I started thinking about the companion animals in my family, and wanted to situate farmed animals in relation to my companions, and the idea of "companion animal" ... I basically wanted to create a valentine to them, in the spirit of children's handmade valentines with red, pink, and white colours, and paper doilies ... also representing the rainbow bridge, the*

symbol of heaven or other world where animals who have died go, and, as the story goes, humans can reunite with their loved ones when they too die. I also think about the lives of animals used for food, and I think about the animals I ate before I was vegan. Within the context of this collage, I wondered about those animals used for food, crossing the rainbow bridge. I thought about them meeting "companion animals," I thought about meeting them all there.

The rainbow has dual significance, though.

The rainbow as a queer symbol represents multi-species relationships and chosen family, relationships that are socially regarded as a phase or immature … The rainbow also splays apart and begins to disintegrate on one side. That's a lot of things, the inconsistency of its application by society – companions are elevated to the rainbow bridge, but in global minority culture, they don't think about animals they eat as having "souls," or what the idea of soul implies – being someone with an emotional and cognitive life, caring for family from whom they were taken (standard practice in animal agriculture), and companions or "families of circumstance."

Queer animal activists and theorists have described the transgressive nature of affections that are not deemed "natural," garnering hostility and state-sanctioned violence from those who seek to maintain the human-heteronormative status quo. As Dell-Aversano (2019) stated, "like lesbian feminism, animal queer is about political choice and emotional preference" (p. 15). The essence of this collage was succinctly captured by Ramirez (2020), a bi disabled woman of colour and animal rights activist: love is not scarce; it is not a finite commodity. Love can be shared with all species and all genders; caring about one justice issue – queer, animal, racial, disability, etc. – can open one up to other justice issues.

Body and Physicality

Relationality of *Bisexual Invisibility* (Figure 3.1) is intertwined with body and physicality, as represented by the image of the embracing couple, but I also wanted to depict physical pleasure as an experience that is not dependent on a partner, regardless of gender.

The hand gripping the sheet is the only photo of a person solely situated in the "private" sphere, but it's also about fantasy, and what isn't seen, as well as lived experience.

Body and physicality was also an integral theme of the collages about T1D. Some of the meaning modules for those collages referred to the "nuts and bolts" of diabetes management, which I associated with the body. The process of creating *Carb Counting* (Figure 3.4) was a metaphor for T1D management.

Collecting the labels and gluing them, moving labels around as if I was putting a puzzle together, a puzzle without a clear finished image to reference, is also a metaphor for dietary management with T1D, the repetitiveness of it, the labour with a notion of what it should or could look like – the health outcomes, in medical parlance – but a lot of making it up as I go, the inexactitude, and hoping it all comes together.

I selected the quote collaged onto *Bleeding* (Figure 3.3) – "I really expected to be dead by now!" – because I have been confronted by my mortality since I was very young.

The line, I thought I would be dead, is true. When I was very young, that was the expectation, that people with T1D just didn't live into old age – not that I've made it to old age yet – but we weren't supposed to live that long, and towards the end, we would inevitably experience all manner of disabling diabetes complications.

Bodies were central to *That Ham Had Friends* (Figure 3.2), but my reflections do not specify bodies. During content analysis, I realized I was preoccupied that the pig collage would undermine this project as a whole, given evidence of hostility and microaggressions towards vegans (Cole & Morgan, 2011; Lerette, 2014; MacInnis & Hodson, 2017); if allyship with animals is read as illegitimate, what concern is there for the bodies?

"Well, she's an animal rights extremist, so what does she know?"

The following excerpt does not name bodies but refers to what happens to bodies.

I'm still on the question of what this piece could be, what I'm trying to do. I want to show the animals who get invisibilized, and I want to represent that process. I need that to be authentic and true, and the violence is part of that.

Fernandez (2021) investigated the use of images to challenge the human–animal binary and engage people involved in other social justice movements and concluded that images visibilizing violence against animal bodies are most effective in combination with positive images of animals. *Valentine to My Loves* (Figure 3.5) depicts animals whose bodily autonomy and integrity are respected. I was particularly interested in representing disability, given my experience with invisible disability.

Although not obvious, I also wanted to represent disability by including images of my companions who are disabled – a dog with one eye, and a sparrow with no eyes – and Fawn (top left), a cow who was rescued from a dairy farm, and wore front leg braces during her life at a sanctuary.

Conclusion

Invisibility begets invisibility. Visibility begets visibility. While neither is always good or always bad – i.e., safety-motivated queer invisibility strategies – in my experience, bisexual invisibility and invisible illness have often been detrimental, whereas visibility has usually offered flexibility, authenticity, and healing. Invisibilizing animals harms them and me; visibilizing them has been liberating and is consistent with destabilizing binaries and hierarchies. One question that emerges is, what were the mechanisms that enabled the shift from invisibilizing to visibilizing? The answer is unclear, but perhaps the themes identified here – presentation and visibility, identity and psychological experience, relationality, and body and physicality – might be a starting point. Lastly, artmaking was the foundational component to this project, and its particular value in the exploration of phenomena characterized by invisibilizing is unique and compelling.

References

Adams, C. J., & Gruen, L. (2014). Groundwork. In C. J. Adams & L. Gruen (Eds.), *Feminist intersections with other animals and the earth* (pp. 7–36). Bloomsbury.

Arcari, P., Probyn-Rapsey, F., & Singer, H. (2021). Where species don't meet: Invisibilized animals, urban nature and city limits [Article]. *Environment & Planning E: Nature & Space*, *4*(3), 940–965.

Cole, M., & Morgan, K. (2011). Vegaphobia: Derogatory discourses of veganism and the reproduction of speciesism in UK national newspapers. *British Journal of Sociology*, *62*(1), 134.

Daly, S. J. (2018). *A rock and a hard place: A hermeneutic phenomenological exploration into the lived experience of bisexual women in monogamous relationships.* Doctoral thesis, University of Huddersfield. Huddersfield, West Yorkshire, England.

Dell'Aversano, C. (2019). The love whose name cannot be spoken: Queering the human-animal bond. In A. J. Nocella & A. E. George (Eds.), *Intersectionality of critical animal studies: A historical collection* (pp. 11–47). Peter Lang Publishing, Inc.

Feinstein, B. A., Dyar, C., Milstone, J. S., Jabbour, J., & Davila, J. (2021). Use of different strategies to make one's bisexual+ identity visible: Associations with dimensions of identity, minority stress, and health. *Stigma and Health*, *6*(2), 184–191.

Fernandez, L. (2021). Images that liberate: Moral shock and strategic visual communication in animal liberation activism. *Journal of Communication Inquiry*, *45*(2), 138–158.

Hayfield, N. (2021). *Bisexual and pansexual identities: Exploring and challenging invisibility and invalidation.* Routledge.

Holman Jones, S., & Harris, A. M. (2019). *Queering autoethnography.* Routledge.

Honneth, A., & Margalit, A. (2001). Recognition. *Proceedings of the Aristotelian Society, Supplementary Volumes*, *75*, 111–139.

Lerette, D. E. (2014). *Stories of microaggressions directed toward vegans and vegetarians in social settings* (Publication Number 3615270) Fielding Graduate University].

Lucherini, M. (2016). Performing diabetes: Felt surveillance and discreet self-management [Article]. *Surveillance & Society*, *14*(2), 259–276.

MacInnis, C. C., & Hodson, G. (2017). It ain't easy eating greens: Evidence of bias toward vegetarians and vegans from both source and target. *Group Processes & Intergroup Relations*, *20*(6), 721–744.

Maliepaard, E. (2018). Disclosing bisexuality or coming out? Two different realities for bisexual people in the Netherlands. *Journal of Bisexuality*, *18*(2), 145–167.

McNiff, S. (2011). Artistic expressions as primary modes of inquiry. *British Journal of Guidance & Counselling, 29*(5), 385–396.

Ramirez, J. (2020). Love isn't scarce. In J. Feliz Brueck & Z. McNeill (Eds.), *Queer and trans voices: Achieving liberation through consistent anti-oppression* (pp. 81–88). Sanctuary Publishers.

Rowe, B. D. (2011). Understanding animals-becoming-meat: Embracing a disturbing education. *Critical Education, 2*(7), 1–24.

Sanders, T., Elliott, J., Norman, P., Jonson, B., & Heller, S. (2019). Disruptive illness contexts and liminality in the accounts of young people with type 1 diabetes. *Sociology of Health & Illness, 41*(7), 1289–1304.

Schapiro, M., & Meyer, M. (2015). Waste not, want not: An inquiry into what women saved and assembled — femmage. *Artcritical: The Online Magazine of Art and Ideas.* https://artcritical.com/2015/06/24/femmage-by-miriam-schapiro-and-melissa-meyer/

Syma, C. (2019). Invisible disabilities: Perceptions and barriers to reasonable accommodations in the workplace. *Library Management, 40*(1), 113–120.

Yoshino, K. (2000). The epistemic contract of bisexual erasure [research-article]. *Stanford Law Review, 52*(2), 353–461.

4 Out of the Closet, Into Some Other Kind of Prison

One Gay Asian Man's Journey Finding Self-Worth While Navigating Body Image and Eating Disorders

Jeffrey Sotto

NO FATTIES, NO FEMMES, NO FISH.

Those words captioned a Grindr profile I came across in 2010, written just as above, in capital letters. They emphatically summarized the narrow – literal and figurative – gay space which I had tried to navigate since coming out at 21 years old in 2002.

My mind strolled the years leading up to this moment.

As a teenager, I weighed 140 pounds standing at five feet and three quarters of an inch. I didn't consider myself huge, but I was just past the scale of a normal BMI at 26.4. Atop my pudgy body was my very unchiselled face. The fullness of my cheeks enhanced the naturally round bone structure of my Filipino features. Once, an aunt pinched my chest through my shirt and said, "You have suso, Jeffrey." "Suso" means breasts in Tagalog. "Be careful you don't turn into a woman," she giggled, thinking it was harmless. As with most awkward teens, I was not comfortable in my body. I often hid myself in oversized clothes.

That wasn't the only thing I was hiding. I'd been bullied since grade school for being too girly and not wanting to play with other boys. I was, as it used to be casually said without the blink of an eye in the late 80s and early 90s, a faggot. Ashamed and thinking I was going to hell – my family was devoutly Catholic; my father told me that gay people were abnormal because their chromosomes were backwards, then urged me to stop playing with dolls – I kept the secret to myself and tried to get through my adolescence as inconspicuously as possible.

Then came Ellen DeGeneres. "I'm gay." Those were the words that Ellen's character famously confessed in her eponymously titled sitcom in 1997 (Black et al., 1997).

If you were gay, you knew that scene. Ellen – tormented by her desire for another female character – finally said it out loud into a microphone at an airport. My closeted 16-year-old self, along with many others in the queer community, finally felt some validation at being able to identify with someone on mainstream television. And we braced ourselves to see how our families and friends would react seeing the same thing. Her show was cancelled soon after.

DOI: 10.4324/9781003217121-5

There was *Will & Grace* (Barr et al., 1998–2006 & 2017–2020) in 1998. Again, gay people saw themselves depicted on the small screen. Will Truman and Jack McFarlane respectively represented the gay man – but not *too* gay – that could pass as straight, and the flamboyant and sassy but ultimately harmless queen. As ground-breaking as it was at the time, these portrayals of the queer community were sanitized, digestible … safe. For myself, and others, wanting to see more realistic characters with agency, much was left to be desired.

The turmoil of coming to terms with my sexuality was exacerbated by my life circumstances: my father left our family, my sister moved away, and, when I was 19, my mother died of cancer eight months after diagnosis, during which I was her primary caregiver. I was alone, still in my closet, but now there was nobody else in the house.

It wasn't until 2001 when I stumbled upon the American version of *Queer as Folk* (Cowen et al., 2000–2005) that I started to think about what my gay life might look like. Here were young, unapologetic, and sexually liberated gay men, living their best gay lives.

After devouring each episode, I was always left with a desperate sense of longing. I wanted to live the lives of Brian, Michael, and especially the young and newly out Justin. They went out. They drank. They danced under disco balls and flirted with boys and laughed without a care in the world. They had lots of sex. To me, then 20 and still closeted – often coping with my feelings by eating them – it all seemed so glamourous.

And they were attractive. Worthy of love. Desired.

After finally coming out a year later, I was ready to experience the lives of those boys on the show. I even moved from my dim suburban town of Brampton to the exciting neon city of Toronto to live my best gay life. I wanted to finally lose my virginity, and, or possibly even achieve the ultimate goal of "finding the one." I felt I had a good chance: I had a kind personality; I thought I had nice eyes and a warm smile; I was damn sure I was a good dancer. I still had a bit of that teenage pudge, but otherwise was in "okay" shape. On top of that, the hard part was over: I had come out.

But that wasn't to be. Months and years went by, and I'd leave the bars and clubs wondering why nobody was spinning me around the way Brian did Justin during some romantic song on the centre of the dance floor under a shiny disco ball, like on the TV screen (Cowen et al., 2000–2005). Why didn't my life resemble the television show I clung to every week, the show in which I lived vicariously through its characters?

Eventually, I did start dating someone that I met through friends in 2008. He liked to joke a lot. He'd tease my chubbiness, calling me his "chunky monkey," but he always disclaimed the little extra was "fine" because, on me, it was "cute." He'd call me at work and ask me what I'd had for lunch sometimes:

"Did you have dog for lunch today?" he'd ask.

"I'm sorry, what? *Dog?*" I replied.

"Yeah. 'Cause Filipinos eat dog, right?"

I didn't know how to respond to that. I always thought of myself as being one of those people who saw the humour in all things, but I was confused.

He started laughing. "Kidding. I'm kidding, my little chunky monkey."

We'd often have those kinds of conversations before he dumped me a few months later, claiming that I was uptight.

"Listen, if I can't really be with someone if I can't joke with them. That's just who I am," he said.

Anxiously, I pulled myself together and ventured back into the bars. In the past, I'd sit and nurse a vodka seven for hours as nobody approached me. This time, I looked at the men who attracted the attention, the ones who made everyone's head turn. They looked like the characters on *Queer as Folk* (Cowen et al., 2000–2005) or the impossibly hot guys on the televisions scattered throughout the bar on which gay porn played on a loop. All these particular "desired" men had similar physical attributes: white, six feet or taller, and possessing a body that was either underweight, slim, toned, or extremely muscular. They looked like Ken dolls. This notion was echoed in the online dating and hook-up scene; profiles of tall white men with those body types lined the top "featured profile" border.

I didn't fit any of those criteria.

NO FATTIES, NO FEMMES, NO FISH.

These words years later confirmed why I was alone. Not being super skinny, toned, or muscular, but with a little jiggle, deemed me a "fattie," according to one user. "*NO FEMMES*" could also be written as "*straight-acting only*," or "*masc for masc.*" Gay men wanted "big manly men," so despite being gay, one had to *not act gay* (internalized homophobia, anyone?). Being short and easily identifiable as gay whenever I began talking, I wasn't exactly the pinnacle of masculinity either. Finally, "*NO FISH*" meant no Asians; I, as a person, was reduced to the stereotypical staple of my racial identity's diet.

Like many queer people, my journey through my LGBTQ+ identity ran the gamut of emotions: there was the desperate search to identify other queer people in order to validate myself as "normal"; then, the acceptance of said identity and willingness to share it; the relief I felt letting go of my secret, followed by the desperate need of acceptance from my family and friends; and lastly but certainly not least importantly, there was the immediate sexual liberation I craved after many years of repression. The latter – the final part of my self-actualization as a gay person – pointed to a blaring conundrum: how could I deem myself worthy if I didn't fit within the confines of such desired physical attributes? Within the community I was supposed to belong to. One might hope the queer community could be more accepting, considering the common struggles we face. I realized that I had come out of the closet but entered some other kind of prison.

I then decided that I would work with what I had and alter my body. I knew I'd never be the tall Ken doll that most men wanted or wanted to be. That didn't appeal to me anyway; by that point, I knew that I was a bottom, so I didn't want to come across as the dominant alpha male. Rather, I wanted to be the skinny, smooth, submissive, bottom Asian (who didn't eat dogs) that many fetishized. If I was going to be a stereotype, this was the closest one available to me; I was determined to be the best version of it that I could, which meant I had to lose weight.

In fall 2010, I joined a gym and would do an hour of cardio, four days a week. Ten pounds melted quickly, much to my delight. I then cut my meal portions in half. By the end of the year, I completely cut out carbohydrates. It felt strange not eating rice. As if eliminating it – eliminating my Asian-ness – was required to achieve the new desirable version of myself. Another 20 pounds came off me. By the spring of 2011, I'd cut out dinner completely. At many points, I wanted to cut my wrists; starving and overexercising was misery. But then I wondered, *would that help me get thinner? Probably not.* So bleeding to death wasn't an option.

The hunger pains proved too difficult at times, and I began binging. As I panicked at the thought of gaining weight after another episode one night, I went to the toilet and stuck my finger down my throat. The food came back up; I felt as if I had pressed a magic button. This was a revelation: if I did this all the time, I would never get fat. I could eat what I wanted, as much as I could dream of, and get away with it because I was just going to get rid of it later, like committing a crime and getting off scot-free.

To augment my strategy, I added laxatives, diuretics, and fat burners to my diet. By the end of 2011, I was at 98 pounds. Instead of food, I fed off compliments: "You've lost so much weight, you look amazing!" "Holy shit, you look like a different person!" "What is your secret, you skinny bitch!" people would say to me. If I tipped the scale into triple digits, I'd starve myself, which would eventually cause a binge, which would lead to a purge. The vicious anorexia–bulimia cycle to keep off the weight of my unwanted self was exhausting, but at least I knew that people would be jealous of my size 26 jeans. Someone would be envious of *me*. I felt like I had achieved the validation I had been longing for. Others could have better jobs than me, make more money, or flaunt their statuesque handsome boyfriends – their Ken dolls – to my face or on social media, but I was thin, so I had that. As my body became smaller, my pride only grew.

However, maintaining this worthy version of myself had a cost. As I lost more weight, I felt hungry, cold, and tired all the time. If I got out of bed too quickly or stood up from my chair after sitting for too long, my vision would fade to black. My cuticles were ripped, and my gums bled. Two of my teeth cracked in half, and eventually I had to have them extracted. I'd wake up to patches of my hair on my pillow. My brain functioned at a slower speed, causing my school and work performance to suffer. I'd go to bed early to avoid being awake and feel the hunger pains. Night was my favourite part of the day; I could be unconscious. Free from the uncontrollable mind that had betrayed me. Having been diagnosed with depression and anxiety disorder when my mom died many years before, I already had suicidal ideations; the eating disorder did not help.

My family and friends, concerned about my appearance, confronted me, but I was defensive and told them to mind their own business. Eventually, I couldn't hide it from my family doctor; he then referred me to a psychiatrist, who subsequently sent me for an assessment in an inpatient eating disorder programme. When the programme offered to take me in, I declined, saying I couldn't afford to leave university (I went back to finish my bachelor's degree when I was 30) for two months or else I wouldn't be able to graduate. That was true, but the primary reason why I didn't want to attend was the recovery. It terrified me; "recovery" meant I'd probably gain weight. I continued in my pattern.

But it was only a matter of time. In 2016 at age 35, dumped by another boyfriend and unable to handle the stresses of work, finances, and my already existing mental health struggles, I imploded. I overdosed on a range of medications and was found unconscious in my apartment after not showing up at work. I woke up in Toronto Western hospital to my older sister's very stern words: "I ended your lease. When you get out of here, you're living with me." I was not of sound mind and unable to take care of myself.

I completed an inpatient programme and then went to live with my sister and her family in the suburb of Mississauga. After a week of being in the house, my sister called me over to the kitchen one day. She showed me a doughnut on a plate; the top of the doughnut (where rainbow sprinkles were) was eaten. But the middle and bottom of it still remained. I looked closer: the bite marks along the top were tiny.

"This is a doughnut Gabby ate earlier today," my sister said. Gabby, my niece, was three years old at the time.

My eyes and shoulders lowered. I knew where this was going. *Shit.*

My sister continued. "When I asked her why she ate it like that, she said, 'I saw Uncle Jeff do it'."

Her tone told me enough, but then she said it explicitly: "I will not have you doing this in my house. The kids are watching you."

"Okay, yes," I nodded, unable to look her in the eye.

I was horrified and embarrassed. What if my niece developed the same problem? And because of me?

Perhaps this was where my recovery really began.

I cannot say with more joy that I am a proud uncle. I love my nephew and niece more than anything in the world. It turned out I couldn't do it for myself, but for them, I was able to slowly relearn how to take care of myself, step by step. I worked up to consistently eating and keeping down three meals a day. I continued seeing a psychiatrist, learned about and practiced cognitive behavioural therapy, and participated in eating disorder programmes and support groups, even though I didn't always believe they were working. There was one day in a workshop when the facilitator asked us to colour on a circle graph the portion of the value in which we place our appearance and weight in. I hated doing it, but I was honest and coloured my portion in; it took up about 70% of my circle. Then the facilitator asked us, "if you look back at the end of your life, is this how you want to measure your own self-worth?" I haven't forgotten that day.

As I worked toward my recovery, I was glad to see the LGBTQ+ community has and continues to slowly but surely make steps toward accepting and embracing all bodies. Larger figures are celebrated through famous advocates like Sam Smith and Demi Lovato and popular television shows such as *RuPaul's Drag Race*. But along with a handful of queer body positive social media influencers – less famous and mainstream than the likes of Sam Smith and Demi Lovato – there is not much more in terms of visibility. Roxane Gay, author of *Hunger: A Memoir of (My) Body*, may be the only well-known queer writer to discuss pervasive fat-phobia in and out of the community. And though hopeful as healthcare providers (in Toronto, anyway) have created more resources for the queer community including transgender members through outreach and presentations of marginalized and minority individuals, we often only see these depictions in spaces where trauma has already occurred and immediate help is needed asap.

Conversely, in queer spaces outside of healthcare facilities such as the glittery lit streets of Toronto's gay village, it is likely that one will *not* see many overweight bodies among those in the lines of the bars or on the dancefloor, but rather on the drag stages. Though drag performers – many in larger bodies – are celebrated during the spectacle of performance, it is not the same on gay dating/hook-up apps or even in everyday life. There is a way to go.

As for myself, I continued working toward my wellbeing and eventually moved out of my sister's home and back on my own. Even today, it isn't always easy; although I have naturally gained some weight during my recovery, the fear of gaining more lingers. For the most part, I have not slipped into my past patterns. I always loved writing, having journaled since I was young, and I thought I might put together my diary entries and experiences into a book. Much hard work and a few years later, I published it – a novel called *Cloud Cover*. I had to make sense of what I had gone through; I had to make it mean something. So I thought – and then decided – that the meaning of it all was to share my story, and maybe someone going through something similar could relate and perhaps feel less alone. Since the book's publication in 2019, many people, particularly men, have reached out to me to share their experiences. I frequently speak about my journey with various organizations and am a peer mentor for people with eating disorders at a not-for-profit called Eating Disorders Nova Scotia (EDNS). Recalling that day in the workshop when I sadly stared at my self-worth pie chart, I'm happy to say that my validation no longer depends on my appearance and weight. It now lies in my resilience, kindness, empathy, and most prominently, the connections I've made with others as a result of my experiences.

References

Barr, A., Burrows, J., Flebotte, D., Greenstein, J., Herschlag, A., Janetti, G., Kinnally, J., Kohan, D., Malins, G., Martin, S., Marchinko, J., Mutchnick, M., Poust, T., Quaintance, J., & Wrubel, B. (Executive Producers). (1998–2006 & 2017–2020). *Will & Grace*. [TV series]. 3 Princesses and a P Productions; 3 Sisters Entertainment; KoMut Entertainment; NBC Studios (1998–2004); NBCUniversal Television Studio (2004–2006); Universal Television.

Black, C., DeGeneres, E., Driscoll, M., Marlens, N., Newman, T., Rosenthal, D.S., Savel, D., Stark, J. (Writers), & Junger, G. (Director). (1997, April 30). The puppy episode (season 4, episodes 22/23) [TV series episode]. In M. Driscoll & V. Kaplan (Executive

Producers). (Eds.), *Ellen*. The Black/Marlens Company; Touchstone Television. https://www.imdb.com/title/tt0570077/

Cowen, R., Jonas, T., & Lipman, D. (Executive Producers). (2000–2005). *Queer as folk* [TV series]. Channel 4; Cowlip Productions; Showtime Networks Temple Street Productions; Tony Jonas Productions.

Gay, R. (2017). *Hunger: A memoir of (my) body*. HarperCollins.

5 Fermentating Trans Care

Embracing Animacy as a Life-Affirming Alternative to Nutritionism

Esther Kaner

My gut speaks to me as I write. I am sometimes overwhelmed by her visceral cries, unable to confidently understand her repertoire of rumbles and gurgles. She makes me anxious, triggering cycles of confusion and distress that render these signals even more indeterminable. But still, I listen in the hope that we might find a way to placate each other. Such is life with irritable bowel syndrome, a common functional gastrointestinal disorder with no clear pathophysiology (Enck et al., 2016). I am lucky to have mild symptoms, but my gut has always been sensitive to upsets. I suffered from long undiagnosed infant pyloric stenosis as a child, a condition that can become life-threatening if untreated (Parnall et al., 2016). Following an eventual operation at the age of two, I developed an intense phobia of eating during my early childhood, having previously been unable to ingest most solid foods without vomiting. I remember my parents and siblings holding my hands and eating with me as I cautiously chewed my meals, convinced that I might be poisoned unless they proved the food's safety for themselves.

Through familial support, I came to love food. My tastes were ambitious; I was unbeholden by the fussiness usually expected of British children. I came to be accused of overeating, evidenced by the accumulation of fat in places unexpected for my assigned sex. My body soon came to be regulated according to racial-gendered logics of compulsory whiteness and cisnormativity (Brewis, 2011); I was regularly teased in early adolescence for my wide hips and girlish gait. I was fat in a purportedly feminine way. I began to experience bouts of diarrhoea, abdominal discomfort, and gassiness around this time. Trips to the doctor were unyielding, but my symptoms would stabilize intermittently. I was also severely depressed but buried my pain in studiousness, only for it to be displaced as intense health anxiety and fatigue.

When I left home for university, I developed frequent cravings. Food came to represent a mitigator against social anxiety and feelings of displacement. My depression worsened, and I began to receive psychiatric treatment in the form of anti-depressant medications. Food was both a source of care and morbid fantasy. I regularly imagined gorging myself to death and would spend evenings furtively stuffing my face with a plethora of snacks. My gut wasn't happy – I would spend hours lying bloated and cramping – and yet food continued to soothe me, to offer a sensorial pleasure and alertness that otherwise felt ineffable.

DOI: 10.4324/9781003217121-6

I began to socially transition at the age of 19, four years ago now. I commenced feminizing hormone therapy ten months ago, privileged enough to temporarily access private care but delayed by patchy access to fertility preservation. Pearce (2018) describes how a British landscape of enormous treatment delays leaves trans people "bound up in the temporal and emotional disjuncture of waiting time," unsure when this period of anticipation will cease; even in private care, there are numerous disjunctures and delays. For me, this involved a period of experimentation, of finding ways to affirmatively reinterpret my gendered embodiment through an embrace of fatness. My relationship with food changed as my curves no longer substantiated a view of myself as the grotesque assemblage of bulbous, tumescent fat that I had imaginatively constructed. Instead, I could begin to reimagine my body as feminine and voluptuous, which, in the absence of overt physiological changes, is made phenomenologically real through an interpretive reformulation of embodied meanings and sensuous attachments. Or in Salamon's (2010) terms, I strove for my body "to be situated at materiality's threshold of possibility rather than caught within a materiality that is at its core constricted, constrictive, and determining" (p. 92).

In *Gut Feminism* Wilson (2015) argues that "mood is not added onto the gut secondarily, disrupting its proper function; rather, temper, like digestion, is one of the events to which enteric substrata are naturally (originally) inclined" (p. 66). Here the gut is not controlled or coordinated by a separated brain or mind but expresses its own moods, desires, and intentions. By emphasizing the extensiveness of the enteric nervous system and the gut's perceptual faculties, Wilson imbues the gut with psychic agency. Further apparent is the gut's configuration as a porous site capable of ingesting and absorbing its surrounding ecology. This corresponds to a recent turn in the social sciences and science studies to challenge the supposed boundedness of the body. Roberts (2008), for example, examines contemporary anxieties surrounding the threat of xenoestrogens, a "sea of toxic chemicals," against which the body must be defended. While such discourse constructs the body as under threat of increased permeability, we might ask ourselves what it would like to accept or perhaps embrace ecological perviousness.

Chen (2012) offers some answers by considering how their experience of intimacy is sensorially transformed by living with multiple chemical sensitivity. Daily chemical exposures incur proprioceptive readjustments that blur the boundaries between human and non-human touch, making it difficult to distinguish between the warm embrace of their partner and the comfort of sinking into their sofa. This phenomenological landscape thus disrupts the hierarchies of animacy that strip the non-human of agency, vibrancy, and intimate potential. How might we extend this blurriness and porosity to the gut, whose very existence is marked by the absorption of external substances?

Before continuing this line of thought, it is worth exploring its potential foreclosure by nutritional science and biomedicine. Nutritionism is a term deployed by Scrinis (2017) to describe the nutritional reductionism that has come to dominate scientific, and often popular, understandings of food. At its core is the notion that food can be reduced to biochemical constituents that act distinctly upon the body. Missing is relationality: how nutrients interact with each other and with the body;

the body itself is always "situated" and biosocially contingent (see: Lock, 2017); the biosocial contexts in which food is actually consumed; the animacy of the food itself, or rather its own history of biosocial contingency; and the meanings given to foods by individuals, communities and peoples. In *The Weight of Obesity*, Yates-Doerr (2015) offers insight into how nutritionism operates in practice. She highlights how nutritionists in Guatemala define foods as "good" or "bad" to create a prescriptive map for weight loss. Yet the vicissitudes of everyday life complicate the simplicity of such a mapping process, which at its core, assumes that weight is a direct consequence of individualized choice. Fresh vegetables are encouraged, but the high presence of pathogens in the water supply wards against their use. One woman surprised clinicians when she admitted to adding vast amounts of sugar to her coffee as it was fortified with vitamin D, a substance deemed "healthy" in consultations. For many, the prescriptivism with which foods were assigned value, contrasted heavily with a culture of communal eating that was not orientated around medicalized understandings of health. Failure to adhere to nutritional advice was not a matter of ignorance or non-compliance but rather the failure of the nutritionism paradigm to account for the complexities of living.

As suggested, nutritional reductionism is mobilized as part of a broader "war on fat" that has come to characterize much of global and public health policy (Guthman, 2011). This war is articulated in largely affective terms; fatness is rendered a source of shame, a marker of indolence and self-neglect that is assumed to mirror an uncaring relationship to others and the state (Abbots et al., 2020). Under a neoliberal logic, health is again seen as the preserve of individual choices where failure to be slender means failure to be a good "biocitizen" (Greenhalgh & Carney, 2014). Is obesity simply a matter of choice or lifestyle? To suggest so is to ignore the complex multitude of biological, social, and ecological relations that influence our metabolism in sometimes unexpected ways (Yates-Doerr, 2020).

We never eat alone. Our guts are teeming with microorganisms and bacterial critters that challenge the very terms of human selfhood (Rees et al., 2018). Our foodstuffs are primarily derived from living matter that too is brimming with microbes, no less embedded in rich webs of relations. As Yates-Doerr (2015) suggests, eating is "dependent on the negotiations and considerations of the many relational bodies responsible for producing, procuring, and consuming foods" (p. 178). How might we then foster this engagement with others in our understandings of eating? Fournier (2020) offers fermentation as a feminist praxis with transformative potential. The selective cultivation of microorganisms in and upon food products to enhance their flavour and nutritional value is "a process that both begins with, and continually engenders, vital matter: matter that actively alters the world around it" (Fournier, 2020, p. 94). In fermentation the unruliness of this living matter resists determinacy. Its protracted and unpredictable nature demands careful attention to ecological conditions as its products take on the flavour of the world around them.

Fermentation is not accessible to everyone; it demands patience that many are not afforded. It is not a solution to the structural violence and inequalities that undergird many experiences of obesity. A focus on any one mode of food preparation might also be co-opted by the reductive division of food by nutritional value, further entrenching inequalities of taste (Guthman, 2011). Similarly, an excessive focus on microorganisms may also align with broader processes of medicalization and "molecuralization" that partition the body into a set of decontextualized components (Rose, 2007). But as it inspires us to attend to vibrant others, "an ethics of fermentation" might ward against simple solutions of consumption and choice, instead of alerting us to the contingency and relationality of bodies and eating. Fermentation demands humility and patience by virtue of its "durational needs" (Fournier, 2020, p. 108). Its very reliance upon microbial others requires openness to experimentation and collaboration across difference. Fermentation may then constitute a form of slow care, a set of practices and conditions that liberate eating from the logics of capitalist consumption and extractivism.

Mol (2008) draws a distinction between "the logic of care" and "the logic of choice." While the latter sees health as reckoned through individual choices, where technologies and clinicians serve a clear, delimited purpose, the former operates through slow processes of collaborative "tinkering" and "attending to the body" that allow for the unexpected. Care recognizes that not all bodies operate in the same way; that health always involves the collective negotiation of multiple needs, priorities, and conditions; and that determinate outcomes and "cures" are frequently elusive. Care is about making life more liveable in conditions of uncertainty and insecurity, even where that entails difficulty and compromise. Malatino (2020) describes how trans communities form "care webs" around each other in the face of "affective and practical disinvestment" that effectively denies us access to normative support structures and state care. This "trans care" is manifest as alternative forms of kinship and horizontal mutual aid that keep us going in times of waiting and abandonment. It adapts continually to fluctuating needs and conditions. This is, of course, idealistic; some trans people are afforded more care than others and the resilience of any supportive web is limited by the limited capacities and competing interests of those involved. Even still, we might take inspiration from trans care's proliferation, not least for its potential to foster affective bonds in the face of neglect.

I commenced this chapter with an account of my complex relationship with food and my gut and its imbrication with my gendered embodiment. A popular view of gender transition assumes a kind of linearity, whereby treatments are accrued additively and result in the eventual dissipation of dysphoria. In reality the experience of gendered embodiment rarely reaches such an apotheosis or point of conscious absence. Instead, it shifts in and out of awareness as we are enlisted to perform gender in various ways. The impossibility of a complete performance demands a perpetual attendance to, and thus caring for, our gendered bodies (Salamon, 2010). And for me this is bound up with the chronicity of caring for my vocal and disorderly gut. Fermentation has, at times, been an aspect of this labour; cultivating sourdough bread has been a great source of psycho-enteric relief. By adopting this patient practice, I have found new ways to care for myself, to feel somewhat more comfortable in my embodiment by building the mental resilience to expand its phenomenological limits. I don't always manage. I struggled to regularly feed my last "mother dough" – a charming term commonly used in baking to describe sourdough pre-ferments, further imbuing these bubbling, doughy assemblages with a sense of animacy and generativity – and she was over-come by bacteria and fungi that I would be best to avoid eating. But fermentation allowed me to appreciate food's animacies and thus to develop new forms of caring relations with what I eat. Insofar as it imagines a counterpoint to the anti-social, reductive logics of nutritionism and its associates, fermentation might make trans life feel more liveable.

References

Abbots, E.-J., Eli, K., & Ulijaszek, S. (2020). Toward an affective political ecology of obesity. *Cultural Politics, 16*(3), 346–366.

Brewis, A. A. (2011). *Obesity: Cultural and biocultural perspectives.* Rutgers University Press.

Chen, M. Y. (2012). *Animacies: Biopolitics, racial mattering, and queer affect.* Duke University Press.

Enck, P., Aziz, Q., Barbara, G., Farmer, A. D., Fukudo, S., Mayer, E. A., Niesler, B., Quigley, E. M. M., Rajilić-Stojanović, M., Schemann, M., Schwille-Kiuntke, J., Simren, M., Zipfel, S., & Spiller, R. C. (2016). Irritable bowel syndrome. *Nature Reviews Disease Primers, 2*(1), 16014.

Fournier, L. (2020). Fermenting feminism as methodology and metaphor approaching transnational feminist practices through microbial transformation. *Environmental Humanities, 12*(1), 88–112.

Greenhalgh, S., & Carney, M. (2014). Bad biocitizens?: Latinos and the US "obesity epidemic". *Human Organization, 73*(3), 267–276.

Guthman, J. (2011). *Weighing in: Obesity, food justice, and the limits of capitalism.* University of California Press.

Lock, M. (2017). Recovering the body. *Annual Review of Anthropology, 46*(1), 1–14.

Malatino, H. (2020). *Trans care,* University of Minnesota Press.

Mol, A. (2008). *The logic of care: Health and the problems of patient choice.* Routledge.

Parnall, T., Caldwell, K., Noel, J. M., Russell, J., & Reyes, C. (2016). Hypertrophic pyloric stenosis in a 15-year-old male. *Journal of Pediatric Surgery Case Reports, 15*, 33–36.

Pearce, R. (2018). *Understanding Trans Health: Discourse, Power and Possibility.* Bristol University Press.

Rees, T., Bosch, T., & Douglas, A. E. (2018). How the microbiome challenges our concept of self. *PLoS Biology, 16*(2), 1–7.

Roberts, C. (2008). Fluid ecologies: Changing hormonal systems of embodied difference. In Lykke, N. and Smelik, A. (Eds.), *Bits of life: Feminism at the intersections of media, bioscience, and technology* (pp. 45–60). University of Washington Press.

Rose, N. (2007). *The politics of life itself: Biomedicine, power, and subjectivity in the twenty-first century.* Princeton University Press.

Salamon, G. (2010). *Assuming a body.* Columbia University Press.

Scrinis, G. (2017). On the ideology of nutritionism. *Food History: Critical and Primary Sources, 8*(1), 405–421.

Wilson, E. A. (2015). *Gut feminism.* Duke University Press.

Yates-Doerr, E. (2015). *The weight of obesity: Hunger and global health in postwar Guatemala.* https://ebookcentral.proquest.com/lib/ucl/detail.action?docID=2025593#

Yates-Doerr, E. (2020). Reworking the social determinants of health: Responding to material-semiotic indeterminacy in public health interventions. *Medical Anthropology Quarterly, 34*(3), 378–397.

6 Thirst Trap

Fran Lawn

> *Gay culture is unforgiving of aging. It highly prizes sexual potency, perfect bodies, and youth. This is for a good reason; any signs of vulnerability and imperfection feel dangerous in a heteronormative world where there is a high likelihood to be rejected and criticised.*
>
> (Neves, 2021).

Thirst is a universal human experience. Within the English language the word thirst can be used literally to refer to the biological sensation to drink but it can also be used figuratively to refer to wants, desires, and needs (Merriam Webster, 2022). A person may have a thirst for wisdom, knowledge, power, or the affections of others. The term "thirst trap" emerged as a product of selfie culture and was first defined to be an image within social media designed to entice people sexually, to draw attention to oneself and to create a "thirst" in the viewer (Merriam Webster, 2022).

I want to explore, as a gay man, how I view and experience shame as part of my sexuality, body, and health within the construct of gay culture. With these images, my intention is to play off the idea of the "thirst trap." In these images, I represent the socially constructed labels for gay men as the masks I wear. My intent is to explore the influence of such labels on how I see myself, how I am seen by others, especially in the context of social media and dating (hook-up) apps, and how my experiences with my health, body, and food are shaped (Figure 6.1).

My work is influenced by the expectations of masculinity and the restrictive nature of stereotypes within gay culture, reproduced through social media, which promotes a standard of perfection that excludes many men. With so much of this focus on short-term fixes and physical attractiveness over long-term health and healthy bodies, it makes it harder for ageing gay men of different body sizes to see themselves positively. This can lead to low self-esteem, disordered eating, body dysmorphia, anxiety, and depression (Griffiths et al., 2018; Parker and Harriger, 2020).

DOI: 10.4324/9781003217121-7

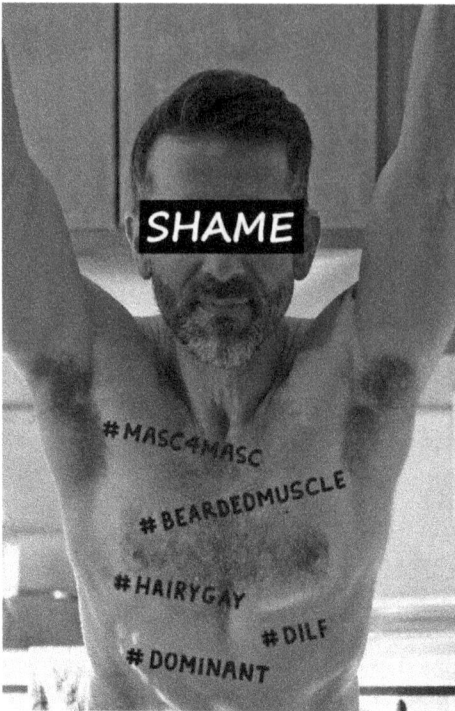

Figure 6.1 Mask of Shame. Photographed by David de Leyser @2021.

I want to move beyond #labels that define and limit us, to move from a place of shame towards authenticity and vulnerability (see Figures 6.2–6.6). I want to challenge the idea of ageing as undesirable and to build more awareness in the gay community around long-term health. I want people to begin to move the focus away from diet culture promoting "perfection" towards a focus on healthy, balanced lifestyles that supports gay men of any size and age.

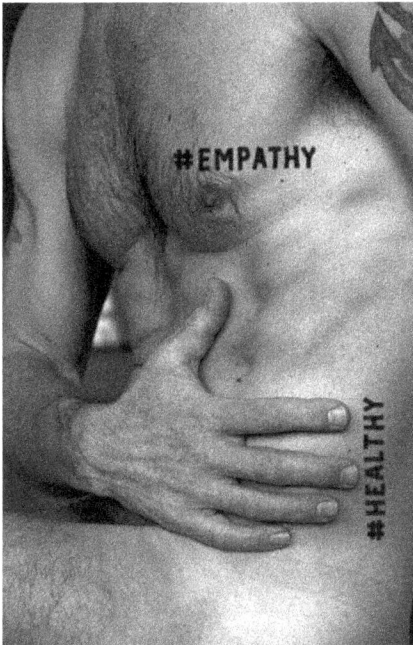

Figure 6.2 Health. Photographed by David de Leyser @2021.

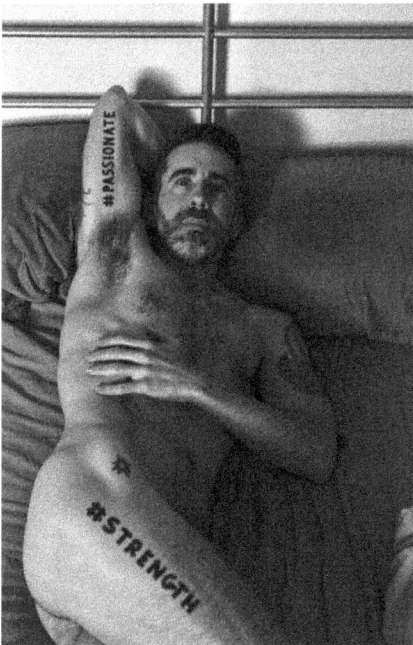

Figure 6.3 In Bed. Photographed by David de Leyser @2021.

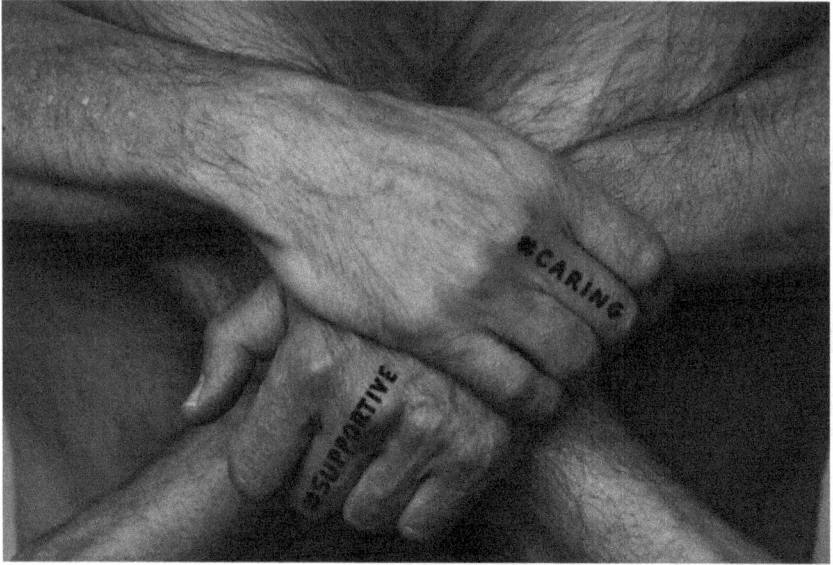

Figure 6.4 Caring. Photographed by David de Leyser @2021.

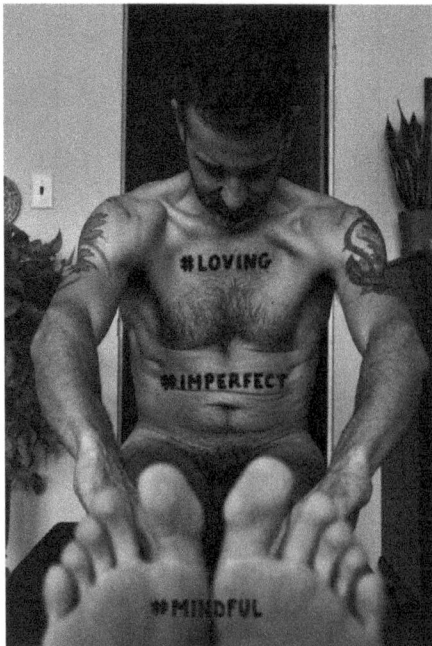

Figure 6.5 Stretched Out. Photographed by David de Leyser @2021.

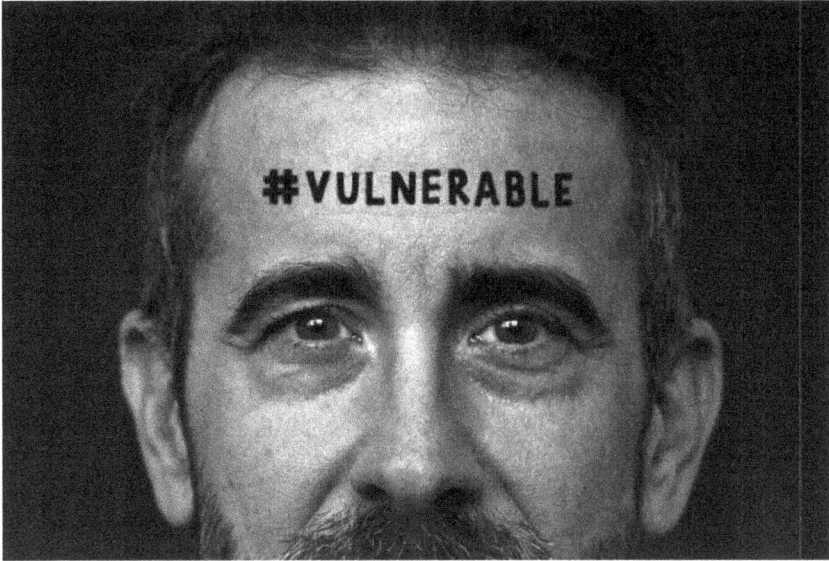

Figure 6.6 Eyes Looking Out. Photographed by David de Leyser @2021.

References

Griffiths, S., Murray, S. B., Krug, I., & McLean, S. A. (2018). The contribution of social media to body dissatisfaction, eating disorder symptoms, and anabolic steroid use among sexual minority men. *Cyberpsychology, Behavior, and Social Networking, 21*(3), 149–156.

Merriam Webster. (2022). *What is a 'thirst trap'? A tall drink of water.* https://www.merriamwebster.com/words-at-play/what-is-a-thirst-trap

Neves, S. (2021). Gay men and aging: When you're a gay man, aging is complicated. *Psychology Today.* https://www.psychologytoday.com/us/blog/talking-sex-and-relationships/202103/gay-men-and-aging

Parker, L. L., & Harriger, J. A. (2020). Eating disorders and disordered eating behaviors in the LGBT population: A review of the literature. *Journal of Eating Disorders, 8*(1), 1–20.

7 Coming Together over Food

Coalitional Possibilities Surfacing in/through (Un)Healthy Queerness

Emerson "Kai" Armstrong and Shinsuke Eguchi

For this chapter, we share our stories as a critical cultural methodology (Boylorn, 2021; Johnson, 2008) to showcase how our relationships with food represent ongoing negotiations of queerness in/across the lines of differences (e.g., race, ethnicity, gender, sexuality, class, and the body). By queerness, we mean a temporal paradox of de/reconstructing the normalized conditions and structures of power materialized through heteronormativity, cisgenderism, patriarchy, ableism, fatphobia, whiteness, and/or capitalism (Muñoz, 2009). Specifically, this chapter is about the collaboration happening between Kai as a white transmasculine queer person and Shinsuke as an Asian cismale effeminate queer person. Inspired by LeMaster and Stephenson (2021), we believe in the political significance of seeking out (im)possibilities that work towards remedying the lack of coalitions within/among trans and non-trans queer people. Because queer coalitions are extremely challenging practices, we emphasize both possibilities and impossibilities of the ways we move towards coalition-building. Here, we are reminded of Anzaldúa (1991), arguing that "queer is used as a false unifying umbrella which all 'queers' of all races, ethnicities, and classes are shored under" (p. 250). Hence, in/through the sharing of our narratives that signal two different queered experiences of being (un)healthy, we come together over food to unpack brief moments of coalitional (im)possibilities between us.

The rationale behind the emergence of our collaboration is that the practices of food and nutrition, performed by queer people like us, implicate our (dis)identifications with the politics of healthism that privilege the normative power relations. Our meaning of (dis)identifications comes from Muñoz's (1999) theorizing of disidentification through which minoritized queer subjects engage in everyday life performances that work *on* and *against* the normal and the ordinary. However, we are also dissatisfied with how cultural nuances of queerness working with the consumption of food and nutrition remain overlooked in the academy. As a consequence, we are committed to the sharing of our narratives that centre our bodies as social and performative platforms to fill a gap of knowledge concerning these neglected topics. In doing so, we together question how everyday operations of healthism shape and reshape our embodied performances of queerness in/across two different social contexts. By writing this essay, we gesture towards reviving multidimensional queer politics that offer moments of coalitional (im)possibilities among trans and non-trans people.

DOI: 10.4324/9781003217121-8

In what follows, we begin this chapter by showing how Kai makes sense of his transmasculine body that implicates his negotiation of queerness working with the politics of food, nutrition, and health(ism). Then, we turn the attention to the way Shinsuke develops and negotiates their relationships to food nutrition and health(ism) in/through the embodied performance of racialized non-trans queerness over time. After presenting our narrative separately, we end this chapter by collaboratively returning to discuss how juxtaposing our differences of queerness points to temporal moments of coalitional (im)possibilities among trans and non-trans people like us.

It Always Seems to Start in a Girls Bathroom

I [Kai] used to stand in front of my mirror naked, a masochistic part of myself staring and wondering what I could do to fix my body. By the end of summer, after being outside all day, my skin was a deep tan, but my breasts and genitals, always covered, were bright white, an uncomfortable highlight of what I hated most about my body. I would pull at my breasts, pushing them up, to the side, flat against my chest, all in the hope of seeing what I could look like without them. I would pinch the fat at my hips and think about what I could do to make them disappear, and that maybe if I ate better and worked out, I would lose all the fat that signalled to others my assigned femininity. Femininity that I never felt right in, and I know now this was dangerous and looming dysphoria, "Chest dysphoria is the distress or discomfort one feels because of chest tissue that has developed after undergoing an endogenous female puberty" (Julian et al., 2021, p. 1130).

I've had these feelings ever since puberty. In middle school, I was in the restroom with my friend and told her I felt fat. She assured me I wasn't, but a part of me didn't believe it. I'd look at the boys with their flat chests and think that was how I wanted to look. Growing up as someone perceived as a girl, my body, like many women and young girls, was often centralized and sexualized (Wright et al., 2015), and that had a direct implication on my relationship with my body and food. I was an athlete, playing all manner of sports starting at five years old, until I reached college. My after-school activities always involved me running around, playing, and engaging in athletics and sports. Because of this I had a huge appetite and was always eating, but I never gained weight. I was often called pretty in relation to my thinness. I was told by my mother and others that it was good. I was so pretty because I wasn't as smart as my younger sister.

"*Skinny as a stick and as dumb as one too.*" My sister would throw this jest at me for years; I wasn't more than eight years old when it started. While my sister was taunting me, my mother would look on and laugh with her, making comments about how much I ate. My childhood, whether I knew it or not, was about surviving. Surviving in a body I couldn't describe or feel comfortable in and surviving the external abuse and bullying of a toxic home and school. Many transgender people have struggles surviving in their bodies, and their relationship with food suffers (Obarzanek & Munyan, 2021).

Returning to the conversation in the girl's bathroom, I continued, saying that I was going to hell, for being a bad person. She probed deeper, asking why, and I gave reasons about being a sinner, very tied to my learned white Catholic guilt. But what I didn't tell her was I was thinking of lunch that day and how someone had explained to me what a lesbian was and that it was a sin. I struggled the rest of the day feeling like my body was wrong like I was wrong. My stomach was in knots, and I felt sick. I was critiquing my body because I didn't have the terms to understand who I was, and so I turned to calling myself fat and sinful. But the "fat" that I was was the breasts that were just starting to grow, my hips starting to fill out. Otherwise, I was just as skinny as I had always been; I just didn't have the words to explain the feelings I was experiencing. Gender dysphoria was not something that I had ever heard of, so I used the only negative word I knew to describe my feelings towards my body, and that was centred on a deep fatphobia, and so I used the language of dysmorphia rather than dysphoria.

Comments about my body started in my youth and have never stopped. When I got mono in my undergraduate year, I lost 20 pounds over a week due to my illness. So many people gave me positive comments about my weight and jokingly asked me to give them mono. I was stunned; here I was barely surviving after multiple trips to the ER, and they wanted my unhealthy body. White skinny femininity was an ideal that others wanted to obtain, ignorant of the fact I lost my health for my thinness. It took me years to get any type of weight back, and a large portion of that weight came from my anti-depressants. This weight was in exchange for the years of suicidal thoughts I had held. And still comments came, even from therapists and doctors, about how I could lose weight if I just stopped taking them.

After my top surgery, I was stunned by how joyous I felt in my body and how I can now ignore commentary about my weight. I'm not alone in these feelings; reconstructive chest surgery is a permanent solution many seek to lessen or eliminate chest dysphoria (Julian et al., 2021). I am the healthiest I have ever been, but nowhere near the smallest I have ever been. With the (literal) weight off my chest, I feel free. I am no longer as skinny as a stick, but I am more happy, confident, and emotionally intelligent. This isn't to say there was a magic fix. I have dog ears, or skin and fat deposits on the sides of my chest that require a revision surgery. I wear baggy shirts to hide these, because I still tie feelings of fatness and unhealthiness to the breast tissue my body has. These are feelings I work every day to interrupt and investigate, looking towards a future of radical self-love and acceptance.

Trying (and Trying) to be Queer-as-Fuck

A few times a month, I [Shinsuke] struggle with my urge to eat a basket of KFC original, dark meat fried chicken by myself. Yes, once in a while I end up eating them all. However, when I do so, I feel guilty eating heavy fast foods, which any fitness trainer would tell me to stay away from. I regret my choice to not resist my temptation. Still, my feeling points to the simultaneous operations of differences that produce the paradox of my knowing, acting, and being.

Born and raised in Japan, I internalized the nuance of fatphobia through which the social institutions circulate the ideal images of the cisgender male slender and toned body. Growing up, I was taught not to be like a fat sumo wrestler who needs to eat a lot. Non-fat, healthy cismale appearance was the beauty standard I was subjected to aspiring to become and be. Hence, there was no need for me to unfollow "proper" dietary practices. Here, it is important to connect my social learning to Japan's cultural value of social conformity. Becoming and being just like everyone else is Japan's normative cultural ideal (Toyosaki, 2011). The individualistic logic of standing out that disrupts relational and communal harmony isn't a preferable characteristic. Hence, children and teens are taught neither to be too skinny nor too fat. Because the physical examinations suggested I was much smaller than the standard cisgender boy throughout my schooling, I knew I had to eat more. Still, no matter how much I ate, I didn't gain weight. So, I developed the self-concept as a skinny boy prior to my relocation.

Throughout my US-based undergraduate and graduate education, I, for sure, capitalized my skinny-boy status as I participated in gay sexual cultures across San Francisco, New York, and Washington DC. While gay sexual cultural norms that worship the youthful white masculine ideal marginalize people of colour (Han, 2021), there is a subcultural space of paradox through which "feminized" and "diminutive" Asian cismale subjects are sexually fetishized (Nguyen, 2014). So, I played along with the racialized gender stereotype to get by, while embodying my knowledge(s) of resistance against the aesthetic standards of cisgender whiteness seen in/across gay sexual cultures. I went to bars and clubs, drank cocktails, and ate junk food without thinking about exercise and physical fitness even though gay sexual cultures reify fat stigmas. Nothing I did for my *gay city life* changed how I appeared. However, going into my 30s with the professoriate job in Albuquerque changed my relationship with the body because of my increasing stressors, especially caused by the pressure for tenure and promotion. Indeed, academia is a toxic industry, especially for queer people of colour who do not subscribe to the logic of cis-hetero-whiteness as an embodied code of conduct (Calafell, 2007). Hence, I had to find a way to *feel good* in my personal times. Going to non-queer bars and clubs, drinking cocktails, and eating junk food were not helping me. So, I have gradually developed an interest in improving my health.

Still, I cannot get away from the present produced by the episodes of my past habits, despite having known my significantly high levels of triglyceride through my bloodwork. In late January 2020, I got gout. *Oh my god, it was so painful!* Literally, I could not walk as if my bones were broken. The urgent care doctor told me that I must have been eating high cholesterol foods during the holidays. So, I have been trying to eat healthier than before. I never again want to experience the speechless pain. Yet, multiple episodes of discourses around incidents under the pandemic (e.g., Black Lives Matter, Anti-Asian hate, the insurrection at the US Capitol, and the withdrawal of US troops from Afghanistan) are not helping me. *My anxiety is ultra-high!* I worry about my future.

The reason I stay in the US is my desire to have my *queer-as-fuck* life I thought I would not be able to have in Japan. A part of my social aspiration implicates the logic of homonationalism that conflates cisgender gay rights as the US nationalist ideology (Puar, 2007). Still, my body is a product of queerness that requires immediate attention to food and nutrition. Of course, I want to ignore that I am ageing, so I can eat whatever I want. But I want to live longer to achieve my *queer-as-fuck* life. My body experiencing high levels of anxiety tells me to stop eating whatever I want. I can't let my dietary practices cause any severe medical conditions in my body. Hence, while I hate going along with the normative social construct of what being healthy means, I am staying away from a basket of fried chicken as much as I can so I can continue trying to live *queer-as-fuck*. As Muñoz (2009) reminds, "We may never touch queerness, but we can feel it as the warm illumination of a horizon imbued with potentiality" (p. 1).

Coming Together over Food

Despite our two different queered stories remaining individual and culturally specific to each of our lived experiences, we believe brief moments of coalitional (im) possibilities within our sharing of narratives exist. But these queer coalitions begin with the need for a radical self-acceptance and love that stems from Black feminist thought (Taylor, 2018). By this, we mean a critical acceptance that is inclusive of every person's body, translating back to a radical self-acceptance that then reciprocally goes back to inclusive community-making. We are different kinds of queers; still, we share critical dissatisfactions with the normative power relations that possibly (dis)connect our differences.

In looking at Kai's struggle that surrounded feelings of dysphoria and the harmful, toxic, commentary surrounding their body, moments of radical self-acceptance would have drastically changed his life. By having a radical self-acceptance as a transgender person in a transphobic society, Kai now loves the transformative parts of who they are despite marginalization by a cisheteropatriarchical society. But, he also has learned to recognize the power that whiteness has afforded him. These two aspects involve a love that is inclusive of all body types, before or after or never having surgery or starting hormones. A love that is inclusive of transgender bodies that perform multiple versions of queerness. A self-acceptance that is rooted in coalitional possibilities and allyship.

Shinsuke's narrative that suggests their ongoing tensions around Japanese conformity values that compete with the US-American logic of individualism is further replicated in white cisnormative homonationalist ideals. Problematizing the aesthetical standards of cisgender whiteness seen in/across gay sexual cultures, Shinsuke's radical self-acceptance of queerness as a cismale Japanese American person not only chooses a self-love that is a disruption to the hegemonic US-America. But it also requires their critical awareness of cisgender advantages. There is a gay subcultural space where Shinsuke can play along with the racialized Asian stereotype to get by. Still, in unveiling the toxic industry of academia, societal, and international tensions, Shinsuke's desire for self-acceptance of queerness rooted in a coalition of allyship begs to solve not just individual issues but more wide-sweeping cultural concerns. A self-acceptance that is rooted in coalitional possibilities and allyship.

Hence, in understanding our singular stories and need for radical acceptance, we come together to recognize the relevance of our differing queerness. We recognize that our stories contend with a need for a greater alliance among differences of queerness that make up the LGBTQ+ community. We use the multidimensional queer politics of Ferguson (2019), which argues against the mainstream commodification of the LGBTQ+ community as a product of US nationalism. Further, he argues towards working with intersectional aspects of queer liberation as well as a return to the multidimensionally informed movement that came primarily from queer trans women of colour. It takes a radical love to be able to accept oneself in a society that is actively violent towards and lethal to marginalizations of queerness in/across the lines of differences. Ultimately, this love extends from the self towards family, community, and society at large. Therefore, *how can we accept and love our own bodies' variances and differences of size, queerness, and gender with deep-seated fatphobic rhetoric echoed by ourselves and society?* Likewise, *how can we use self-love to return to multidimensional queer politics with the inclusion of all bodies, thin or fat?* In returning to multidimensional queer politics, we desire to create coalitions that recognize differences of queerness exemplified in our relationships to food and nutrition. Building on the theory of disidentification (Muñoz, 1999) that extrapolates (im)possibilities of shared critical dissatisfactions that we have with others and with mainstream political spheres, together we can better challenge hegemonic structures. Hence, we call to empathize with those who we may see as polarized or completely unlike ourselves by seeing (im)possibilities of queerness as sites of commonalities and shared lived experiences.

References

Anzaldúa, G. (1991). To(o) queer the writer: Loca, escrita y chicana. In B. Warland (Ed.), *Inversions: Writing by dykes, queers, and lesbians* (pp. 251–273). Press Gang.

Boylorn, R. M. (2021). Visual voices and aural (auto)ethnographies: The personal, political, and polysemic value of storytelling and/in communication. *Review of Communication, 21*(1), 1–8.

Calafell, B. M. (2007). Mentoring and love: An open letter. *Cultural Studies <=> Critical Methodologies, 7*(5), 425–441.

Ferguson, R. A. (2019). *One-dimensional queer.* Polity Press. Cambridge UK.

Han, C. W. (2021). *Racial erotics: Gay men of color, sexual racism, and the politics of desire.* University of Washington Press.

Johnson, A. (2008). Quare/kuaer/queer/(e)ntersectionality: An invitational rhetoric of possibility. *Cross Currents, 68*(4), 500–514.

Julian, J. M., Salvetti, B., Held, J. I., Murray, P. M., Lara-Rojas, L., & Olson-Kennedy, J. (2021). The impact of chest binding in transgender and gender diverse youth and young adults. *The Journal of Adolescent Health: Official Publication of the Society for Adolescent Medicine, 68*(6), 1129–1134.

LeMaster, B., & Stephenson, M. (2021). Trans (gender) trouble. *Communication and Critical/Cultural Studies, 18*(2), 190–195.

Munoz, J. E. (1999). *Disidentifications: Queers of color and the performance of politics.* University of Minnesota Press.

Muñoz, J. E. (2009). *Cruising Utopia: The then and there of queer futurity*. New York University Press.

Nguyen, H. T. (2014). *A view from the bottom: Asian American masculinity and sexual representation*. Duke University Press.

Obarzanek, L., & Munyan, K. (2021). Eating disorder behaviors among transgender individuals: Exploring the literature. *Journal of the American Psychiatric Nurses Association, 27*(3), 203–212. https://doi.org/10.1177/1078390320921948

Puar, J. K. (2007). *Terrorist assemblages: Homonationalism in queer times*. Duke University Press.

Taylor, S. R. (2018). *The body is not an apology*. Berrett-Koehler Publishers.

Toyosaki, S. (2011). Critical complete-member ethnography: Theorizing dialectics of consensus and conflict in intercultural communication. *Journal of International and Intercultural Communication, 4*(1), 62–80.

Wright, P. J., Arroyo, A., & Bae, S. (2015). An experimental analysis of young women's attitude toward the male gaze following exposure to centerfold images of varying explicitness. *Communication Reports, 28*(1), 1–11.

8 Queer(y)ing Foodways

An Agrifood Feminist Killjoy Critique of Narratives Dominating Foodways

Michaela Hoffelmeyer

Bodies need to be nourished and fed. Feminism too can be thought of as a diet; a feminist diet is how we are nourished by feminisms. In my killjoy survival kit, I would have a bag of fresh chilies … I am not saying chilies are little feminists. But you would have in your kit whatever you tend to add to things; however, you adapt dishes to your own requirements. If we have a diversity of bodies, we have a diversity of requirements.

(Ahmed, 2017, p. 247)

In this quote from Sara Ahmed's book, *Living a Feminist Life*, readers are reminded of the reciprocal nature of food and feminisms; both can keep one surviving. Ahmed's concept of the feminist killjoy describes a form of embodiment and being in which the feminist killjoy *exposes* problems and, in that process, *becomes* a problem. The problems that feminist killjoys expose include racism, sexism, and heterosexism. Ahmed's feminist killjoy takes shape first around the kitchen table when interrupting dinner to name racism, sexism, and heterosexism. The killjoy refuses to be satisfied with a world that perpetuates these inequalities. However, refusing to accept social requirements and interrupting others' "happiness" wears on the body and mind; thus, a killjoy survival kit helps maintain this embodiment. Ahmed's chilies packed in her survival kit, I argue, symbolize foodways. I suggest foodways are necessary for survival, and queer peoples' survival through food must be recentred as a core piece of the queer liberation movement.

In this chapter, I bring the idea of the feminist killjoy into agrifood studies through queer foodways. I invite the feminist killjoy to our proverbial kitchen table and ask her to offer a queer(y)ing of foodways. I borrow the term queer(y) ing from Sandilands (1994), wherein query (or to question) intertwines with queer, showing how a critical lens is inherent in a queer approach. At this dinner, my agrifood feminist killjoy is interested in exposing four problems: (1) the lack of focus on food as a feminist and queer issue, (2) the assumption that in order to "feed the world" we need increased food production, (3) "the home" is the ideal place to intervene in food consumption, (4) non-dominant communities' foodways are responsible for unhealthy outcomes, and these foodways require outside intervention to correct eating habits.

DOI: 10.4324/9781003217121-9

Foodways refer to the practical processes and cultural meanings involved in food production, preparation, and provisioning (Garcia et al., 2017). Further, foodways demonstrate "struggles and adaptations, oppressions and innovations, customs and cultures" which characterize the way people eat (Garcia et al., 2017, p. 2). Foodways combine the pragmatic means of growing, cooking, and consuming food to examine how such practices are shaped across generations. A queering of foodways then explores how foodways may serve as a form of oppression and colonization. At the same time, foodways are a source of freedom for communities to retain cultural practices.

Appetizers: Who Is at the Table?

The feminist killjoy can kill "feminist joy" (Ahmed, 2017, p. 177), meaning that the killjoy may name problems inherent to the feminist movement. Sachs and Patel-Campillo (2014) noted that despite the gendered and racialized implications for food and hunger, feminist scholars and activists rarely consider this area core to mainstream feminist work. Similarly, Mikki Kendall's book *Hood Feminism* argued that alleviating hunger is rarely conceived of as a feminist issue. Kendall (2020) asked what it would mean for feminists to rally around hunger in the same way feminists have fought for equal pay and reproductive rights. Sachs and Patel-Campillo (2014) suggested the disconnect between food and feminism is due to the connection of food to the domestic sphere, which has historically reinforced women's subordination. In a similar fashion to the feminist movement, the queer liberation movement has largely disregarded food-related issues as queer issues. The lasting legacy of the division of food work embedded in traditional gender roles remains equally enmeshed in compulsory heterosexuality, thereby limiting our understanding of queer food production and consumption.

To queer foodways, the feminist killjoy asserts that food access is inherently a feminist and queer issue. Gender and sexual minorities experience disproportionate levels of food insecurity as heterosexism creates barriers for these communities to access healthy, affordable, and nutrient-dense food (Brown et al., 2016). Food insecurity among queer communities of colour is further intensified (Brown et al., 2016). While mainstream queer rights efforts have centred around issues of marriage equality, queer liberation requires a more capacious understanding of queer issues. As a basic need, food is necessary for survival, and queer life is constantly under attack, albeit differently based on race, class, and location. Food sustains people and allows communities to engage in political action (Kendall, 2020). The broader issue of lack of access to food through poverty remains an essential queer issue deserving greater attention.

Further, these inequalities in food access demonstrate the continued false narrative that more food production will solve hunger. The agrifood feminist killjoy recognizes this narrative perpetuates the unsustainability of capital-intensive agricultural production without recognizing the inequality in food distribution. Food access goes hand in hand with economic and housing security as food remains a more elastic cost. The world already produces enough food to feed the world's population (Holt-Giménez et al., 2012). Instead, issues of economic inequity, exemplified through housing, health care, and low wages, show that increased food production will not solve economic inequities. The agrifood feminist killjoy connects how economic inequities surrounding housing, wages, and healthcare are intertwined and play out in foodways.

Entrée: Who Are Queer Foodways Feeding?

Writers, such as Michael Pollen, have suggested that if we can only cook at home more often and have "family" dinners (read as white, cisheteronuclear), then our relationship with food would be healthier (Bowen et al., 2019). Focusing on the home as a place for nutritional (foodway) intervention is tempting in a neoliberal society that privileges the individual above all else. However, an agrifood feminist killjoy rejects this notion of individualistic education as solving nutritional issues. This narrative ignores the economic disparities which leave people with less time, resources, and access to cooking. Bowen et al. (2019) covered these issues at length in their book *Pressure Cooker*. Focusing only on the home does little to confront the historical injustices regarding how foodways have been appropriated and stripped from their original form, allowing certain communities to be pathologized, which I return to in the final section.

Instead of outside "experts" offering input on potentially unfamiliar foodways, reclaiming foodways can be a powerful source of literal and figurative nourishment. In *The Cooking Gene,* Michael Twitty, a Black, queer, Jewish chef, explored the powerful healing that cooking the food of his ancestors facilitates. Twitty (2017) works as an agrifood feminist killjoy by rejecting the dominant narrative of the "unhealthiness" of Soul Food by highlighting his ancestors' culinary talent in the face of racism. It is no coincidence that just as Ahmed's killjoy formed around the kitchen table, Michael Twitty first came out to his mother at their family's kitchen table. Similarly, Black queer chef Lazarus Lynch described how on Juneteenth, barbequing and preparing Soul Food offers a connection with the loss of Black lives in the United States of America (Lynch, 2020). As chefs Michael Twitty and Lazarus Lynch highlight, food can be a place of nourishment and survival through cultural embodiment. This approach to celebrating and reconnecting with traditional food demonstrates how cooking at home is not simply an individual act; instead, foodways facilitate a meaningful connection to the community.

Producing food also facilitates a reclaiming of power around foodways. For many communities, specifically Black, migrant, and Indigenous communities, being excluded from the global agrifood system has meant that production and consumption go hand in hand (Minkoff-Zern, 2017; White, 2018). Activists and scholars in the food justice and food sovereignty movements challenge the departure from agrarian livelihoods as empowering (Holt-Giménez, 2010). The practice of food production and cultivation is political, as it has the potential for communities to regain power over foodways and reject displacement from land

(Minkoff-Zern, 2017; White, 2018). In this way, a feminist agrifood killjoy recognizes a holistic approach to food justice as access to food and the freedom to produce food. I suggest that queer farmers are a crucial linchpin in facilitating queer foodways.

Historically, community-based foodways such as potlucks served as a crucial part of queer movements (Kirkey & Forsyth, 2001). Similarly, queer back-to-the-land movements of the 1970s and 1980s illustrated a sense of power in returning to the land for food cultivation (Anahita, 2009; Sandilands, 2002). Queer agrifood organizations have intentionally recreated agrifood networks around confronting injustices in the food system which exclude queer communities from accessing food and production.

Existing literature in agriculture demonstrates that queer people are active in cultivating food (Hoffelmeyer, 2021; Leslie, 2017). Additionally, queer farmers often go beyond individual household production for business purposes. For example, Sbicca (2012) asserted that through food, "queers can develop community, challenge heteronormativity, and create sustainable alternatives to capitalist modes of industrialized agriculture" (p. 45). Sbicca (2012) found that queer people are working at the intersection of environmental, sexuality, and gender justice to "build community, fight oppression, and/or take better care of the planet and the human body in all its diversity" (pp. 46–47). Similarly, Smith (2019) asserted that Black farmers and queer farmers "create and (re)create emancipatory spaces for farming, food, and community" (p. 9).

As an example of building queer foodways, Rock Steady Farm in rural New York designed their farm to leverage healthy, nutrient-dense food production for low-income and queer communities (Rock Steady Farm, 2020). Recognizing these communities as systematically excluded from food access and production, Rock Steady is building a queer foodway that spans across communities. By implementing a sliding-scale Community Supported Agriculture and Food Sovereignty Fund, Rock Steady is the embodiment of food production, directly confronting injustices in food consumption. Farms such as Rock Steady and scholarship documenting queer farmers' community-oriented foodways demonstrate how a reorientation of queer-liberatory efforts in food production nourishes both bodies and movements toward liberation.

"Brownies" for Dessert

Foodways are shaped and reshaped based on power. Dominant culture often works to stigmatize foodways, only later to appropriate and mainstream the foodway while seeking to strip away the very people associated with the cultural production of food (Massoth, 2017; Minkoff-Zern, 2017). An agrifood feminist killjoy examines how global food systems are viewed as the most efficient way to feed the world, often at the expense of non-dominant foodways. At the same time, many communities are then pathologized for nutritional deficiencies when the dominant foodway replaces or appropriates traditional foodways.

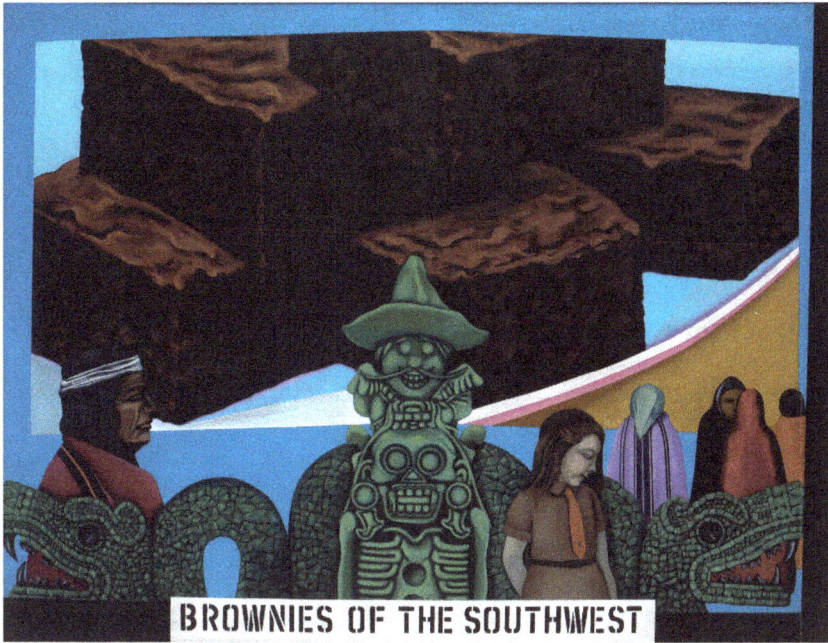

Figure 8.1 Melesio Casas, Humanscape 62, 1970, acrylic on canvas, Smithsonian American Art Museum, museum purchase through the Luisita L. and Franz H. Denghausen Endowment, 2012.37, © 1970, the Casas Family.

The appropriation of foodways in the painting *Brownies of the Southwest* (Figure 8.1) exemplifies "colonizing the colon" (Garcia et al., 2017). This painting portrays US and Chicano cultural imagery and stereotypes (SAAM, n.d.). In the foreground, a young Girl Scout (colloquially called a "Brownie") stands in front of Native American or Mexican American people of the Southwest. In the background stands a stack of brownies, which highlights the erasure of Mexican culture in the US (SAAM, n.d.). Also depicted is the Frito Bandito, which was the Frito-Lay corn chip icon during the 1960s. The mascot portrayed Mexican culture associated with laziness and theft (SAAM, n.d.). Although Frito-Lay eventually retired the mascot after pushback (SAAM, n.d.), the Frito Bandito is not the only case of cultural appropriation and stereotyping by multinational companies, as the Chiquita banana was also used to sexualize women of colour and sell bananas (Enloe, 2014).

By calling attention to the strategic use of foodways by agribusiness through appropriation and stereotyping, this painting begins to *queer* foodways. The porosity of foodways illustrates how pieces of food cultures can be retooled; however, when done by certain actors in the agrifood system, these actions undermine cultural practices. Any approach to queering foodways requires a re-examination of the agrifood system predicated on the devaluation of certain cultures and bodies, primarily non-white bodies.

Conclusion: Digestif

The power to build, shape, and enact foodways offers insights into society, thereby offering scholars and practitioners meaningful ways to engage with issues of power and inequity. Although food at a basic level is required for living, foodways recognize the deeper meaning behind nourishment. Numerous agrifood feminist killjoy organizations exist worldwide, such as United Farmworkers and La Vía Campesina. These organizations include queer people (European Coordination Vía Campesina, 2021) and employ killjoy approaches to challenge norms and power in the agrifood system. When the survival of communities and foodways is at stake, one can hardly not afford to be a killjoy. But by *exposing* problems, these organizations and individuals *become* problems for powerful actors in the agrifood system. As such, foodways – as a piece of killjoy survival kits – remain a core queer and feminist issue deserving greater attention and focus.

Several avenues related to queering foodways emerge through this initial stocktaking. First, queerness transcends culture, ethnicity, and geographic region. Some foodways are in tension with one another, such as veganism and some Indigenous foodways which value meat consumption. This tension, among others, questions how issues of privilege and power may be embedded in certain queer foodways. Second, while foodways often entail a diasporic or historical connection to family, many queer communities form chosen families rooted in acceptance rather than blood (Weston, 1991). How are chosen families bringing together their collective histories to adapt dishes and provide sustenance for one another? Finally, how are organizations actively working to develop queer foodways? Connections to our queer elders are challenging due to heterosexism, which silenced our queer ancestors. Nevertheless, today organizations such as the Queer Food Foundation may show ways to connect across cultures, generations, and histories through queer foodways (https://queerfoodfoundation.org/, n.d.). Just as Ahmed carries chilies to maintain energy and strength in the painful and exhausting fight against racism, sexism, and heterosexism, queer liberation movements must recentre food – particularly diverse and culturally appropriate food – as a way to maintain political and activist energy toward justice and equity.

References

Ahmed, S. (2017). *Living a feminist life*. Duke University Press.

Anahita, S. (2009). Nestled into niches: Prefigurative communities on lesbian land. *Journal of Homosexuality*, *56*(6), 719–737. https://doi.org/10.1080/00918360903054186

Bowen, S., Brenton, J., & Elliott, S. (2019). *Pressure cooker: Why home cooking won't solve our problems and what we can do about it*. Oxford University Press.

Brown, T. N. T., Romero, A. P., & Gates, G. J. (2016). Food insecurity and SNAP participation in the LGBT community. http://williamsinstitute.law.ucla.edu/wp-content/uploads/Food-Insecurity-and-SNAP-Participation-in-the-LGBT-Community.pdf

Enloe, C. (2014). Going bananas! Where are women in the international politics of bananas? In Cynthia Enloe (Eds.), *Bananas, beaches and bases: Making feminist sense of international politics* (pp. 208–241). University of California Press.

European Coordination Via Campesina. (2021). *Embracing rural diversity: Genders and sexualities in the peasant movement.* https://www.eurovia.org/wp-content/uploads/2021/06/MEP _ENG_web.pdf

Garcia, M., DuPuis, M. E., & Mitchell, D. (2017). *Food across borders* (M. Garcia, M. E. DuPuis, & D. Mitchell, Eds.). Rutgers University Press.

Hoffelmeyer, M. (2021). "Out" on the farm: Queer farmers maneuvering heterosexism and visibility. *Rural Sociology*, 86(4), 752–776.

Holt-Giménez, E. (2010). Food security, food justice, or food sovereignty? *Food First, 16*(4). http://www.foodfirst.org/sites/www.foodfirst.org/files/pdf/Food_Movements _Winter_2010_bckgrndr.pdf

Holt-Giménez, E., Shattuck, A., Altieri, M., Herren, H., & Gliessman, S. (2012). We already grow enough food for 10 billion people… and still can't end hunger. *Journal of Sustainable Agriculture*, 36(6), 595–598. https://doi.org/10.1080/10440046.2012.695331

Kendall, M. (2020). *Hood feminism: Notes from the women that a movement forgot.* Penguin.

Kirkey, K., & Forsyth, A. (2001). Men in the valley: Gay male life on the suburban-rural fringe. *Journal of Rural Studies*, 17(4), 421–441. https://doi.org/10.1016/S0743 -0167(01)00007-9

Leslie, I. S. (2017). Queer farmers: Sexuality and the transition to sustainable agriculture. *Rural Sociology*, 82(4), 747–771. https://doi.org/10.1111/ruso.12153

Lynch, L. (2020). This Juneteenth, I don't feel like celebrating. Instead, I'm cooking barbecue in memory of Black lives lost. https://www.washingtonpost.com/news/ voraciously/wp/2020/06/16/this-juneteenth-i-dont-feel-like-celebrating-instead-im -cooking-barbecue-in-memory-of-black-lives-lost/

Massoth, K. (2017). "Mexican cookery that belongs to the United States": Evolving boundaries of whiteness in new Mexican kitchens. In M. Garcia, E. Melanie DuPuis and D. Mitchell (Eds.), *Food across borders* (pp. 44–63). Rutgers University Press.

Minkoff-Zern, L.-A. (2017). Crossing borders, overcoming boundaries: Latino immigrant farmers and a new sense of home in the United States. In M. Garcia, M. E. DuPuis, & D. Mitchell (Eds.), *Food across borders* (pp. 219–235). Rutgers University Press.

Rock Steady Farms. (2020). https://www.rocksteadyfarm.com

SAAM (Smithsonian American Art Museum). (n.d.). Cultural imagery and stereotypes. Retrieved February 4, 2020, from https://americanexperience.si.edu/historical-eras/ contemporary-united-states/pair-humanscape-diary-december-12/

Sachs, C., & Patel-Campillo, A. (2014). Feminist food justice: Crafting a new vision. *Feminist Studies*, 40(2), 396–410.

Sandilands, C. (1994). Lavender's Green? Some thoughts on queer(y)ing environmental. *UnderCurrents: Journal of Critical Environmental Studies*, 6, 20–25.

Sandilands, C. (2002). Lesbian separatist communities and the experience of nature. *Organization & Environment*, 15(2), 131–163.

Sbicca, J. (2012). Eco-queer movement(s) challenging heteronormative space through (re) imagining nature and food. *European Journal of Ecopsychology*, 3, 33–52.

Smith, B. J. (2019). Food justice, intersectional agriculture, and the triple food movement. *Agriculture and Human Values*, 36(4), 1–11. https://doi.org/10.1007/s10460-019-09945-y

Twitty, M. (2017). *The cooking gene: A journey through African American culinary history in the old south.* Amistad.

Weston, K. (1991). *Families we choose: Lesbians, gays, kinship.* Columbia University Press.

White, M. (2018). *Freedom farmers: Agricultural resistance and the black freedom movement.* University of North Carolina Press.

9 Styling Flesh

Queer and Trans Bodies and the
Neoliberal Commodification
of Health Veganism

Fergal Ó Baoill

When I think of veganism, I think of activism, street protests, and political demon-strations. My mind goes to environmentalism, animal rights, and even an ambition for societal improvement. When I consider a vegan, I also find myself associating this person with queerness and feminism. Granted, this is a biased perception, but there is something politicized, socially engaged, and defiant about the image of the vegan in my mind – perhaps something a bit "punk." Yet when I speak to people about eating vegan and vegetarian, topics of conversation tend towards body and appearance: whether my hair has gotten so much healthier, my skin so much clearer, or if I've lost weight. These same themes dominate many vegan food blogs, even just searching for a recipe. *Health veganism*, a diet for the purpose of bettering oneself, overshadows my own assumptions of the phenomenon in contemporary culture. This incongruity creates a fruitful terrain for investigating the relationship of queer and trans people and their bodies to the neoliberal com-modification of veganism. By outlining the perpetuation of cis- and heteronorma-tive body ideals by veganism that prioritizes improvement of appearance, we can explore the potential harms experienced by queer and trans people.

Health Veganism

There seem to be more vegans or more people "eating vegan" than ever. According to the preliminary results of a cross-Canadian study of consumer attitudes to meat eating, 1.1% of the sample population identified as vegan, while an estimated 6.4 million people in the country are making efforts to reduce or eliminate meat from their diet (Charlebois et al., 2018). This increased interest in veganism may be due to a growing consciousness of the harmful effects of meat and dairy consumption on the environment, largely credited to popular mainstream documentaries and the striking, widely published results of an enormous study on almost 40,000 farms (Poore & Nemecek, 2018).

However, an association between veganism and improved health dominates representations of the diet. Moreover, improved appearance is often implied by this subjective form of better health. As Bratman (2017) writes, "the term fitness, which once meant 'an ability to walk up hills without getting short of breath' now also describes the 'fit' body type" (p. 384).

DOI: 10.4324/9781003217121-10

The commodification of this veganism is evident in online spaces. Some of the most frequently recurring Instagram posts retrieved by the search, #vegan, show aesthetically pleasing plant-based meals, pre- and post-diet comparisons, and thin or gym-fit bodies. Many of these social media users represent a growing number of vegan nutritionists, health gurus, and personal trainers who are using their own image to sell vegan diet plans, workout routines, fitness paraphernalia, and, ultimately, a body ideal. The product the person is selling is indistinguishable from the seller themself. By buying into this individual's brand, the consumer is led to believe they can achieve their same body. Health veganism, in this way, is marketed like many other diets and takes advantage of the expectation of continuous self-improvement that neoliberalism has fostered. In this culture, we have "become responsible for the design of our bodies" (Giddens, 1991, p. 102). The successful commodification of veganism, as a diet or fitness plan marketed primarily for the improvement of appearance, is an exemplary product of late capitalist culture.

The Gendered Body

By approaching a queer and trans experience of the *body* (its perception and nourishment), we may better understand the relevance that eating habits bear to the queer and trans experience of gender. In their commendation of Simone de Beauvoir's vision of the body and the distinctions she establishes between sex and gender in *The Second Sex* (1972), Judith Butler argues the centrality of the body, and our behaviours surrounding it, in the construction of gender differences. Elaborating a description of "gender as choice," Butler (1986) writes that "the body becomes a choice, a mode of enacting and reenacting received gender norms which surface as so many styles of the flesh" (p. 48). A person's diet and relationship with food can play a symbiotic role in one's attitude to their body. Queer and trans people have respectively unique experiences with the societal perception of their bodies. The gendered contemporary representation of health veganism may therefore impact queer and trans people in unique ways.

This gendered approach to the body is not a universal truth, however, and nor does it bear universal significance. The establishment of gender as a category which is distinct to, but constructed upon, "biological sex" derives from a Eurocentric understanding of the world that places the visual body at the centre of human experience. This disregards non-Western characterizations of masculinity and femininity. Oyěwùmí outlines this exaggerated importance of the visual in criticism of Butler's conceptions of sex and gender (1997, pp. 1–30). Bearing in mind the limitations of this perspective, the feminist scholarship that has arisen in this framework provides useful tools for surveying the landscape of neoliberal commodification ideology. Visual appearance will later be established as crucial in the perpetuation of binary male and female body ideals by health veganism. I will also explore the potential of centring personal feeling and social responsibility on vegan eating behaviours as a means for queer and trans people to escape the resultant conceptions of masculinity and femininity.

Queer and Trans Negotiations of "The Binary"

Queer and trans people negotiate the physicality of a perceived gender binary in daily life. This isn't to say that cisgender or heterosexual people are less impacted than queer or trans people by the constructed opposition of masculinity and femininity. Rather, trans and queer people embody identities that disrupt the expectations of such an opposition. Historically, homosexuality and identities to which we now refer to as transgender were somewhat conflated under the term "sexual inversion" (Prosser, 1998; Stryker, 2006). Transness was eclipsed by homosexuality until the later studies of "transvestism" and "transsexualism" in the field of sexology (Hirschfeld, 1991; Benjamin, 1966). These "deviances" were grouped together for a shared failure to adhere to the expectations of masculinity and femininity. Such an opposition lies at the ontological root of Western homosexuality and transgender identity (against which the concepts of heterosexuality and cisgender identity were defined and established as dominant). Queer and trans people may have reactionarily internalized these binary characteristics in ways that impact their relationships to their physical bodies.

Queer tendencies towards bodily dissatisfaction have been explored by various research studies and queer theorists alike. The heightened desire among gay men to achieve a thin or muscular body, for example, has attracted interrogation over the past 30 years (Gettelman & Thompson, 1993; Strong et al., 2000). More recently, studies of gay dating app activity have shown the muscular body type as a perceived signifier of masculinity and an active, insertive, or "top" position in sex role enactment (Moskowitz & Hart, 2011). Meanwhile, there seems to be a societal fixation on the "construction" of masculinity and femininity in the identities of trans men and women. Serano (2007) explores the notion of "feminization" that appears in real and fictional depictions of trans women, where the *act* of becoming feminine (dressing, applying makeup) is privileged over simply showing trans women already in feminine clothing or wearing makeup. This may lead to what Serano calls "ungendering," an undoing of a trans person's gender identity based on some incongruencies or discrepancies in appearance that would typically be overlooked in a person who is presumed to be cisgender. Conversely, within the queer community, pressure is sometimes placed upon trans people to deconstruct binary gender by actively rejecting normative standards of masculine and feminine appearance. Regardless of trans people's own conceptualization of their masculinity or femininity, a societal obsession with this binary is projected onto their bodies.

Vegan Body Ideals

Health veganism for the purpose of improving one's appearance represents an aforementioned consumer choice and a bodily manifestation of neoliberal self-regulation. There is a distinct opposition between males and females in the representation of the ideal vegan body, although the expected behaviour to adhere to both ideals is similar and they often go hand in hand (quite literally, given the number of vegan fitness influencer couples). Thinness and a more recent gym-fit combination of a cinched waist and appropriately womanly curves have become standards of normative feminine beauty. Vegan dieting, which mandates food *restriction*, becomes an extension of consumerist, beauty-oriented, feminine identity construction (Lazar, 2013). The goal of health veganism for women "is to have the outer self match the inner, where the inner is a (thin) beautiful, self-contained woman who does not struggle with food or her desires to eat, and always eats the perfect amount" (Dean, 2014, p. 132). This ideal may not be readily accessible for queer and trans women (as well as women of colour, differently abled women, or women with different body types). Moreover, this and the following male ideal are entirely exclusionary to non-binary people.

The health-vegan man presents another narrative. While femininity may be perceived as self-control, masculinity is often associated with the exertion of control over others. In *The Sexual Politics of Meat,* Adams (2000) establishes a connection between masculinity and the consumption of meat, arguing that "manhood is constructed in our culture, in part, by access to meat eating and control of other bodies" (p. xxvii). Yet men who consume a meat-free or vegan diet for health motivations don't seem to contradict this image. In fact, there is a growing number of health-conscious male vegans and, especially, vegan bodybuilders who uphold the ideal of masculinity "despite being vegan" (Greenebaum & Dexter, 2018). When these men sell their version of veganism, they emphasize the means of consuming as much protein as possible in their diet and highlight their own muscularity in the process. As Wright (2015, p. 126) puts it, "they are so ultra-masculine as to be able to be vegan and to make that dietary choice manly as well." The ideal neoliberal man appears to be muscle-building, while the ideal neoliberal woman is self-restricting. Veganism, in this sense, is sold as a technique for the 21st-century consumer to adhere both to normative binary body standards and to the role of the ideal subject of neoliberalism, who continuously self-improves. Undertaking veganism for this purpose may lead to harmful eating behaviours, especially among queer and trans people.

Self-Regulation and Disordered Eating

Neoliberalism can be understood increasingly as "constructing individuals as entrepreneurial actors who are rational, calculating and self-regulating" (Gill, 2007, p. 163). The ideal neoliberal individual is primarily concerned with their own wellbeing, as a means of bettering the economy and society. The phenomenon represents a "mobile, calculated technology for governing subjects who are constituted as self-managing, autonomous and enterprising" (Gill & Scharff, 2013, p. 5). Health veganism may offer queer and trans people a means of self-surveillance and regulation to adhere to these neoliberal ideals with the goal of achieving the aforementioned *body* ideals. If a Foucauldian "panoptical male connoisseur resides within the consciousness of most women," is it not also true that a panoptical cisgender or heterosexual connoisseur resides within the consciousness of most trans or queer people (Bartky, 1997, p. 140)? When queer and trans people are predisposed to embodied negotiations of the opposition of masculinity and femininity, there are greater potential harms in exposure to the binary ideals that veganism propagates.

Due to the strict dietary limitations of veganism, when it is undertaken for concerns with appearance and health, self-regulation may quickly decline into disordered eating. Steven Bratman coined the term *orthorexia nervosa* to refer to a "pathological fixation on eating proper food" (1997, p. 42). "Proper food" for the health vegan might mean low-calorie food for weight loss, high-protein food for muscle-building, or any plant-based products with vitamins directly associated with better skin, hair, and nails. A study carried out at Heinrich Heine University, Düsseldorf, found that both vegans and vegetarians were more likely to display orthorexic eating behaviour than meat eaters (Barthels et al., 2018). I argue that this likelihood may increase in the case of the queer or trans health vegan. When a societally driven focus on adherence to normative standards of masculinity and femininity is combined with restrictive eating practices that may help one achieve those normative body ideals, orthorexic eating may arise more easily for queer and trans vegans. This is an area that warrants illumination with focused qualitative and quantitative research.

Conclusion: Vegan Alternatives

In the above reflections, I have explored health veganism as a harmful perpetuator of the neoliberal incentive to self-improve among queer and trans people. As Bordo wrote of the effect of diet culture on women, health vegans are rendered "less socially oriented and more centripetally focused on self-modification" (1993, p. 166). However, I do not wish to present socially motivated veganism alone as an antidote to this damaging inward focus, nor as without fault. Vegan activism sometimes risks practising neocolonialism and replicating eurocentrism in the imposition of its values on Indigenous communities, as has been the case in certain Canadian regions (Donaldson & Kymlicka, 2011; Legge & Taha, 2019). Environmental and animal rights veganism also encourages a devout commitment to the cause that may foster an absolutism, in turn provoking harmfully restrictive eating habits in a similar manner to health veganism.

How then do queer or trans people participate in veganism without falling into orthorexic eating behaviours? We must seek to reaffirm our motivations to pursue veganism "for the sake of something other than the ideal feminine [or masculine] body" and reinstate that image of the socially disruptive vegan (Dean, 2014). Within these social movements however, and within the context of neoliberal commodification of health veganism, we must centre the experience of queer and trans people, as the above explorations have attempted. By turning our attention towards our *feelings*, the visual element of the body is demoted and instead *sensing* what feels good for our bodies gains more importance. The question shifts from "am I being good?" to "is it good for me?", meaning not only "is it healthy?" but also "does it *feel* good?" (Vogel & Mol, 2014). This allows us to make decisions for ourselves; to "eat vegan" one day, and not the next, while understanding that our actions can still bear significance to the wider environmentalist movement, for example. By prioritizing personal experience and feeling, space is created in veganism for nuance and escape from an absolutism that can lead to moral imperialism and to unhealthy eating habits. Centring our queer and trans identities in the repoliticization of veganism not only steers us away from these potential harms but may also contribute to a positive development of environmentally motivated vegan activism.

References

Adams, C. J. (2000). *The sexual politics of meat: A feminist-vegetarian critical theory*. Bloomsbury.

Barthels, F., Meyer, F., & Pietrowsky, R. (2018). Orthorexic and restrained eating behaviours in vegans, vegetarians and individuals on a diet. *Eating and Weight Disorders – Studies on Anorexia, Bulimia and Obesity, 23*(2), 159–166. https://doi.org/10.1007/s40519-018-0479-0

Bartky, S. L. (1997). 'Foucault femininity and the modernisation of patriarchal power'. In K. Conboy, N. Medina, & S. Stanbury (Eds.), *Writing on the body: Female embodiment and feminist theory* (pp. 129–154). Columbia University Press.

Benjamin, H. (1966). *The transsexual phenomenon*. Julian Press.

Bordo, S. (1993). *Unbearable weight: Feminism, western culture, and the body*. University of California Press.

Bratman, S. (1997). Health food junkie. *Yoga Journal, 136*, 42–44.

Bratman, S. (2017). Orthorexia vs. theories of healthy eating. *Eating and Weight Disorders – Studies on Anorexia, Bulimia and Obesity, 22*, 381–385. https://doi.org/10.1007/s40519-017-0417-6

Butler, J. (1986). Sex and gender in Simone de Beauvoir's Second Sex. *Yale French Studies, 72*, 35–49. https://doi.org/10.2307/2930225

Charlebois, S., Somogyi, S., & Music, J. (2018). *Plant-based dieting and meat attachment: Protein wars and the changing Canadian consumer (preliminary results)*. Dalhousie University.

de Beauvoir, S. (1972). *The second sex*. Penguin Books. Orig. pub, 1949; H. M. Parshley (Trans.).

Dean, M. A. (2014). You are *how* you eat? Femininity, normalization, and veganism as an ethical practice of freedom. *Societies, 4*(2), 127–147. https://doi.org/10.3390/soc4020127

Donaldson, S., & Kymlicka, W. (2011). *Zoopolis: A political theory of animal rights*. Oxford University Press.

Gettelman, T. E., & Thompson, J. K. (1993). Actual differences and stereotypical perceptions in body image and eating disturbance: A comparison of male and female heterosexual and homosexual samples. *Sex Roles, 29*, 545–562. http://doi.org/10.1007/BF00289327

Giddens, A. (1991). *Modernity and self-identity: Self and society in the late modern age*. Stanford University Press.

Gill, R. (2007). Postfeminist media culture: Elements of a sensibility. *The European Journal of Cultural Studies, 10*(2), 147–166. https://doi.org/10.1177%2F1367549407075898

Gill, R., & Scharff, C. (2013). Introduction. In R. Gill & C. Scharff (Eds.), *New femininities: Postfeminism, neoliberalism and subjectivity* (pp. 1–20). Springer.

Greenebaum, J., & Dexter, B. (2018). Vegan men and hybrid masculinity. *Journal of Gender Studies, 27*(6), 637–648. https://doi.org/10.1080/09589236.2017.1287064

Hirschfeld, M. (1991). *Transvestites: The erotic drive to cross-dress*. Prometheus Books. Orig. pub. Berlin, 1910; Michael A. Lombardi-Nash (Trans.).

Lazar, M. M. (2013). The right to be beautiful: Postfeminist identity and consumer beauty advertising. In R. Gill & C. Scharff (Eds.), *New femininities: Postfeminism, neoliberalism and subjectivity* (pp. 37–51). Springer.

Legge, M. M., & Taha, R. (2019). "Fake vegans": Indigenous solidarity and animal liberation activism. *Journal of Indigenous Social Development, 6*(1), 63–81.

Moskowitz, D. A., & Hart, T. A. (2011). The influence of physical body traits and masculinity on anal sex roles in gay and bisexual men. *Archives of Sexual Behavior, 40*(4), 835–841. https://doi.org/10.1007/s10508-011-9754-0

Oyěwùmí, O. (1997). *The invention of women: Making an African sense of western gender discourses*. University of Minnesota Press.

Poore, J., & Nemecek, T. (2018). Reducing food's environmental impact through producers and consumers. *Science, 360*(6392), 987–992. https://doi.org/10.1126/science.aaq0216

Prosser, J. (1998). Transsexuals and the transsexologists: Inversion and the emergence of transsexual subjectivity. In L. Bland & L. Doan (Eds.), *Sexology in culture: Labeling bodies and desires* (pp. 116–131). Polity Press.

Serano, J. (2007). *Whipping girl: A transsexual woman on sexism and the scapegoating of femininity*. Seal Press.

Strong, S. M., Singh, D., & Randall, P. K. (2000). Childhood gender nonconformity and body dissatisfaction in gay and heterosexual men. *Sex Roles, 43*, 427–439. https://doi.org/10.1023/A:1007126814910

Stryker, S. (2006). (De)subjugated knowledges: An introduction to transgender studies. In S. Stryker & S. Whittle (Eds.), *The transgender studies reader* (pp. 1–15). Routledge.

Vogel, E., & Mol, A. (2014). Enjoy your food: On losing weight and taking pleasure. *Sociology of Health & Illness, 36*(2), 305–317. https://doi.org/10.1111/1467-9566.12116

Wright, L. (2015). *The vegan studies project: Food, animals, and gender in the age of terror*. University of Georgia Press.

10 How Sociocultural Structures Shape Body Image and Dietary Practices among Gay, Bisexual, and Queer Men's Communities

Adam W.J. Davies, Dalia El Khoury,
Nathan Lachowsky, David J. Brennan, and Ben Klassen

Gay, bisexual, and queer (GBQ) men – both cisgender and transgender – experience enormous pressures to conform to hegemonic norms for masculinities within and outside of GBQ communities (Davies, 2021a, 2021b; Wood, 2004). Such pressures can result in body image norms that encourage dysregulated eating habits and over-exercising (Brewster et al., 2017). Involved in these pressures are GBQ men's dieting habits and supplemental uptake regimes, which are influenced through heteronormative ideals for masculinity and body image pressures from within GBQ communities that constitute idealized bodies (Joy & Numer, 2018a). Such pressures to conform to dominant ideals propagated through normative notions of masculinized gay bodies can cultivate shame in GBQ men about their own bodies (Davies, 2021a; Downs, 2012; Joy et al., 2021). As such, the dietary intake habits of GBQ men and how such habits are influenced by constructions of GBQ masculinities are of critical importance to dietitians, health promoters, and healthcare professionals.

Yet, there is only emerging work in nutritional sciences and dietetics that specifically focuses on the needs of GBQ communities by ensuring practitioners receive appropriate training to develop cultural competencies for working with GBQ individuals (Joy & Numer, 2018b). Following calls for more inclusivity in dietetic practices and training (e.g., Dhami, 2018; Joy & Numer, 2018b) and work in critical dietetics (Brady & Gingras, 2019), we call for future work in the dietetic profession to consider the specific sociocultural influences on GBQ men's dietary supplement uptake, such as normative constructions of GBQ masculinities and femmephobia, through a harm-reduction approach that centres anti-oppression and intersectional practices within psychosocial and ecological analytics. As such, this chapter proposes new considerations for working with GBQ clients in the field of dietetics with specific mentioning of emerging arts-based approaches (e.g., Joy & Neish, 2021). Our hope is that through this chapter, further attention can be paid to the specific needs of GBQ men's communities in dietetics through an anti-oppression and harm-reduction lens.

DOI: 10.4324/9781003217121-11

Critical Dietetics: A Necessary Intervention

Focused on social justice and anti-oppression by bridging dietetics with the social sciences and humanities in a transdisciplinary manner, critical dietetics orients itself politically towards equity and liberation by emphasizing how systems of oppression interact with the dietary habits of marginalized individuals (Brady & Gingras, 2019). Critical dietetics situates how the dietetics field is implicated within structures and systems that pathologize and subjugate marginalized communities (Gingras & Brady, 2019). Employing critical social theory, critical dietetics uses theory to analyze systems of oppression in an intersectional (Crenshaw, 1991) fashion. In this sense, social theories are crucial for critical dietetics in understanding how norms are involved in processes that inform dietary supplement uptake and how such processes are constituted through power dynamics and hierarchies (Brady & Gingras, 2019).

Anti-oppressive practices within dietitians' work emphasize how issues of power and privilege inform the relationships between dietitians and clients, name and address systems of oppression, acknowledge and amplify the lived experiences of marginalized communities, and actively advocate for social change, both societally and within the health and food sciences (Ng & Wai, 2021). All these considerations are important when working with GBQ men's communities, which have experienced extensive surveillance and regulation by medical, public health, and legal systems (Davies et al., 2019; Dean, 2009). In what follows, we outline the sociocultural importance of considering constructions of GBQ masculinities in dietetic practice with GBQ men's communities and future considerations for the field.

GBQ Masculinities: Considerations for Dietic Practices

The influence of gender and sexuality (as well as other identity markers) on dietary practices and supplement uptake is relevant for considering how understandings of masculinities inform GBQ men's supplement uptake practices. Theorizing masculinity as a sociocultural relationship consisting of gendered and racialized hierarchies, the sociologist Raewyn Connell (1995) described how hegemonic masculinity situates men within hierarchies of masculinities whereby they are positioned vis-à-vis other men in relations of domination and subjugation (Jewkes et al., 2015). Importantly, while GBQ men are traditionally viewed as "failed men" who are marginalized and subjugated vis-à-vis hegemonic masculinity, there are complicated gendered, classed, and racialized dynamics with GBQ men that position some men closer to hegemonic masculinity and reproduce dynamics of domination and subjugation amongst men (Connell, 1995; Davies, 2020, 2021a, 2021b; Edwards, 2005). Edwards (2005) describes how constructions of gay masculinities have focused on markers of hypermasculinity throughout the development of the Gay Liberation era, specifically emphasizing a masculinized aesthetic featuring leather, a moustache, a muscular toned body and hypersexualized self-presentation. Other productions of gay masculinities, such as young, feminine "twinks" or larger "bears" with facial and body hair, are all subjugated and positioned within hierarchies of GBQ masculinities (Davies, 2020; Unsain et al., 2020, 2021). Such emphases on hypermasculinity have remained within GBQ men's communities in current times, impacting body image ideals and self-conceptions of GBQ men who experience immense pressures to continually tone their bodies and build muscles to attract other men (Joy et al., 2020, 2021). These norms produce psychosocial pressures from within GBQ men's communities to employ muscularity to attract the attention of other men and gendered power relations that constitute hierarchies of desire that subordinate GBQ men who are feminized (Davies, 2020, 2021a, 2021b; Wood, 2004). Importantly, these issues of GBQ masculinities intersect with racial fetishization and stereotyping to reinforce white heteromasculinity as the ideal while men racialized as non-white are encouraged to either reinforce dominant archetypes or distance themselves from colonial forms of feminization (Yep & Elia, 2012) or hypermasculinization (Watts & Bentley, 2021).

Work in the field of dietetics is just beginning to analyze GBQ men's dietary habits (e.g., Unsain et al., 2020, 2021). Halkitis et al. (2008) describe how hegemonic constructions of masculinities – defined by steroid users as physical appearance and social behaviour – are involved in the self-definition of GBQ men, meaning that steroid consumption is a component of how GBQ men might conceptualize a masculinized form of self-presentation. Due to pressures from within GBQ communities to present as masculine and muscular to attract potential sexual and/or romantic partners, some GBQ men consume anabolic steroids to change their bodies (Sánchez et al., 2009). It is important to consider both the social and ecological factors that might influence dietary supplement usage. As such, we propose the implementation of critical ecological theory (Rothery, 2017) through a critical dietetic lens (Brady & Gingras, 2019) as a useful approach to understanding what influences GBQ men's body image pressures and dietary supplement practices.

A Critical Ecological Approach to GBQ Dietary Supplement Usage

Work currently in existence researching determinants of dietary supplement usage in different communities has yet to employ both social and ecological approaches to understanding the consumption of dietary supplements (e.g., El Khoury & Antoine-Jonville, 2012; El Khoury et al., 2019; El Khoury et al., 2020; Roy et al., 2021). Ecological approaches to analyzing phenomena draw from social work literature that considers how psychological, social, economic, and political factors impact the actions of individuals and how larger community norms impact social actors (Jack, 2012; Pardeck, 1988). Such an approach is highly consistent with critical dietetic practice, which aims to consider how social and structural systems interact with systems of oppression (Brady & Gingras, 2019). Ecological approaches are influenced by the work of Bronfenbrenner (1979) in how they consider both the macro and micro factors of individuals' quality of life and overall behaviours (Pardeck, 1988). Devine et al. (2004) theorize an ecological model for dietitians' professional practice that is explicitly grounded in environmental factors and contextual issues that impact dietitians' practices. Important work has begun to illustrate how social pressures and the attitudes towards individuals in social circles towards dietary supplements can influence uptake (e.g., El Khoury et al., 2021). However, when considering motivational factors for supplement usage, it is imperative to move beyond a strictly cognitive or psychological model that predominately focuses on interior motivations. It is necessary to consider sociological, ecological, and structural factors for why people in certain populations such as GBQ men may exhibit certain dietary practices. As will be discussed, arts-based approaches to understanding GBQ body image influences and nutritional uptake motivators can be considered in combination with a critical dietetics and critical ecological approach to ensure a depathologizing approach to understanding GBQ nutrition (see Joy et al., 2020; Joy & Neish, 2021).

Critical Ecological Approaches

Critical ecological approaches expand from ecological systems theory to bring into conversation how behaviours are impacted by structural systems of oppression and how marginalized individuals navigate systems where choice is limited (Rothery, 2017). In this sense, critical ecological approaches emphasize the social justice aims of ecological approaches by refusing to blame or responsibilize individual actors and considering the structural and sociological factors that inform how an individual makes their decisions (Rothery, 2017). For example, GBQ men are positioned as subordinated within heteropatriarchal hierarchies for masculinities (Connell, 1995). As such, while consuming anabolic steroids could position GBQ men as "unhealthy," there are power structures that inform such decisions that are necessary to consider.

Critical ecological approaches have been embraced within the human services professions, such as social work, and are commonly used in alignment with harm-reduction principles (Bigler, 2005). Although ecological approaches have been critiqued for being too theoretical and abstract (Rothery, 2017), this is not the case when placed in tandem with harm-reduction approaches, which value the holistic humanity of individuals, consider the various risk factors that contribute to behaviours, and engage with community activism to promote safer practices and risk reduction (Matto, 2012). Ecological approaches emphasize agency and how individuals engage in reflective practices and meaning-making regarding how they are positioned in structures (Rothery, 2017). This is highly consistent with work in arts-based approaches, which aim to provide space for individuals to engage in self-reflection and employ arts to challenge hegemonic norms that subjugate their agency (Joy & Neish, 2021). Current work in arts-based approaches to GBQ embodiment and nutrition (Joy et al., 2020; Joy & Neish, 2021) exemplify how critical ecological and critical dietetic approaches are embedded within the frameworks being used in arts-based approaches, which commonly draw from poststructuralism to emphasize the subversion of hegemonic discursive norms (Joy & Numer, 2018a; Joy & Neish, 2021).

Critical ecological approaches argue that when individuals' demands in their environment (in terms of basic needs for survival) outweigh their access to resources (and social community support), it is reasonable that their decision-making is hindered (Rothery, 2017). As well, such approaches consider how to move beyond merely analyzing the interactions between individuals and the environment, which we propose by taking into consideration four structural factors that impact GBQ men's intake of dietary supplements and are associated with structures of GBQ masculinities: (1) fatphobia, (2) femmephobia, (3) heteromasculinity, and (4) structural racism within GBQ communities. We will move to defining each of these structural factors and considerations for dietitians who work with GBQ communities.

(1) **Fatphobia** is the regulation and surveillance of fatness and fat bodies through medical knowledges and discourses of "obesity" (Davies, 2021a; Joy & Numer, 2018a). Fatphobia impacts GBQ men through the drive to diminish visible signs of fatness or to masculinize one's embodiment to disassociate from the feminization that often occurs through visible signifiers of fatness on male bodies (Davies, 2021a; Whietsel, 2014).

(2) **Femmephobia** is the regulation and surveillance of femininity through self-presentation, affect/emotion, and other significations of femininity (Davies, 2020, 2021; Hoskin, 2020). The regulation of femininity within GBQ men commonly takes place through attempts by GBQ men to masculinize embodiment through anabolic steroids, exercise, and nutrition and fitness regimes (Brewster et al., 2017; Davies, 2020, 2021a, 2021b). Body image pressures from within GBQ communities increase the pressure to self-stylize in a masculinized form through "bulking up" (Wood, 2004).

(3) **Heteromasculinity** is the notion that hegemonic masculinity is associated inherently with heterosexuality, thereby othering GBQ men and non-(cis)heterosexual acts and behaviours (Pronger, 1990, cited in Elder et al., 2015). As described by Downs (2012) and Elder et al. (2015), GBQ men might internalize (cis)heteromasculine ideals, which can then lead to emphasizing markers on the body of traditional masculinity, such as muscularity or a spornosexual, "fit" physique (Hakim, 2016).

(4) **Structural racism** within GBQ communities, as well as sexual objectification and fetishization, impact ethnoracialized GBQ men and posit stereotypical ideas of how ethnoracialized and non-white men are expected to present themselves and their respective embodiments (Brennan et al., 2013). As such, men might attempt to masculinize their embodiment to either offset feminization or to combat/reinforce racialized archetypes.

The impact of these structural factors on GBQ body image reaches into supplement usage, with GBQ communities privileging a lean, trim, and muscular masculine embodiment that impacts nutrient and food consumption (Joy & Numer,

2018a). Joy and Numer (2018b) recommend that dietetic training programmes emphasize cultural competencies and create GBQ-specific placement opportunities for students. We emphasize the importance of thinking about these four critical structures – fatphobia, femmephobia, heteromasculinity, and structural racism – within nutritional and dietetic work within GBQ men's communities in a critical ecological manner. There are experiences specific to GBQ men's communities that require addressing in a holistic and depathologizing manner, such as how being HIV-positive historically impacted the body image of GBQ men through the feminization of their embodiment through lipodystrophy syndrome (Power et al., 2003; Tate & George, 2001). Arts-based approaches in dietetics offer opportunities for GBQ to resignify the sociocultural and hegemonic norms imposed on queer bodies, while offering opportunities for reflection and critical deconstruction by both the researcher and participants (Joy & Neish, 2021). Importantly, arts-based approaches in dietary practices can begin to deconstruct binaries between theory and practice, arts and pragmatics, and application and professional practice (Joy & Neish, 2021). In this sense, dietetic practice might be able to move beyond simplistic binaries that consider "theory" as divided from "practice" and "practice" as lacking in ontological assumptions (Britzman, 1991). Arts-based approaches are one creative way to imagine new ways of conducting practice that can challenge dominant sociocultural systems and structures while reimagining practice in itself (Joy & Neish, 2021).

What this chapter advances is the specific necessity of considering how constructions of GBQ masculinities impact GBQ men's body image and ultimately supplement usage. Future work should consider dietetic interventions through a depathologizing, harm-reduction, and ecological approach for GBQ men that acknowledges the structural factors that influence supplement uptake.

Conclusion

The importance of considering the sociocultural and ecological factors that impact GBQ men's supplement uptake cannot be understated. Critical dietetic (Gingras & Brady, 2019) analyses that incorporate understandings of GBQ masculinities and related structures are a necessity to begin to research the specific needs of such communities. Through this work, we hope to have begun conversations about relevant considerations when enacting dietetic work and research with GBQ communities. Future work can pick up these considerations and employ these related frameworks within their respective professional practices.

References

Bigler, M. O. (2005). Harm reduction as a practice and prevention model for social work. *Journal of Baccalaureate Social Work, 10*(2), 69–86. https://doi.org/10.18084/1084-7219 .10.2.69

Brady, J., & Gingras, J. (2019). Critical dietetics: Axiological foundations. In J. Coveney & S. Booth (Eds.), *Critical dietetics and critical nutrition studies* (pp. 15–32). Springer.

Brennan, D. J., Asakura, K., George, C., Newman, P. A., Giwa, S., Hart, T. A., Souleymanov, R., & Betancourt, G. (2013). "Never reflected anywhere": Body image among ethnoracialized gay and bisexual men. *Body Image*, *10*(3), 389–398. https://doi .org/10.1016/j.bodyim.2013.03.006

Brewster, M. E., Sandil, R., DeBlaere, C., Breslow, A., & Eklund, A. (2017). "Do you even lift, bro?" Objectification, minority stress, and body image concerns for sexual minority men. *Psychology of Men & Masculinity*, *18*(2), 87–98. https://doi.org/10.1037/ men0000043

Britzman, D. (1991). *Practice makes practice: A critical study of learning to teach*. State University of New York Press.

Bronfenbrenner, U. (1979). *The ecology of human development: Experiments by nature and design*. Harvard University Press.

Connell, R. W. (1995). *Masculinities*. Polity.

Crenshaw, K. (1991). Mapping the margins: Identity politics, intersectionality, and violence against women. *Stanford Law Review*, *43*(6), 1241–1299. https://doi.org/10 .2307/1229039

Davies, A. W. (2020). "Authentically" effeminate? Bialystok's theorization of authenticity, gay male femmephobia, and personal identity. *Canadian Journal of Family and Youth/Le Journal Canadien de Famille et de la Jeunesse*, *12*(1), 104–123. https://doi.org/10.29173/ cjfy29493

Davies, A. (2021a). Gay fat femininities! A call for fat femininities in research on gay socio-sexual applications. *Fat Studies*, 1–14. https://doi.org/10.1080/21604851.2021 .1948161

Davies, A. W. (2021b). *Queering app-propriate behaviours: The affective politics of gay social-sexual applications in Toronto, Canada* [Unpublished doctoral dissertation]. University of Toronto, Toronto, Canada.

Davies, A. W., Souleymanov, R., & Brennan, D. J. (2019). Imagining online sexual health outreach: A critical investigation into AIDS service organizations workers' notions of 'gay community'. *Social Work in Public Health*, *34*(4), 353–369. https://doi.org/10.1080 /19371918.2019.1606755

Dean, T. (2009). *Unlimited intimacy*. University of Chicago Press.

Devine, C. M., Jastran, M., & Bisogni, C. A. (2004). On the front line: Practice satisfactions and challenges experienced by dietetics and nutrition professionals working in community settings in New York State. *Journal of the American Dietetic Association*, *104*(5), 787–792. https://doi.org/10.1016/j.jada.2004.02.023

Dhami, G. (2018). RE: Inclusive dietetic practice (letter to the editor). *Canadian Journal of Dietetic Practice and Research*, *79*(4), 156. https://doi.org/10.3148/cjdpr-2018-032

Downs, A. (2012). *The velvet rage: Overcoming the pain of growing up gay in a straight man's world*. Da Capo Lifelong Book.

Edwards, T. (2005). Queering the pitch? Gay masculinities. In M. Kimmel, J. Hearn, & R. Connell (Eds.), *Handbook of studies on men and masculinities* (pp. 51–68). SAGE.

Elder, W. B., Morrow, S. L., & Brooks, G. R. (2015). Sexual self-schemas of gay men: A qualitative investigation. *The Counseling Psychologist*, *43*(7), 942–969. https://doi.org/10 .1177/0011000015606222

El Khoury, D., & Jonville, S. A. (2012). Intake of nutritional supplements among people exercising in gyms in Beirut city. *Journal of Nutrition and Metabolism*. https://doi.org/10 .1155/2012/703490

El Khoury, D., Tabakos, M., Dwyer, J. J., & Mountjoy, M. (2021). Determinants of supplementation among Canadian university students: A theory of planned behavior

perspective. *Journal of American College Health*, 1–9. https://doi.org/10.1080/07448481
.2021.1951276

El Khoury, D., Dwyer, J. J., Fein, L., Brauer, P., Brennan, S., & Alfaro, I. (2019).
Understanding the use of dietary supplements among athlete and non-athlete university
students: Development and validation of a questionnaire. *Sports, 7*(7), 166. https://doi
.org/10.3390/sports7070166

El Khoury, D., Hansen, J., Tabakos, M., Spriet, L. L., & Brauer, P. (2020). Dietary
supplement use among non-athlete students at a Canadian university: A pilot-survey.
Nutrients, 12(8), 2284. https://doi.org/10.3390/nu12082284

Gingras, J., & Brady, J. (2019). The history of critical dietetics: The story of finding each
other. In J. Coveney and S. Booth (Eds.), *Critical dietetics and critical nutrition studies* (pp.
1–14). Springer.

Hakim, J. (2016). 'Fit is the new rich': Male embodiment in the age of austerity. *Soundings,
61*(61), 84–94. https://muse.jhu.edu/article/609287/pdf

Halkitis, P. N., Moeller, R. W., & DeRaleau, L. B. (2008). Steroid use in gay, bisexual,
and nonidentified men-who-have-sex-with-men: Relations to masculinity, physical, and
mental health. *Psychology of Men & Masculinity, 9*(2), 106–115. https://doi.org/10.1037
/1524-9220.9.2.106

Hoskin, R. A. (2020). "Femininity? It's the aesthetic of subordination": Examining
femmephobia, the gender binary, and experiences of oppression among sexual and
gender minorities. *Archives of Sexual Behavior, 49*(7). https://doi.org/10.1007/s10508-020
-01641-x

Jack, G. (2012). Ecological perspective. In M. Gray, J. Midgley, & S. A. Webb (Eds.), *The
SAGE handbook of social work*, (pp 129–142). SAGE.

Jewkes, R., Morrell, R., Hearn, J., Lundqvist, E., Quayle, M., Sikweyiya, Y., & Gottzén, L.
(2015). Hegemonic masculinity: Combining theory and practice in gender interventions.
Culture, Health & Sexuality, 17, 112–127. https://doi.org/10.1080/13691058.2015
.1085094

Joy, P., Gauvin, S. E., Aston, M., & Numer, M. (2020). Reflections in comics: The views of
queer artists in producing body image comics and how their work can improve health.
Journal of Graphic Novels and Comics, 1–27. https://doi.org/10.1080/21504857.2020
.1806891

Joy, P., Goldberg, L., Numer, M., Kirk, S., Aston, M., & Rehman, L. (2021). Compassionate
bodies, compassionate practice: Navigating body image tensions among gay men.
Canadian Journal of Dietetic Practice and Research, 82(3), 115–120. https://doi.org/10.3148
/cjdpr-2021-012

Joy, P., & Neish, J. I. (2021). The queen of hearts: Exploring the process of creating queer
art and its use in dietetic research and practice. *Critical Dietetics, 5*(2), 34–40. https://doi
.org/10.32920/cd.v5i2.1414

Joy, P., & Numer, M. (2018a). Constituting the ideal body: A poststructural analysis of
"obesity" discourses among gay men. *Journal of Critical Dietetics, 4*(1), 47–58.

Joy, P., & Numer, M. (2018b). Queering educational practices in dietetics training: A
critical review of LGBTQ inclusion strategies. *Canadian Journal of Dietetic Practice and
Research, 79*(2), 80–85. https://doi.org/10.3148/cjdpr-2018-006

Matto, H. (2012). Chapter 37: Drug and alcohol interventions. In M. Gray, J. Midgley, &
S. A. Webb (Eds.), *The SAGE handbook of social work*, (pp 579–596). SAGE.

Ng, E., & Wai, C. (2021). Towards a definition of anti-oppressive dietetic practice in
Canada. *Critical Dietetics, 5*(2), 10–14. https://doi.org/10.32920/cd.v5i2.1407

Pardeck, J. T. (1988). An ecological approach for social work practice. *Journal of Sociology and Social Welfare, 15*, 133–142.

Power, R., Tate, H. L., McGill, S. M. L., & Taylor, C. (2003). A qualitative study of the psychosocial implications of lipodystrophy syndrome on HIV positive individuals. *Sexually Transmitted Infections, 79*(2), 137–141. https://doi.org/10.1136/sti.79.2.137

Pronger, B. (1990). *The arena of masculinity: Sports, homosexuality, and the meaning of sex.* St. Martin's Press.

Rothery, M. (2017). Critical ecological systems theory. In N. Coady & P. Lehmann (Eds.), *Theoretical perspectives for direct social work practice: A generalist-eclectic approach* (pp. 81–107). Springer.

Roy, K. A., El Khoury, D., Dwyer, J. J., & Mountjoy, M. (2021). Dietary supplementation practices among varsity athletes at a Canadian university. *Journal of Dietary Supplements, 18*(6), 614–629. https://doi.org/10.1080/19390211.2020.1826618

Sánchez, F. J., Greenberg, S. T., Liu, W. M., & Vilain, E. (2009). Reported effects of masculine ideals on gay men. *Psychology of Men & Masculinity, 10*(1), 73–87. https://doi.org/10.1037/a0013513

Tate, H., & George, R. (2001). The effect of weight loss on body image in HIV-positive gay men. *Aids Care, 13*(2), 163–169. https://doi.org/10.1080/09540120020027323

Unsain, R. F., Ulian, M. D., de Morais Sato, P., Sabatini, F., da Silva Oliveira, M. S., & Scagliusi, F. B. (2020). "Macho food": Masculinities, food preferences, eating practices history and commensality among gay bears in São Paulo, Brazil. *Appetite, 144*, 104453. https://doi.org/10.1016/j.appet.2019.104453

Unsain, R. F., de Morais Sato, P., Ulian, M. D., Sabatini, F., Oliveira, M. S., & Scagliusi, F. B. (2021). Triangulation of qualitative and quantitative approaches for the study of gay bears' food intake in São Paulo, Brazil. *Qualitative Research Journal, 21*(4), 444–455. https://doi.org/10.1108/QRJ-04-2020-0034

Watts, K. J., & Bentley, K. J. (2021). Perceptions of gay black men on the social construction of masculinity and its role in mental health. *Journal of Gay & Lesbian Mental Health*, 1–24. https://doi.org/10.1080/19359705.2021.1949422

Whitesel, J. (2014). *Fat gay men.* New York University Press.

Wood, M. J. (2004). The gay male gaze: Body image disturbance and gender oppression among gay men. *Journal of Gay & Lesbian Social Services, 17*(2), 43–62. https://doi.org/10.1300/J041v17n02_03

Yep, G. A., & Elia, J. P. (2012). Racialized masculinities and the new homonormativity in LOGO's *Noah's Arc. Journal of Homosexuality, 59*(7), 890–911. https://doi.org/10.1080/00918369.2012.699827

11 Delicious Queer Bodies

Deonté Lee

My project aimed to photograph queer people of colour in underground nightlife in Los Angeles and New York. The main project question was: how do queer people use nightlife and fabulousness to decompress from societal pressures by uplifting their emotional wellbeing? Fabulousness is considered dangerous, political, and practiced by queer people who make themselves a spectacle because their bodies are constantly suppressed, as stated by Moore (2018) in *Fabulous: The Rise of the Beautiful Eccentric*. The inverted stylized portraits make the subjects appear larger than life and otherworldly because in a sense they are. The individuals within the images live life freely and do not allow the constraints of societal pressures to make them conform. They live their life unapologetically by creating an outwardly tangible artistic expression of what is inside them and makes them happy.

Throughout history, representation of queer people of colour from marginalized, ethnic, and low-income backgrounds has been limited throughout the art world. A recent study of 10,000 artists represented by major US museums found that 85% percent of artists were white while only 1.2% were African American (Topaz et al., 2019). The lack of representation of queer narratives within the art world substantiates the validity and importance of this project. Underground queer nightlife culture and self-styling through fabulousness undermines the hegemonic patriarchal ideologies that promote heterosexuality. Furthermore, the added reality that participation within these spaces could lead to potential violence creates a more complex view of underground nightlife culture. Moore (2018) states style is a form of protest, a revolt against the norms and systems that oppress and torture us all every day, things like white supremacy, misogyny, trans misogyny, patriarchy, toxic masculinity, gender policing, and racism (Moore, 2018). The locations each have thriving underground queer communities, yet with varying forms of oppressive factors such as political homophobia, violence, social trauma, and mental illness. The project examines how different forms of fabulousness in underground spaces are created and used to deal with these societal pressures (Figures 11.1–11.6).

DOI: 10.4324/9781003217121-12

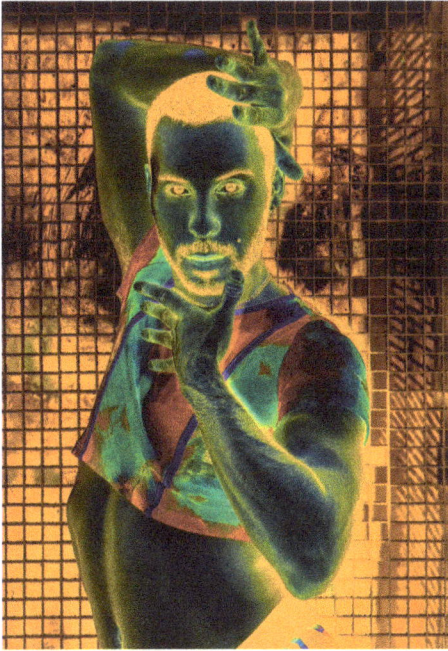

Figure 11.1 Vogue Baby, 2019, New York. Deonté Lee.

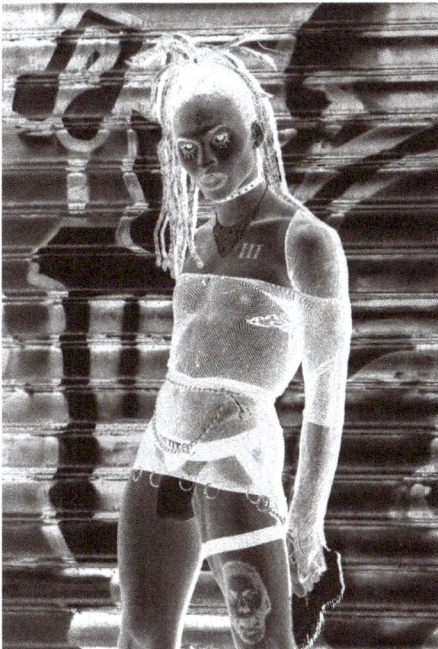

Figure 11.2 Kitty Kat Purr, 2019, New York. Deonté Lee.

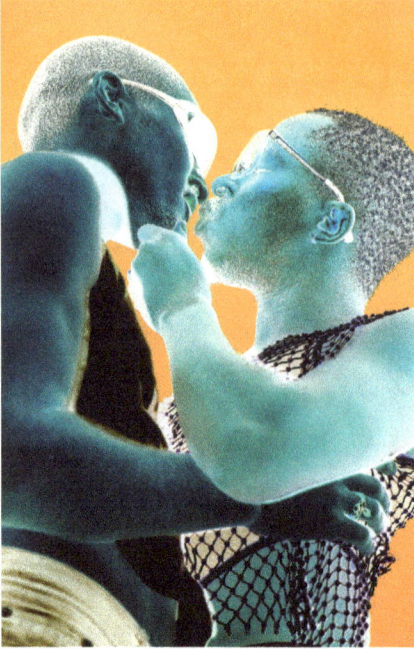

Figure 11.3 Touch Me, 2019, New York. Deonté Lee.

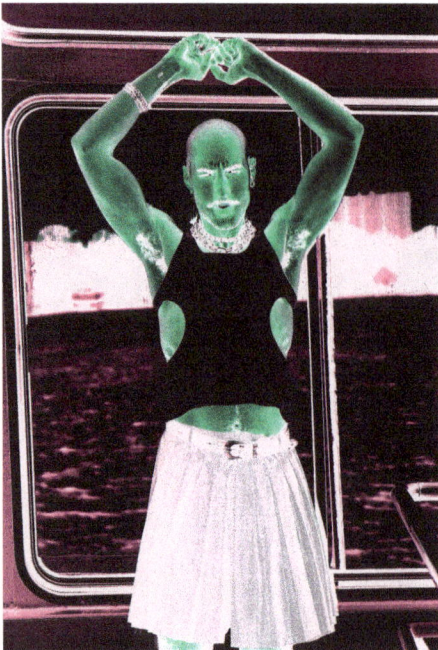

Figure 11.4 Lady Liberty, 2019, New York. Deonté Lee.

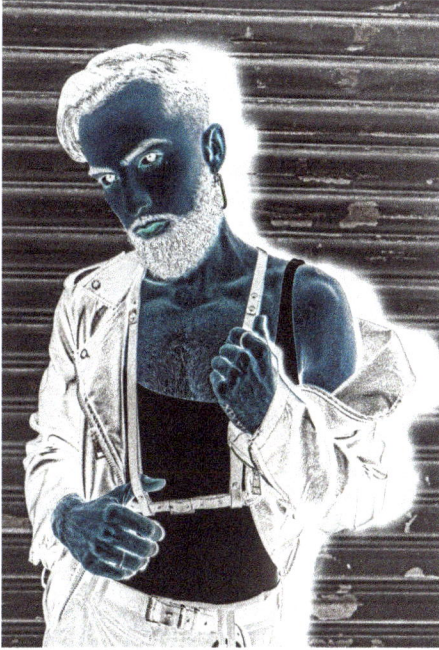

Figure 11.5 Leather Pleasure, 2018, New York. Deonté Lee.

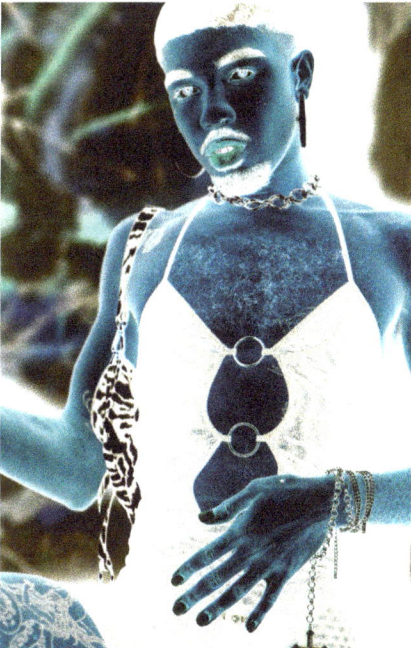

Figure 11.6 Jojo, 2019, New York. Deonté Lee.

References

Moore, M. (2018). *Fabulous: The rise of the beautiful eccentric*. Yale University Press.

Topaz, C. M., Klingenberg, B., Turek, D., Heggeseth, B., Harris, P. E., Blackwood, J. C., Chavoya, C.O., Nelson, S., & Murphy, K. M. (2019). Diversity of artists in major US museums. *PloS One*, *14*(3), e0212852.

12 The Impact of the Outsider's Gaze and Societal Norms around Food and Bodies on Queer Individuals

Alo Greening

Identities and Norms

I guess you can say that I was never the ideal, or even what society deems as "normal," from the start. What those on the outside saw as a "fat" girl playing pretend and acting out what being the ideal wife was from a kid's eyes, was really someone who saw the need to learn societal expectations, both in gender and sexuality, just so they could act those norms out in order to hide. Yes, I wore mostly bright colours, had a typically feminine haircut, liked dolls, and ballet. But honestly, who's to say those things made me a girl?

I went to a small school in the middle of nowhere, which led to me seeing one body and sexuality ideal constantly, that being "skinny and straight," and never anything else. When my friend in middle school, a transfer student, came out to me, my first reaction was surprise that anything outside the expectation was allowed in the first place. You could say that in a sense, it was the first crack in the shell I developed over the years.

Going into high school, I did the typical "person trying to find themselves" move. I read all I could on LGBT topics and settled on a label, pansexual. But something still felt off, so I kept digging and came to the realization that while I understood gender on an academic level, I never really understood it in a personal sense. Who I was and what I felt a connection with was constantly changing, and my labels did too.

In a way, I'm sure my mental health plays a role in my identity and what labels I connect with. Having gone through years of trauma left me with complex post-traumatic stress disorder (C-PTSD), but upon exploring with a therapist and a doctor, it was discovered that I also had dissociative identity disorder (DID) as a result of the trauma. Because of that, my self-identity is constantly in shift, which in turn explains why my gender (and self-image) always feels like it is changing. Because it is, I, as a person, am constantly changing, and while it was startling at the start, and I still have periods of self-doubt (and a lovely belief that I'm faking everything, which people without mental illness don't do), it's something I've slowly started accepting, just like my gender identity.

It is only through accepting these parts of me, and the fact that I will never not be mentally ill, that I can grow, so I do. I work on it every day by making sure to

DOI: 10.4324/9781003217121-13

be open about who I am, and my identity, when it's safe. And sometimes I fail, and hide away from my identity and put on a mask, but then again, is it really a failure when I can get up and try again the next day?

Gaze and Bodies

Before I came out as being what is essentially not cisgender, I knew there were ideals placed on the body. These ideals are enforced by gaze, which is when, through how others see us, we become aware of our self as a subject (Sartre, 1956.) We become aware that we are seen by others, and that how they see us holds weight, thus also impacting how we see our self in turn. It is my belief that this gaze plays a big impact on how we learn to see our self and how we believe we as individuals should be.

Everything in our cisnormative society is placed on extremes, and there are two options: Male or Female. Each option has its own norm. Women are expected to be thin, short, weak, caring, and ideally, someone to protect. Men are expected to be built, tall, unemotional (and if emotional, only in a sense of aggression), strong, and able to protect and provide for their partner (ideally, a wife). More specific norms change with the days, including those such as women being expected to have a big chest and wide hips, but a small waist, while men are expected to have muscles, but not body "fat," and to be over a certain height. These norms are expressed and enforced in media, spread in TV and magazines, and influence which foods and diets become the next trend. This is because gender norms serve as social rules and expectations, that then allow the gender system to stay intact.

But it's those ideals that crush us. While cisgender individuals have those norms placed on them, which for them is just a category in which they are expected to achieve some of the norms or to hold them as goals, the weight of those ideals falls harder on those under the trans umbrella. For those within the binary (male/female) there is an expectation to fit those norms to perfection, or else your gender is questioned, and no one takes you seriously. The world expects you to be the ideal, no matter the cost to achieve them.

For those outside the binary, we are classed as others, which has its own set of expectations with extremes. Either the world wants you to be invisible, to blend into the binary and to choose one gender ideal and stick with it, or you get the third option, which is to be as "genderless" as possible. The popularized ideal for being "genderless" is characterized by being thin, flat-chested and having no prominent hips, all of which can be summarized into an ideal of being small and have no sex markers prominent at all. For those who can't accomplish that, your identity is called into question and is invalidated.

People automatically perceive others within the binary, the brain goes to class people in boxes, and for the perception of gender, it tends to want to class them as either male or female. The lack of sex markers leads to the classification as "genderless" which is popularly assigned to the non-binary umbrella as a whole. However, there is an unease that comes with being misclassed by others.

The concept of dysphoria is something that can sometimes be hard to explain, but simplified to the purest form; it is an unease with perceived gender, which is how people see and assume an individual's gender. This in itself includes how people address us and things that are used in the process of categorization by others such as body characteristics. Personally, things that have always made me dysphoric are my chest, which is prominent, and my voice, which is higher on the register. Their body characteristics tend to be categorized by society as feminine, which in turn can lead to people assuming I'm a woman, which then leads me to get misgendered.

Sometimes that discomfort is small, something I can hide with a baggy sweater or playing it off as a social mistake (when addressed as a woman,) but sometimes, it feels like the world is ending, as if this one thing has ended my life as I know it and leads to me wanting to hide in my room forever. But the biggest impactor of dysphoria, and what makes someone dysphoric, might as well be the dominant binary gender norms within society. Dysphoria in itself is caused by a belief of not fitting a norm. I feel dysphoric about my chest and voice because the norm held for more masculine people is to not have a chest and to have a deeper voice. Because these attributes call my gender into question, I am left with gender dysphoria.

However, if the norms for gender were less rigid, would I be as dysphoric? If I saw more male-identifying people with top surgery scars or with chests, would I be less uncomfortable with my own? If I heard more male-identifying people with higher register voices, would mine make me less likely to want to stop talking entirely? I don't think these are questions I'll ever be able to answer, and the likelihood of me being able to avoid my dysphoria or fix it (even at a high economical and physical cost) is small; my mental illnesses make it hard to qualify for gender reassignment surgeries, and my brain doesn't process hormone changes well, so taking hormones is out of the question. So I'm stuck pondering how to fix society instead of trying to fit a round peg in a square hole.

I know that when people perceive me as the gender I identify with at the time, I feel a wave of euphoria. Simply put, being perceived correctly is the difference between a good and a bad day. Nothing feels better than someone classifying me correctly. And while most people don't do that, I'm lucky enough to have people who not only identify me in a way that makes me euphoric but who are willing to correct others when they misidentify me. But how do we, as a whole, avoid misidentification in the first place? By widening the norms placed on gender.

Norms are heavily influenced by media and representation; by seeing things on a continuous basis, they are normalized within society. This is why representation is important. Specific norms have been influenced by events happening around us, which impact the media both created and consumed. So, if there were more representation, there would be wider norms. And this representation has to be positive; negative representation just creates norms against what is being represented. If people want more trans representation, they are fighting for things outside the negative gaze already set by the cisnormative society we live in (trans women can only be prostitutes, trans men are just lesbians, that type of thing.)

Think about Barbie dolls. The concept behind Barbie is that she can be any-thing, and this belief passes on to other women through her; if Barbie can be anything, so can any girl. If Barbie can be involved in science or politics, so can any girl. Barbie, both as a doll and as a brand, acts as a social vehicle for recreat-ing gender norms. Firstly, with social gender norms, such as what a woman can and can't do, and now, with gendered body norms, with the new line of Barbie dolls who have different body shapes, skin tones, and disabilities. And the concept behind Barbie applies to the representation of different genders in media as a whole. The wider range of representation seen, the more accepted those repre-sented become and the wider societal norms are.

The Impact of Food

Discomfort with how others perceive my body doesn't just stop with gender per-ception. No, because dysphoria wasn't enough, I developed an eating disorder thanks to trauma. This leaves me with a lovely case of dysmorphia on top of my dysphoria. That image of a young "fat" girl? It became the enemy, not just because I was perceived as a girl, but because everyone around me looked like the "skinny" advertisement in the media, and I was deemed the "fat" kid. It haunted me, and eventually, I blamed food and myself instead of society.

From that moment, food became the enemy. The more I saw myself, the more I didn't want to eat, thinking that periods of starvation would make me "skinny," and thus happier. But after starving myself, I'd always binge eat, which would make me feel even worse about myself. The cycle continued for years, with the thought that maybe if I were skinnier, people would see me as more than the "fat" girl, and maybe see me as just a person, never mistaking my gender. There's a problem with that, that the definition of "skinny" and "fat" is constantly changing, and because of that, nothing I ever did would ever be enough to reach that ideal.

Eventually, I internalized a cycle of thought: I had to earn the right to have access to food. In order to earn the food, I had to be "skinny," or not eat much that day, and only then would I deserve to eat. This is only something I have come to discover years later through my recovery. My disorder is not based on a fear of food, but I fear the results I've associated with food: the perception and judgement of others, as well as potential weight gain. This, from an outsider's view, makes no sense because realistically, would you want to be friends with anyone who actually spent time judging you based on what or how you ate? But the concern is always there, that secretly I will make people hate me by how or what I eat.

The fear is that maybe, just maybe, all everyone sees is a "fat" girl just eating non-stop. They don't see the periods of starvation, or the mental calorie counting that goes into every meal; they just see me eating. And that image of a "fat" girl eating is something I've internalized. She was all I saw when I looked in the mir-ror, and I demonized her; I wanted her to disappear. Because even though I know I'm not a girl, and that I eat to survive, I can't help but see her instead of myself. But in recovery, if I'm learning anything at all, it's that there's nothing wrong with that girl; she's just an opportunity to spend time finding pieces of myself that

I love. She isn't evil, I just made her out to be the worst, and even if she isn't me, but an internalization of how I think others perceive me, there's nothing wrong with that. I have to eat to survive, we all do, our bodies need food to live, and there's nothing wrong with anyone, especially myself, for wanting to eat. If I want my friends to eat and stay safe, then I have to practice what I preach, and eat too, because I wouldn't want my friends to not eat because they didn't think they deserved to, or because they were scared of how others perceived them.

Some days are better than others now, sometimes I get days where I can wear a crop top or tight piece of clothing and not cry seeing myself in the mirror, or sometimes I feel like I can see my true self. Some days, if it's a really good day, I just wear whatever I want, and don't think about how others perceive me at all. And those days are, slowly but surely, growing in number the more I work on myself and work towards my eating disorder recovery and therapy.

Through recovery, I'm also coming to realize just how big a connection food and socializing have. Society is shaped in a way that revolves around food, because bodies need food to serve as energy and survive. The problem is that society, instead of seeing food as a need, is selling it as a want, and that instead, is also selling that we need to control our bodies. Society wants us to think we need to fit into this standardized norm, that instead of buying new clothing that fits when we grow, that we need to lose weight to fit in this ideal size. But that's not how bodies work, and it's not healthy to think that that is how we should live.

Many social interactions involve food in some way, it could be going to get coffee, going to see a movie, or just straight up having a meal with someone. Food creeps into the connections we make and if we work to avoid all the social situations involving food, we miss out on forming different social connections, and our social life suffers. I spent years trying to avoid social situations where I would have to eat or worry about "wasted" calories in drinks or prepare for such food by starving myself to "make up" for the consumption. Instead of benefitting me, it left me with a poor social life. This is something I'm noticing more and more in recovery. Food is connected to social life, just as social life is connected to food. Honestly, food is easier to enjoy, and not worry about the calories, when you are having fun with friends and those you cherish. This is especially true when compared to the feeling of eating alone on a kitchen floor at midnight.

Life is more fun sharing food with friends when compared to watching your friends eat while you drink a cup of water. There is this saying in the dieting industry that has stuck around in a lot of people's heads. As noted by Barry (2019), the supermodel Kate Moss was quoted as saying, "nothing tastes as good as skinny feels" (p. 18), but that's not true. When "feeling skinny" becomes associated with eating food you have to pretend to like, you are missing out on social opportunities you wish you could take and has you eating food on the kitchen floor at midnight only to feel shame for eating in the first place, even when you are hungry, then it's not worth it.

Why chase something that only leaves you feeling negative 90% of the time, just to experience brief moments of happiness for the "skinny feeling," especially when that "skinny" ideal is constantly in flux? This is something I had to question in recovery, and I had to decide for myself that the negative feelings I got most of the time weren't worth it. Chasing the "skinny" ideal wasn't worth it. This choice was hard, and sometimes I question it, but I know that the social life and happiness I'm gaining through the connections between food and life are worth way more than chasing "skinny."

I had a shitty past, and it has played an impact on who I am now, and why I am the way I am. But I'm not letting it control my future any longer. I'm working on myself daily, and I like to believe that, yeah, I as a person am growing. I'm in recovery, I'm out about my identity to those I'm close with, I'm learning how to cope with my mental illnesses, and to control my life. I'm actively making a choice to let myself be who I want to be, someone who can eat what they want without feeling guilty, someone who doesn't try to change themself to fit into clothing, but instead simply changes the clothing, someone who corrects people calmly when they are misidentified or mistreated, instead of taking it quietly while feeling terrible. All of that is growth, and I'm proud of it. Maybe one day, I'll be proud of myself as well; I'm working towards that, and know that one day, I'll get there. I also think that while I can be proud of myself for not changing myself to fit into societal norms, it is important to think about why society's norms are the way they are now and go about working towards changing the norms. People shouldn't have to go to extremes to change themselves just to fit the norms; instead, the norms should change to allow everyone to fit within them.

References

Barry, B. (2019). Fabulous masculinities: Refashioning the fat and disabled male body. *Fashion Theory*, 23(2), 275–307.

Sartre, J. P. (1956). The look. In *Being and nothingness* (pp. 284–299). Philosophical Library.

13 Food Has Genders (and Sexualities)

Negotiating Foodways, Bodies, Weight, Health, and Identity

Ramiro Fernandez Unsain, Mariana Dimitrov Ulian, and Fernanda Baeza Scagliusi

In the universe of homoerotic desire, and worldwide, there is a group of individuals who call themselves "bears." They are described (and describe themselves), among other characteristics, as having an ostensible profusion of hair, performing hyperreal masculinity, and having a notably robust body (muscular and adipose), where the belly stands out. This group was first visibilized in the United States between the late 1970s and early 1980s. As the 1990s progressed, other bear groups were organized in various parts of the world (Wright, 1997).

To get a belly that can be erotically appropriated by the members and admirers of this collective, some choose a diet based on carbohydrates and meats, mostly beef, consumed in general in group meetings and bacchanals (Unsain et al., 2020). The intake of these foods will be decisive to build a desirable body and a "masculine" one that differentiates itself, in turn, from other groups of dissident sexualities (Unsain et al., 2021).

In our research, we aimed to comprehend these persons in the context of the city of São Paulo, Brazil, through an ethnographic study. The research objective was to analyze how food, sexuality, and gender were combined, going through the life histories and, especially, the food life histories of the interviewees. The combination of interviews, with other techniques, yielded findings that describe the subjective constructions and intersections between sexuality, gender, and food, as well as class and health, and how this group approaches and, at the same time, distances itself from other groups of dissident sexualities in terms of food.

In this chapter, we seek to describe and analyze how the social construction of bear bodies, based on their weight and body benchmarks, intersects health, identity, and foodways dimensions. It is crucial to understand that, according to our findings, weight and the body shape is a distinct characteristic that overlaps with the ordinary numerical representation to become a diacritical feature. These bear bodies are highly valued and considered masculine and desirable because of their overweight and fat presence, especially in the belly.

In order to own and maintain a body that is labelled as a bear, it is necessary to implement particular eating practices and build a narrative of collective belonging through them. Still, this group perceives that eating abundantly and being

DOI: 10.4324/9781003217121-14

overweight are attributes that can lead to health concerns, some dangerous and potentially life-threatening (Unsain et al., 2020). In this sense, a dilemma arose for the bears interviewed: if they heed the advice of doctors and nutritionists, they could lose weight, but, at the same time, they feared not being identified as bears within their community. The other fear was losing one of the characteristics that separates them from other LGBTQ+ groups: hegemonic masculinity, a social differentiation category they associate with foodways and survival in a highly homophobic country such as Brazil (Gonçalves Pereira, 2021).

Going through life stories and exploring narratives, this research proposes a discussion regarding this apparent contradiction and how the social construction of the bodies of bears can challenge the hegemonic aesthetic standards (Goldenberg & Ramos, 2007) of LGBTQ+ people.

First Things First

We interviewed a total of 35 people who declared themselves to be men, gay, and "bears." As of the beginning of the research, all the interviewed subjects were 30 years old or older. The choice of age was based, firstly, on the reference established by França (2012) regarding the age range of the frequenters of the "Ursound" party, who identify themselves as bears and their considerations in emic terms and, secondly, on the "free observations" (Perlongher, 1999, p. 33), which suggest that a bear, in São Paulo, needs to look like or be 30 or more years old. In addition, being a bear is related to ascribing to the "ursine" (bear) community through the presentation and representation of different diacritics, ways of relating, places to frequent and specific ways of feeding (Wright, 1997).

This research established several locations for both participant and non-participant observations. The first field visit was in the city of São Paulo, in the República neighbourhood, one of the geographic nuclei of reference for this population and other dissident sexuality collectives. The second field visit took place, once a month, at the "Ursound" party, specifically oriented to the collective that defines itself as "bear," but also for their "admirers" and "curious;" these native categories arose in the preliminary observations. The third observational nucleus was in the barbecues organized by the bears and attended by people belonging to this collective and, as in the previous case, by admirers and onlookers. Also, this research conducted a semi-structured and life history interview with each of the participants to understand their ways of constructing meanings about their bodies, food, belongings, and health.

"We Are Family"

This research learned that the bears form a group of belonging ("community" in emic terms). For some, even a family. Through these configurations and the self-ascription by the others, they built a collective with specific characteristics. A specific feeding practice is one of these characteristics, in addition to presenting a specific body type and "masculine" behaviour.

To understand this phenomenon, and in this research, food, or rather a type of food practice, will be thought of as a strategy for the construction and appropriation of identities for collectives that express dissident genders and dissident sexualities.

Regarding the bears, the notion of one's bodyweight concerning food and how this particular variable affected their daily life was common in all the interviews. However, it is essential to emphasize that this variable, a relatively high weight, seemed to be experienced as an element of identity that transcends the ordinary numerical representation to become a diacritical trait, in the sense of situating the individual as having specific characteristics that relate to a way of being for others.

In the same sense, in all the interviews, food practices and food consumption had a common denominator explained by the participants: "abundance." However, this "abundance" did not necessarily have to do with everyday life in the sense of day-to-day food consumption, and it tended to manifest itself mainly on the occasions when there was commensality among equals. Between "machos." Among "bears."

This way of organizing the commensality could be observed in a specific event that the bears organized with a certain regularity, sometimes more than once a month. That was the bear barbecue or "churrasco." The barbecues organized by the bears present a script composed of steps not specifically verbalized but rather embodied in the practices that shape the event as a whole.

During this research, we received invitations to participate in two types of barbecues: one took place in the common area of an apartment building and the other in spaces located in the periphery of the city of São Paulo. We mentioned two types of barbecues because the spatial and behavioural limitations imposed by a barbecue organized in the common area of an apartment building were visible compared to the open space provided by an event organized in a more isolated location. We will focus on the latter. This open and ludic space located in the rural area, in the municipality of Embú das Artes, was 40 kilometres from the city. It was an ample space with a large swimming pool, several soccer fields, and other outdoor games where physical strength and specific skills are necessary.

At noon, there were about 100 people at the site. Moreover, all of them claimed to belong to the bear community or identified themselves as fans. They started playing volleyball and soccer games with a varied number of participants. When someone in these games "broke his wrist," as other players defined the dropping of a hand in some direction imitating a supposedly feminine gesture, he was immediately punished and modified that gesture while laughing at himself.

In this sense, we could identify several tensions between masculine and feminine representations that circulate in the dynamics of the barbecues and in all the bear encounters we attended. These tensions could be summarized in an illuminating expression: "Wow, what the fuck, I have weak hands like a woman." That was exclaimed by a participant, observed by other attendees while eating when an object falls from his hands. Connell (1992) exposes how gender is an arena for relations of domination and subordination, struggles for hegemony, and practices of resistance. For Connell (1992), hegemonic masculinities continue to be valued in subjects whose sexuality is not necessarily hegemonic. Thus, and for Bernstein Sycamore (1992), the men who practice dissident sexualities often present themselves by adopting behaviours that dictate hegemonic masculinity to avoid being discriminated against by a large part of society. That would be a way to defend themselves and survive in a homophobic and hostile context for non-hegemonic sexualities and genders; furthermore, in Brazil's political and social context, whose head of state publicly condemns dissident sexualities by promoting verbal and physical aggression towards these collectives.

However, let us continue with the barbecue. At approximately 1:00 p.m., the organizers started serving the banquet. The meat came out of the grill or barbecue and the people, forming rows, served themselves what they wanted (they chose the cut, or cuts, of meat they desired, as well as the accompaniments or garnishes) to finally sit on the rustic wooden stools that matched the table. All this action took place under a thatched roof. This choreography formed a fascinating gastro-generic process through which participants talked about soccer, sports in general, work, other people's bodies (and bellies), and their own. They also highlighted the abundance of food available at this event because "the important thing is that there never seems to be a shortage of food and drink." That defines a good bear barbecue, which seemed different from other non-bear barbecues and gastronomic events this researcher has witnessed. In almost all of them, abundance was synonymous with a good event, and, in this case, the attitude towards food consumption was exultant and ecstatic. The foundation of this abundance rested on a large amount of meat available on the grill that amalgamates a group of belonging and a specific membership. Fruits and vegetables, though present, were despised and consumed in small quantities. Indeed, a vegetarian bear was "insulted" as a subject that belongs to the feminine world where only fruits and vegetables should be consumed. If in Papua New Guinea, as Kahn (1986) shows for Melanesian societies, men are "taro" and cannot be "rice" because "rice" is for women, in São Paulo, bears are "barbecue" and cannot be "salad" because being "salad" is for women. This article is not saying that bears calculate, in their speech, the way they will verbalize "salad" so as not to appear effeminate. We are simply highlighting what was expressed in the field by all the interviewees: vegetables and fruits are not consumed by bears; men do not consume them; the food of women (and very feminine "queens") is other: fruits and vegetables. The relationships with sweets (basically expressed through desserts) were ambivalent, with some contradictions that emerge in the interviews and the field of events. The preference for sweets can be confused with the feminine universe, and this would not be aligned with the masculinity embodied by bears. So, sweets seemed to be consumed, although they were little present in the conversations, except for chocolate, a product that appeared with a significant frequency among those giving pleasure.

As the afternoon progressed and the action moved to the pool and the park, some bears kissed each other while rubbing their bellies and, especially in the pool, these contacts intensified, involving other parts of the participants' bodies. The pool area was ideal for drinking alcoholic beverages and sugary sodas. As twilight arrived, alcohol was consumed more assiduously (beer, rum, vodka, fruit cocktails, and wine), erotic activity in the pool increased, and at the same time, food and beverages were consumed. Most participants were inside the pool, forming a biotic broth, while other bears had fun and played with giant balls or flotation devices.

The procession to change clothes to return to the city and leave the event began at approximately 7:00 p.m.. As for what the bears consumed, the organizers reported that they calculated between 500 and 600 grams of beef per person, although they assured that they even predicted a kilo per person on other occasions. We must also add 150 sausages, poultry (they did not remember how many pieces), potatoes (five kilos), pieces of cheese (without calculation), two five-kilo bowls of cooked ham, olives, and three bowls of farofa (manioc flour cooked with different ingredients such as bacon and onion). Interestingly, they commented that if there had been women in this or another party, which rarely happens, they would have calculated between 300 and 350 grams for them. Because, as one participant explained: "women do not know how to eat barbecues." In addition, the organizers served 50 kilos of bread, several kilos of white rice (the organizers did not remember exactly how much), and a Greek Gyros grill with more meat, regardless of the specific meat planned for the barbecue.

On the other hand, the organizers catered a pan of about eight litres capacity with spaghetti in tomato sauce. Finally, they served the desserts from 5:30 p.m. onwards: two milk flan bowls, two strawberry mousse bowls, and one lemon tart. It is essential to mention that the food above was almost entirely consumed, leaving a small plastic bag of leftovers offered to the caretakers of the space.

It is important to stress that attending these events requires an investment in money to cover the entrance fee and transport. It is not cheap to be part of these meetings because, besides those mentioned above, one must invest in an appropriate aesthetic. In that sense, attending a bear meeting involves buying clothes and grooming the body hair appropriately, best done by a professional.

When we were leaving the event, one of the bears asked: "Is it possible to receive a woman here in this reunion?" His question was self-responded to before anyone could respond: "They would not understand this ... women have other ways of eating, of being ... just like 'queers' or 'trans' women ..."

In this sense, food, more specifically what bears eat, how they eat, and with whom they eat, seems to be a way by which the construction of these masculinities is achieved, materializing, in the sense of producing erotically desired bodies. Food and food practices, in this case, could be considered as instruments endowed with an agency in dialogue with the subjects and traversing them. From this perspective, food practices and "bear foods" are complex and articulated artifacts.

Final Considerations

These socio-food articulations stress the bear collective. Being at the barbecue is an objective to be achieved to be considered a member of the community. To be there and eat "a lo macho" (like a "macho") is to belong. The above articulations are translated into a fabric of collaborative wefts embodied in specific social relations and crystallized in affinity bonds that, in a way, build a type of non-blood family relationship. These gatherings celebrate bellies and individuals with corpulent, masculine bodies who manage to establish a gastro-erotic bond among themselves.

Finally, it is essential to highlight that obese or corpulent bodies are pleasure and erotic spaces and health concern representations. Furthermore, health is considered more to "take into account after the age of 60" than an asset built through everyday life. Thus, and for this research, the concepts of food and food practices will be thought of as devices that articulate identities, inclusions, exclusions, and belongings. It is crucial to think of these articulations in specific temporal, symbolic, economic, and political contexts because descriptions and explanations are only possible by considering all these dimensions in a dialogical and intersectional manner. In other words, the bears' bodies seem to be products in dialogue with these articulating devices that arise in a field of struggle and conflict, placing otherness in the arena of negotiation. Likewise, these obese and corpulent bodies are adorned with diacritics that suggest the idea that masculinity, corpulence, and belly and adipose tissue can be "dressed" in a seductive, provocative, and desired manner.

These bellies, these fleshy legs, these abundant arms, and these generous hairs tell a story that refers to a universe whose gateway, in this research, was food in dialogue with health, masculinity, sexuality, and identity. In this sense, these bodies are fields of narrative disputes about masculinities, food, and health, forming spaces of rich ethnographic intervention to think about the proposed objectives and raise new questions.

References

Bernstein Sycamore, M. (1992). *Why Faggots are so afraid of faggots*. AK Press.

Connell, R. (1992). A very straight gay: Masculinity, homosexual experience, and the dynamics of gender. *American Sociological Review, 57*(6), 735–751.

Goldenberg, M., & Ramos, M. (2007). A civilização das formas: o corpo como valor. In M. Goldenberg (Org.), *Nu e vestido: dez antropologos revelam a cultura do corpo carioca* (pp. 19–40). Record.

Gonçalves Pereira, A. (2021). Violência, Homofobia, Saúde, Minorias Sexuais e de Gênero. *Brazilian Journal of Health Review, 4*(3), 10937–10948. https://doi.org/10.34119/bjhrv4n3-104

Kahn, M. (1986). *Always hungry, never greedy: Food and the expression of gender in a melanesian society.* Cambridge University Press.

Lins França, I. (2012). *Consumindo lugares, consumindo nos lugares: homossexualidade, consumo e subjetividades na cidade de São Paulo.* EDUERJ.

Perlongher, N. (1999). *El negocio del deseo. La prostitución masculina en San Pablo.* Paidós.

Unsain, R. F., de Morais Sato, P., Ulian, M. D., Sabatini, F., da Silva Oliveira, M. S. & Scagliusi, F. B. (2021). Triangulation of qualitative and quantitative approaches for the study of gay bears' food intake in São Paulo, Brazil. *Qualitative Research Journal, 21*(4), 444–455. https://doi.org/10.1108/QRJ-04-2020-0034

Unsain, R. F., Ulian, M. D., de Morais Sato, P., Sabatini, F., da Silva Oliveira, M. S., & Scagliusi, F. B. (2020). "Macho food": Masculinities, food preferences, eating practices history and commensality among gay bears in São Paulo, Brazil. *Appetite, 144*, 104453. https://doi.org/10.1016/j.appet.2019.104453

Wright, L. (1997). *The bear book, readings in the history and evolution of a gay male subculture.* Harrington Park Press.

14 My Daily Meal

Michelle Forrest

As part of my doctoral dissertation in the philosophy of education on the value of imposing chance into the curriculum to make it an "open" work that challenges one's pedagogical intentions and inventiveness, I responded to a notice on an art gallery bulletin board calling for photos of food for an art exhibition entitled "Daily Meals" (Forrest, 1997, Forrest et al., 2010). The openness of the project intrigued me, seeing as the unpredictable range of submissions would likely test any curator's intentions. I shot 12 black-and-white photos of my cereal bowl, as I ate its contents, and sent them in (Figure 14.1).

Though I did not hear back or see any sign the exhibition took place, the experience served my purpose of participating in an "open" artwork so that I could explain and demonstrate in my thesis what distinguishes this concept of radical openness, theorized by Umberto Eco (1967, 1989), from the typical sense of the term whereby a work is open to interpretation, reception, and analysis; not open to chance or aleatory (L. *aleator* dice player) additions to the originally conceived work. My dissertation is in the philosophy of education, and I see it now as auto-theoretical in that it draws variously from descriptions and images of my daily experience, allows viewers glimpses into my environment, and makes theoretical claims regarding the value of imposing a radical form of openness into teaching and research. Hidden in plain view, even from me at the time, was a shameful story behind why I followed this unvarying breakfast routine. There was a significant truth beyond the facts I presented that has taken me decades to recognize and acknowledge.

Little did I know when I depicted my personal surroundings in the work that initiated my career in the philosophy of education, that years later I would see it differently on account of having been influenced by feminist and queer theory in the interim. In the wake of some of my recent work using autoethnography to revisit a humiliating episode from grade school (Forrest & Joy, 2021), I now see my doctoral experiments through a feminist lens informed by queer theory. Making my personal story political brings me to the gist of this essay: my struggle with food and what it means to me today.

. . . . .

I was fortunate to have loving and supportive parents who worked hard to provide for the middle-class small-town life I grew up in, coming as they did from

DOI: 10.4324/9781003217121-15

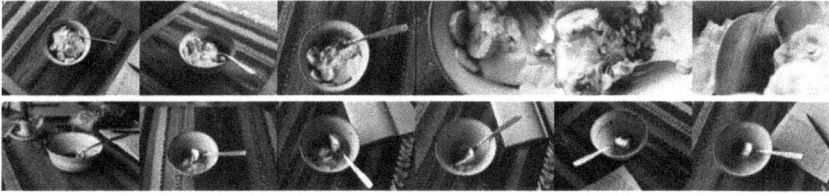

Figure 14.1 My Daily Meal, contact sheet. Photographs by Michelle Forrest.

working-class rural roots and not having had the advantage of finishing school. Like me, they had no idea about the complexities involved in "making it" in the multi-genre art form of grand opera. This was the career I set my sights on during university, influenced by a sophisticated "upper-Canadian" woman with whom I had become enamoured. Mine was too late a start for entering such a competitive world of classical music, as I was to discover. I was not unlike the protagonist, Monica Gall, in Davies's (1958) novel *A Mixture of Frailties*: a small-town Canadian girl, with a clear, naturally well-placed, but unschooled soprano voice, who goes to England to study singing supported by a trust. In my case, the trust did not pay the lion's share of expenses, however. These were paid for by my parents with minimal help from the little I earned doing secretarial and waitress work, which went towards shabby bedsit lodgings with shared bathroom facilities. My winning the talent trust award encouraged my parents, my singing teacher, and me to believe I had sufficient potential to head over the pond to London.

Living in the sprawling metropolis of Greater London in very basic digs, taking singing lessons once a week, and finding poorly paid part-time work was more than a bit disorienting. My letters home, full of anecdotes and experiences leading folks to imagine me living my best life, hid the grim reality because I didn't want them to worry. I was miserably adrift and out of my depth, barely able to practice enough to make any progress with my studies. In those letters, my escapades must have sounded like the stuff anyone would envy. Yes, I was practising at the BBC Maida Vale Studios, but only because my cafeteria job washing dishes and slopping custard onto the puddings of famous British entertainers at the New Bond Street Studios meant I had a BBC photo identification card. With this I was able to sneak into the BBC sound studio close to where I lived, use the piano, and pretend I had a right to be there. As for the famous British pub life one might think any 20-something student would relish, it was off-limits. The pubs were so smoke-filled and noisy back then that any time spent there gave me a sore throat and raspy voice for days. I led a solitary existence, saving enough from my weekly wages to afford cheap seats to the occasional concert at glamorous venues like The Royal Festival Hall and Covent Garden, but only after I'd learned how to navigate public transport and felt confident coming home late at night on the bus or tube.

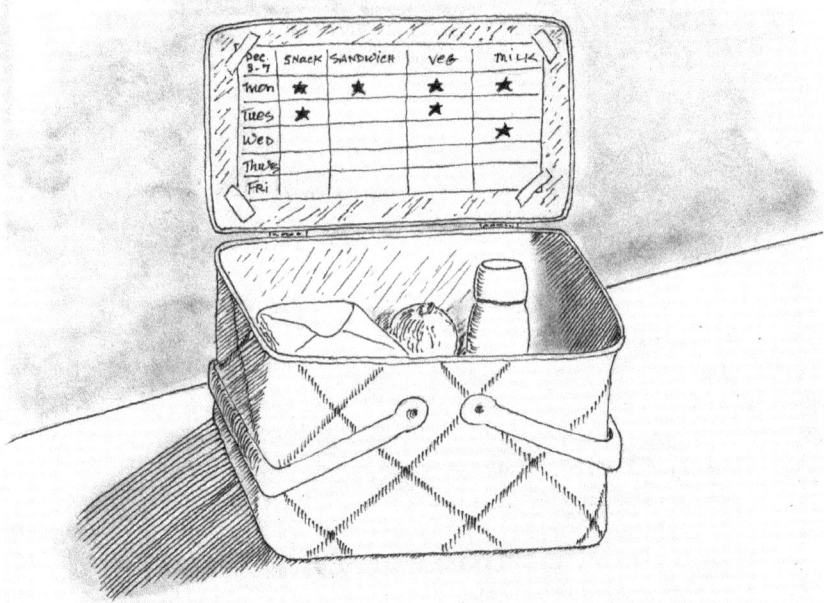

Figure 14.2 Child's open lunchbox with food chart and food items. Line drawing by Michelle Forrest.

As for cooking for myself, I had only basic skills because growing up I had had no interest in learning to cook. Being outside was far more appealing, playing ball, climbing trees, or riding my bike. I took for granted what my mother produced day after day, and, as a child, I had been a "poor eater," preferring raw vegetables to anything else. Many times I was made to stay at the table until I had finished everything on my plate. Early schooling involved a long walk each day, which meant I had to take a lunch. I must have come home too often without eating much because my mother and my grade one teacher worked out a system whereby they pasted a chart inside the yellow lid of my plaid lunchbox (Figure 14.2). It showed the different food groups with days of the week and blocks that the well-intentioned teacher filled with stars to assure my mother when I had eaten everything. The memory is vague but strikes me now as a perfect formula for a child to develop a troublesome relationship with food.

Revisiting my disordered eating in light of its larger history revealed a strong connection to religious beliefs and practices, which reminded me of my parochial school education, steeped in fasting. We fasted before receiving "holy communion," abstained from eating meat on Fridays, and gave up a favourite food – mine was always candy – for the 40 days of Lent starting each February. Though I went to Catholic school, our neighbourhood was predominantly Protestant, which meant that friends' birthday parties, typically held on Fridays, often involved hot dogs or hamburgers. My practically minded mother explained that I should eat whatever was being served and that God would not mind. Nonetheless, to me those experiences marked my difference from friends on our street and from my Catholic friends whose mothers were not as liberal-minded as mine.

In reviewing the literature on eating disorders and religiosity, Weinberger-Litman et al. (2011) recount a long history of the intersections of food, sexuality, and shame within religious tradition. In Genesis, in the Torah of Hebrew Scriptures and the Old Testament of the Christian Bible, it is woman who is depicted as eating the forbidden fruit and giving it to man, after which their eyes are opened, and they see themselves as naked. This early representation of humans' first revelation of sexuality is represented as linked with food, leading them to feel shame and try to hide from their god (p. 110). Although in the classical period there is little evidence of self-starvation, in the Roman world gnostic attitudes to the body as evil obstacles to salvation influenced Christianity and infused European culture in the centuries to follow (Witztum et al., 2011, p. 63). Self-fasting was common among women of the elite in medieval times, to escape parentally imposed marriages as well as for religious purification. The term "anorexia mirabilis" (anorexia – L. from Greek, without appetite (anorexia 2021)) or "holy anorexia" referred to the miraculous loss of appetite experienced by fasting women, which was taken as a sign of sanctity (Weinberger-Litman et al., 2011, p. 110). Complete denial of the flesh was described as a form of hysteria in 1689 and named "anorexia nervosa" in 1874 (p. 111). "Bulimia nervosa," (bulimia – L. from Greek, ravenous appetite; literally "ox-eating" (bulimia 2021)), characterized by bingeing and purging, appears to be a more modern phenomenon stemming from fear of fatness and the obsessive need to emulate an aesthetic ideal of beauty (Witztum et al., 2011, p. 61) and was coined as a diagnostic term in 1979 (p. 68).

My childhood practices of religious observance, however engrained back then, fell by the wayside when I left home to go to university, where I lived initially in residence, eating over-cooked cafeteria fare, and filling up on snack food with friends as we crammed for tests and exams into the wee hours. The sports I had done all through school also ceased. This combined with unhealthy eating and the sedentary life of studying had me overly conscious and displeased with my appearance as I tried to fit in with the worldly-wise young women I'd befriended in residence. I became infatuated with a flamboyant free spirit who played classical piano and encouraged me to have aspirations as a singer, but I was eventually rejected by her when she came face to face with her latent lesbianism, which likely contributed to my tendency to "eat my feelings." My newly acquired patterns of eating, concern over body image, and pain from being rejected by her fostered a sense of shame for being queer – an identifier I would never have used in those days – and for the fact that I fasted and overate in ways I knew to be detrimental but could not stop.

This shame over my self-humiliation remained past graduation through two years studying singing in Toronto, after which I worked as an administrative assistant in Halifax in a government office, where avoiding inappropriate advances from my boss was a continual struggle. I hadn't the nerve to tell him point-blank that his "cuddly" attitude was inappropriate. There seemed little point in complaining about it. This was long before the Me-Too movement (#meetoo) gave many women the courage to speak out, though harassment and abuse still abound. As Ahmed (2021, p. 108) says, even not complaining about harassment "changes your relationship to yourself and to the world around you." You no longer trust your own judgement and can end up feeling that you have betrayed yourself (p. 108). So, I continued with vocal studies and eventually won the first of two Portia White Talent Trust awards that supported my move to England.

Until recently it was thought that women from sexual minorities were less prone to disordered eating than cisheterosexual women, the presumption having been that lesbians' rejection of traditional sex roles and dominant beauty "ideals" served as a protective function (Fallon et al., 1994). More recent findings indicate, however, that persons from sexual minorities are disproportionately adversely affected by concerns and behaviours accruing from disordered body image (Convertinoa et al., 2021; Jones & Malson, 2013). As a queer woman trying to establish a career in the 1970s in a context where openly admitting to queerness was unthinkable, it is only recently that I have reconsidered how hiding my minority status affected my general wellbeing. Even though recent research has brought to light the extent to which disordered eating affects sexual minority women, there are still few findings that lead to recommendations for targeted prevention and intervention programmes (Watson et al., 2017). Not having disclosed my queerness as a part of coming of age, I can now reassess experiences that affected me growing up as they pertain to my sexual orientation and the complex feelings I carry along with that history.

The phrase "compulsory heterosexuality" was coined by Adrienne Rich in 1980, who claims that it sets up a hierarchy "through which lesbian experience is perceived on a scale ranging from deviant to abhorrent, or simply rendered invisible" (p. 632). Rich (1980) pointed out the ironic fact that much of feminist theory was "stranded on this shoal" (p. 632) and she called for feminist critique of the taken-for-granted prescription toward heterosexuality as a political institution, along with recognition that lesbian sexuality was incorrectly subsumed under the category of male homosexuality (p. 637). Rejecting the clinical sounding term "lesbianism," Rich (1980) opted to use "lesbian existence" and "lesbian continuum" to refer to the broad range of "woman-identified" experience that includes "primary intensity between and among women" that may or may not involve intimate sexual relations and that entails "sharing of a rich inner life, the bonding against male tyranny, the giving and receiving of practical and political support" (p. 649). In short, she reconceptualized the common stereotype of lesbian experience as either exotic or perverse, by incorporating the lesbian continuum into the complex radical history of female resistance.

My interest in singing the great roles of the operatic stage was fed by the incomparable feeling of expressing *fortissimo* my innermost feelings. I had no inkling of compulsory heterosexuality and how traditional opera reinforced its systemic nature. The famous arias in my repertoire are almost all soliloquies; the audience listens in on the soprano's heterosexual hopes and dreams, usually unfulfilled, as she longs for the departed lover to return (*Madama Butterfly*), wonders in torment over what she did wrong to lose her beloved (Countess in *Marriage of Figaro*, Desdemona in *Othello*), or remembers early days of blissful love irredeemably lost (Violetta in *La Traviata*). There were two roles I particularly enjoyed singing, likely because these were strong women, not mere ciphers of female victimhood. Fiorgiligi (*Così fan Tutti*) outsmarted all the male forces pitted against her and Tosca lived for art and love (Visi d'arte, visit d'amore), duping Scarpia out of having his way with her, the bargain she made to save her lover from the firing squad. Her escape was death by her own hand, but she had triumphed over all the political forces mustered against her.

As a result of writing this chapter, I have researched names of operas that defy the tropes of compulsory heterosexuality that ground the history of most Western opera. A lesbian-themed opera was unheard of in the 1970s, though operas with travesty roles – women playing young men (e.g., *Der Rosenkavalier*) – featured female voices proclaiming their love for each other. Had an opera like Paula Simpers' *Patience and Sarah* (1998), featuring a lesbian love story (Salazar 2017), existed when I was singing opera, it is unlikely I would have been drawn to it since that would have marginalized me even more in that competitive artistic environment.

The training of opera singers in London in the 1970s is the context for my "toughing it out" on the audition circuit, despite the emotional toll of continually being rejected. Aspiring operatic sopranos were a dime a dozen, which meant many were driven to extremes to be chosen for a plum role, including dieting to look the part and putting up with the bullying tactics of some teachers and vocal coaches. Sopranos were lined up to take over from anyone who failed to excel immediately, as I soon discovered. I was about to perform my first major role in the college opera school – Violetta in Act 2 of *La Traviata* – when I began to experience vocal difficulties. My singing teacher was caring and old-school, very protective of his singers' voices. Suspecting infection, he sent me to a Harley Street specialist who still practiced in the tried-and-true way, using nothing strong to numb my larynx to examine it. He darkened the room, numbed only my palate, placed a strong light at the back of my throat, and saw from outside the profile of the vocal cords. He diagnosed infection and prescribed complete vocal rest for at least two weeks to prevent the infection around the cords from developing into nodes, which typically need surgery and risk changing one's vocal quality irreparably. This meant no talking and definitely no whispering, which is more harmful because it rubs the cords together. Singing was out of the question. The artistic director of the opera school was not impressed and made me feel like a coward for backing out, even though I had an understudy. Other students told stories of their teachers pushing them to take the drugs prescribed by the newer Harley Street specialists to help them sing on top of an infection. My teacher warned that this was not the best option for long-term vocal health. I took his advice and missed singing my first starring role, in front of critics and opera company recruiters.

Fortunately, my singing teacher did not teach through humiliation and bullying, which I had experienced with my first teacher in Toronto and in a masterclass with a famous conductor, who shall remain nameless, rest his soul. In my final year at the London college, I managed to arrange a session with a renowned vocal coach, who worked on repertoire with sopranos at the Royal Opera House, Covent Garden. My enthusiasm was soon dashed, when I brought in my favourite aria, "Visi d'arte, visi d'amore," for his guidance. The hour-long session was a nightmare. He played and I sang the first lines of that aria over and over with him yelling at me to correct my vowel colour, dynamics, vibrato, and interpretation as I tried to project through the window to the famous concert hall across the street. Incorporating everything he insisted on was a lost cause but trying not to cry was the most difficult part. As the throat begins to constrict with genuine emotion singing is impossible. "I live for art; I live for love" sings Tosca. The irony of that scene is vivid. His appalling pedagogy taught me to hate the aria I had loved and struck a lasting blow to my dream of singing opera professionally. Nonetheless, I lived to sing another day, though I learned through bitter experience that I would have needed intense musical training from an early age plus thicker skin to compete successfully in that ruthless environment.

Pressures like that – having to choose between singing a leading role and seriously damaging my vocal cords – doubtless takes a toll on one's self-confidence and overall wellbeing. The legendary operatic diva, Maria Callas, lost megapounds later in her career, a move that is still debated as to the toll it took on her voice. Her weight loss was part of a general trend in the mid-20th century towards far greater emphasis on an ideal of thinness among women in the Western world, which shifted attitudes in the opera world, from prizing the quality of the voice above all to valuing how one looked in the costume and matched the visual stereotype of the heroine. On top of my insecurities as a queer soprano passing as straight and pretending to have more musical training than I had, there was the general pressure of looking the part and competing against sopranos with more training and sight-singing ability. Fasting, over-eating and purging in the vain hope of landing a starring role made shame into my state of being.

All that my parents and I had gone through to get me here at the epicentre of the English-speaking opera world was at stake, in my mind. Yet, I didn't know how to let it go, return home, and find another path. Describing the fate of Stephen Mary Gordon in the most famous "lesbian" novel, *The Well of Loneliness* (Hall, 1990), Kathryn Stockton (2006, p. 49) says that for this protagonist "fantasy splutters; sacrifice fails. There is, finally, only loneliness." This describes my situation; like Stephen, I had "no social holdings (no public structures) [...] to make her self-humiliation into a social solitude." Despite the reality that homosexuality in private was decriminalized in Britain in 1967 and by the mid-1970s the British Sociology Association had called for the establishment of a gay archive to document discrimination, I was oblivious to these milestones and to the first UK gay pride march held in central London in 1972 (Donnelly, 2008). I had no community to help mitigate my shame, so I assumed it was mine alone. Social holdings, says Stockton (2006, p. 27), refer to the "range of people holding people in their arms and in their minds, even in astonishing scenes of debasement."

Returning to my daily meal and how it became a kind of ritual, the worst of my eating disorder ended suddenly when I saw a made-for-TV drama about a suburban woman with an apparently "perfect" life who hides her bulimic behaviour (Seidelman, 1986). Though my condition was not as extreme as that depicted in the film, seeing the double life led by the protagonist as she maintained a seemingly happy existence while hiding her uncontrollable bingeing and purging, was my turning point. Prior to that, I had no knowledge of any such condition, had never heard the term "bulimia," and assumed the reason for my shame was unique to me. Although the extreme behaviour ended, this did not mean my relationship with food was somehow "fixed." I had been around various diet regimes since adolescence; my mother and her sisters were influenced by the Weight Watchers peer support approach (Hendley, 2003). I tried it, as well as a calorie counter diet from a self-help book and became vegetarian for a time in London. Eventually, taking into account the best regime for my own digestive health, I stuck to wholegrain fibre each day, which I ate at breakfast in the form of granola with plain yogurt for active bacillus, and banana for potassium. These comprise the contents of the bowl in the photos (Figure 14.1 and Figures 14.3–14.6).

The series is in black and white for practical reasons. It was uncommon in the 1990s for a dissertation in Education to include personal photo images and I felt certain the university would not agree to printing anything in colour. As I reinterpret them through feminist eyes, the starkness of the greyscale is telling because the photos do not depict my breakfast regime accurately. I set the table with a placemat and used a special bowl for the shoot, whereas normally I ate

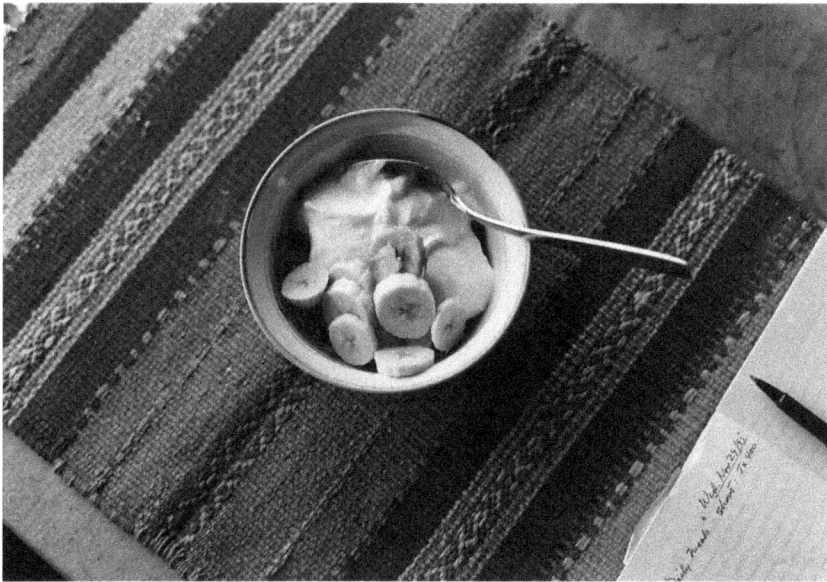

Figure 14.3 My Daily Meal # 1. Full cereal bowl with spoon; notepad and pen with date and title of photo shoot. Photographs by Michelle Forrest.

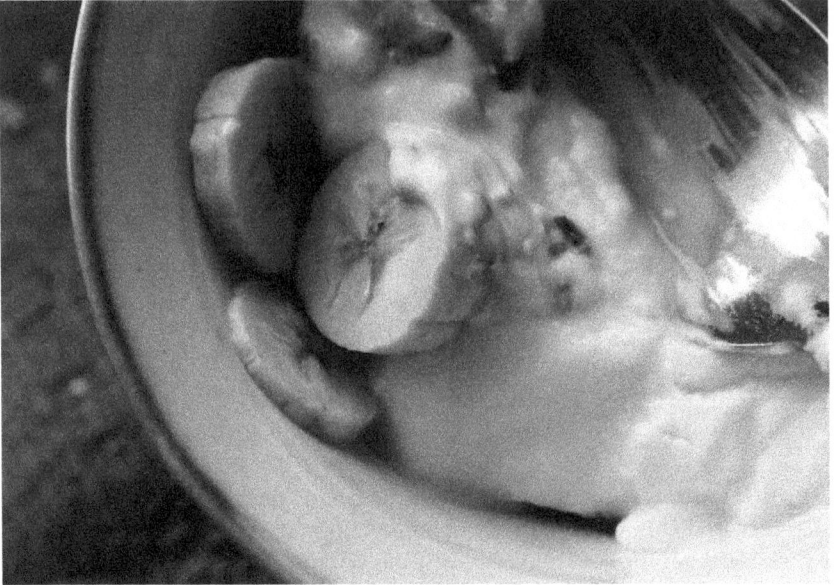

Figure 14.4 My Daily Meal #4. Close-up of bowl rim and spoon with granola and bananas. Photographs by Michelle Forrest.

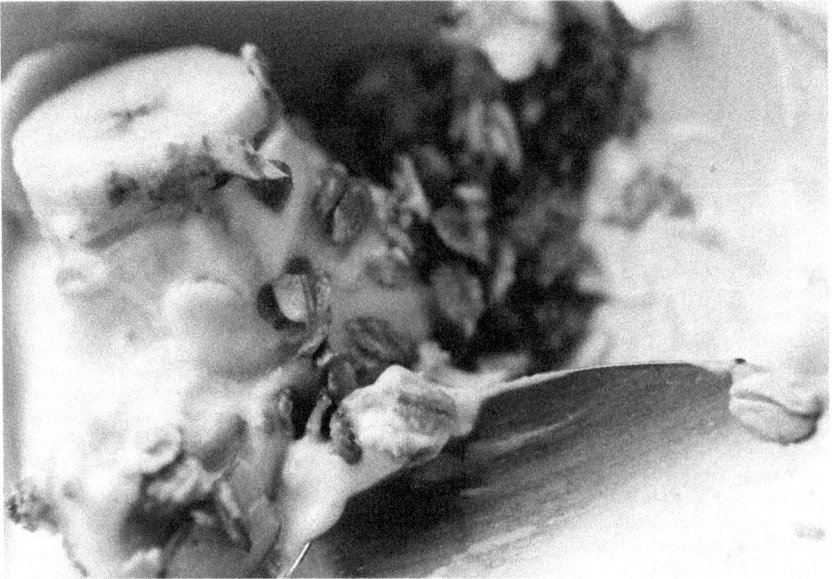

Figure 14.5 My Daily Meal # 5. Close-up of bowl contents with edge of spoon. Photographs by Michelle Forrest.

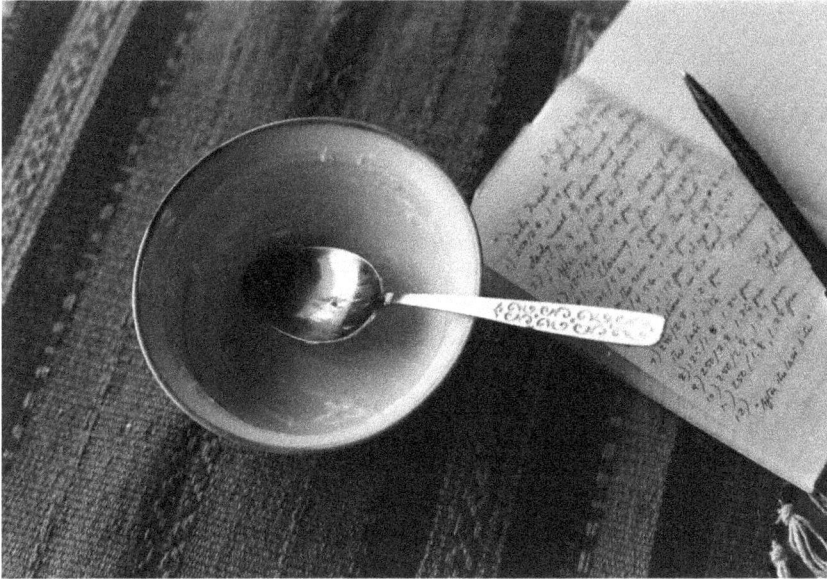

Figure 14.6 My Daily Meal # 12. Empty cereal bowl and spoon with yogurt traces; pen on notepad page full of annotations on photo shoot. Photographs by Michelle Forrest.

breakfast on the move, going about other tasks, not sitting formally at the table or using a special, hand-painted bowl. My everyday bowl would end up in different spots, depending on what I was doing when I finished eating. The fake set-up for the photoshoot was like my seemingly glamourous life in London, hiding the real circumstances of my daily life.

Naming myself as this or that ontological being has never come easily, perhaps as a result of being an only child and not seeing myself as necessarily one of any group, and likely because the heterosexual orientation I was assumed to have never fit my reality. My otherwise privileged life has always been a bit off-kilter or queer. According to Mayhew (2006), Ahmed (2006) "approaches queerness not as a condition of being, but specifically as phenomenology, a means of experiencing the world that is both destabilising and optimistic" (p. 242). In other words, "queerness" for Ahmed is not a fixed ontology but happens in the flux of experience, in how one reacts to the world and to the extent that one can still be hopeful in the face of opposing forces. As I approach the end of my academic career, I believe that in spite of, and possibly because of, living my life slantwise from the norm, I remain hopeful and try to embody optimism from day to day. Seeing each moment as another chance to make things better may be akin to what Ahmed (2006, p. 2) describes as the contribution of phenomenology to queer studies. It "can offer a resource [...] insofar as it emphasizes the importance of lived experience, the intentionality of the consciousness, the significance of nearness or what is ready-to-hand, and the role of repeated and habitual actions in shaping bodies and worlds."

. . . . .

Looking at these photos of my daily meal after so many years of disordered eating, I could not be re-evaluating their relation to my queer self at a more fitting time. Major surgery recently prompted me to reconsider my come-what-may attitude to life, which brings me back to the food chart in my lunchbox (Figure 14.2). This time round – I feel I've been granted a second chance – I try to be grateful for each bite I consume, assured my mother rests in peace knowing her ingenuity has succeeded. As a teacher educator, I have known in theory that early schooling is where one learns one has a public identity (Rodriguez, 1982). It has taken me a lifetime, however, living in the only body I'll ever get, to realize how many interlocked societal norms pressured me from the start to conform to what did not fit – compulsory heterosexuality, ubiquitous archetypes of female perfection, feast-or-fast puritanical ethos of purity – and led me toward self-destructive behaviour, spitting me out all these years later. Am I wiser? That is not for me to say. But I am acutely aware of the precious quotient of time remaining. One of my mother's sayings, "the longest way round is the shortest way home" (Joyce, 1937), made no sense to me as a literal-minded child. Ironically, it has fulfilled its promise. The secret of any paradox is that it must be lived to be understood, something my mother knew well enough to bestow that puzzle on me. I would describe my eating now as careful, not obsessive; healthy, not puritanical. As for my queerness, my parents took Wittgenstein's tack – "what we cannot speak about we must pass over in silence" (2004, p. 89) – while gracing me with boundless love and support.

When he defended his thesis in 1980, 25 years after he began, Derrida said, "never have I felt so young and so old at the same time" (Derrida 1983, p. 34). The series of chance occurrences leading me to write this essay in which I reinterpret work I did 25 years ago makes me feel old in having sufficiently reconciled with the past to describe it here and young in hope for having laid that chaos to rest and seen how fortunate I have been. In my doctorate, I learned from Derrida about the paradox of the trace, "which in order to take actual form must erase itself and produce itself at the price of this self-erasure" (Derrida 1983). Inspired by his example, I wrote a dissertation about its own "performative structure" (Derrida 1983), erasing and reinscribing itself as it progressed, which was a way of "queering" the thesis form, although I did not call my method "queer" at the time. Like him, 25 years after beginning, I see that this "strategy is a strategy without finality," one that "holds me in its grip, the aleatory strategy of someone who admits that [s]he does not know where [s]he is going" (Derrida 1983). Truth is a kind of trace and has a funny way of reappearing when I least expect it.

References

Ahmed, S. (2006). *Queer phenomenology: Or242ientations, objects, others*. Duke University Press.
Ahmed, S. (2021). *Complaint!* Duke University Press.

'anorexia'. (2021). Online etymology dictionary. Retrieved October 16, 2021, from https://www.etymonline.com/word/anorexia

'bulimia'. (2021). Online etymology dictionary. Retrieved October 16, 2021, from https://www.etymonline.com/search?q=bulimia

Convertinoa, A. D., Bradya, J. P., Albright, C. A., Gonzales, M., & Blashill, A. J. (2021). The role of sexual minority stress and community involvement on disordered eating, dysmorphic concerns and appearance- and performance-enhancing drug misuse. *Body Image 36*, 53–63.

Derrida, J. (1983). The time of a thesis: Punctuations. In A. Montefiore (Ed.), *Philosophy in France today*, (pp. 34–50). Cambridge University Press.

Donnelly, S. (2008). Coming out in the archives: The hall-carpenter archives at the London school of economics. *History Workshop Journal, 66*(1), 180–184.

Eco, U. (1967). Formes et Communication. *Revue Internationale de Philosophie, 21*, 231–251.

Eco, U. (1989). *The open work (1962–68)*. A. Cangogni (Trans.). Harvard University Press.

Fallon, P., Katzman, M. A., & Wooley, S. C. (Eds.). (1994). *Feminist perspectives on eating disorders*. Guilford.

Forrest, M. (1997). 'No ordinary chaos': Heuretics for media work in education [PhD dissertation]. Dalhousie University.

Forrest, M., Cooley, M., & Wheeldon, L. (2010). Mapping the movement of invention: Collaboration as rhizome in teaching and research. *Power and Education, 2*(1), 31–47.

Forrest, M., & Joy, P. (2021). Out of the closet and into quarantine: Stories of isolation and teaching. *Atlantis: Critical Studies in Gender, Culture & Social Justice, 42*(1) (Special Section: COVID & the Academy), 31–46.

Hall, Radclyffe (1990). *The Well of Loneliness*. New York: Anchor Books (original work published 1928).

Hendley, J. (2003). Weight watchers at forty: A celebration. *Gastronomica, 3*(1), 16–21.

Joyce, J. (1937). *Ulysses*. The Bodley Head.

Jones, R., & Malson, H. (2013). A critical exploration of lesbian perspectives on eating disorders. *Psychology & Sexuality, 4*(1), 62–74.

Mayhew, M. (2006). Discomforting delights (review of Ahmed's *queer phenomenology*). *Cultural Studies Review, 13*(2), 242–246.

Rich, A. (1980). Compulsory heterosexuality and lesbian existence. *Signs: Journal of Women in Culture and Society, 5*(4), 631–660.

Rodriguez, R. (1982). *Hunger of memory: The education of Richard Rodriguez: An autobiography*. Bantam Books.

Salazar, F. (2017). Pride month 2017: A look at the LGBT operas in history. *Opera Wire*. June 2017. Retrieved October 31, 2021, from https://operawire.com/pride-month-2017-a-look-at-the-lgbt-operas-in-history/

Seidelman, A. A. (Dir.) (1986). *Kate's secret* (Film). IMDb.

Stockton, Kathryn (2006). *Beautiful Bottom, Beautiful Shame. Where "Black" Meets "Queer"*. Durham and London: Duke University Press.

Watson, R. J., Adjei, J., Saewyc, E., Homma, Y., & Goodenow, C. (2017). Trends and disparities in disordered eating among heterosexual and sexual minority adolescents. *International Journal of Eating Disorders, 50*, 22–31.

Weinberger-Litman, S., Latzer, Y., & Stein, D. (2011). A historical, cultural and empirical look at eating disorders and religiosity among jewish women. In Y. Latzer, J. Merrick, & D. Stein (Eds.), *Understanding eating disorders: Integrating culture, psychology, and biology* (pp. 109–122). Nova Science Publishers.

Wittgenstein, L. (2004, c2001). *Tractatus logico philosophicus.* D. F. Pears & B. F. McGuinness (Trans.). Routledge.

Witztum, E., Latzer, Y., & Stein, D. (2011). A historical background to current formulations of eating disorders. In Y. Latzer, J. Merrick, & D. Stein (Eds.), *Understanding eating disorders: Integrating culture, psychology, and biology* (pp. 61–76). Nova Science Publishers.

Part 2

Communities, Connections, and Celebrations

15 The Eating Test

Notes from a Jewish Lesbian Omnivore

Bonnie J. Morris

> *But where is the writer who has done justice to the glories of white stewed fish as it appears on the Passover table? Golden balls, of delicate flavor, surmounting slices of the whitest halibut; cayenne peppers, with circles of lemon, adding brilliant color and spicy taste to the compound; over all the yellow sauce, almost jelly-like in consistence. Those who have spoken of Judaism as a "kitchen religion" lose sight of the fact that spirit and body are equally in need of nourishment.*
>
> Mary Cohen, "The Influence of the Jewish Religion in the Home," 1893

Few of us get to have our love of eating tested, measured, and marked down in the annals of science, but I did. In the mid-1980s I paid my way through graduate school as a volunteer patient in food studies at the National Institutes of Health (NIH). For several summers I served as a "normal" eater in a treatment programme for women with eating disorders. I personally knew several friends who struggled with anorexia or bulimia and had followed with keen interest the new body image literature in feminist scholarship and arts activism – from *Our Bodies, Ourselves* to *Shadow on a Tightrope: Writings by Women on Fat Oppression*. Out and proud since age 18, I wanted to make sure the NIH incorporated lesbian bodies in its health studies. That same cultural moment saw a surge in Jewish lesbian literature, starting with Evelyn Torton Beck's 1982 volume *Nice Jewish Girls*, plus Leslea Newman's novel *Good Enough to Eat*, leading many of us to Jewish lesbian discussion groups about food, ethnicity, and the body throughout the 1980s. I thought I might expand upon these themes while completing NIH hospital tests, perhaps writing an article about the experience. I did indeed publish my very first scholarly article (in *Feminist Issues*) about my summers at NIH, but not before I was dismissed from the eating study for being too "radical," having alienated the medical patriarchy by smuggling in a copy of *Our Bodies, Ourselves* to share with the patients. I had time, in that hospital bed, to ponder ways in which we use food as seduction, comfort, taste; and to question whether anyone ill could rekindle their love of eating while dining on hospital food. The truly radical act was having my lesbian body inscribed in the record as *normal*.

I'd completed my first year of graduate school with a long hot summer ahead, full of difficult books to read for my MA exam in the fall. Hoping to study in a

DOI: 10.4324/9781003217121-17

quiet place, serve society, and save up tuition money, I applied to my employer from college years – NIH. There, simple possession of *mens sana corpore sano* enabled one to earn thousands of dollars being a "normal volunteer" in research studies. As a college undergraduate in search of easy money, I'd done it all: eye-hand coordination tests, IQ tests, sleep pattern and aging studies, even an interesting hypnosis experiment that uncovered memories from second grade. Now I boldly signed up to be the control subject in an experimental, long-term eating disorders unit. No one else wanted this job, which required spending overnights in a locked ward, where women on suicide watch ate three meals a day under medical supervision. I joined their table; I became their friend. I never met another "normal" volunteer there.

Every week of that summer, I spent two or three days and nights in a hospital bed in the NIH complex in Bethesda, dutifully eating symbolic calories from a medical tray while my blood, urine, and hormonal reactions to hospital food were measured in comparison with the other patients around me. I soon neglected my planned reading list (Clark's *Working Life of Women in the Seventeenth Century*, Kraditor's *The Ideas of the Woman Suffrage Movement*, and Ruether's *Religion and Sexism*) as I became fascinated by the real women's history unspooling right in my face. What were the mixed messages to women that made thinness a measure of beauty in my era? In those clinic hours I had plenty of time to ponder how my vibrantly healthy body was helping to normalize homosexuality, which until 1973 had been classified as an illness in the Diagnostic and Statistical Manual (DSM) of the American Psychiatric Association. Here, barely a dozen years later, I was the good specimen, my cheery, 144-pound feminism a slap in the face to centuries of homophobic science. NIH was not interested in "curing" my queerness or making me straight, but, instead, had enlisted me to assist in studying why educated young women were starving themselves to death. Then there was the whole Jewish thing, too. Not too terribly long ago the Nazis had experimented horribly on Jewish women's captive bodies, as well as torturing homosexuals; yet in 1984 at NIH I was the sample supergirl, offered up as anything but victim. And all around me, girls were self-emaciating to the point of resembling concentration camp survivors. Hitler, looking in, would have seen his ideology in tatters, a Jewish lesbian eating the lion's share of food. That awareness of history, of my own ancestors' martyrdom, did have the power to make me lose my appetite.

Some of the tests I participated in seemed dubious, at best. For instance, the binge study. As I was not a habitual binger or purger, I was simply instructed to eat as much as I could in a timed session. Fine. Bring it on. I knew from past experience at grad student potlucks and Jewish brunches that, given the right buffet, I could eat potato salad, macaroni and cheese, or lox and blintzes for hours. But the binge study was built on *hospital food*, spooky trays of mystery-meat burger, air-whipped artificial potato, and cardboardy cups of stale vanilla ice cream, of which I was encouraged to consume all I desired. And I *desired* none of it. The test lacked any element of sexual, secretive, covetous desire, titillating no appetite. Had NIH shuttled me to Georgetown with a credit card, I could have raised the bar of "normal eater" statistics by traipsing through the menus of my favourite restaurants: American Café, Sarinah Satay, La Chaumiere, the Vietnam Georgetown, Booeymonger's. This approach wasn't in the protocol, alas. I failed the binge test, miserably poking at the hospital tray and offering excuses. Other tests were similarly uninspiring: I was shown three different trays and told to select one for that day's lunch. The first tray contained thinned cottage cheese and a lettuce leaf; the second, only sweets and desserts; the third, a high-protein sandwich and whole milk. Gee, could they possibly represent *anorexic, bulimic, healthy choice?*

As a volunteer, I alone was free: free to come and go, unlike the very ill. Yet I stayed in the clinic, befriending patients, talking one-on-one about the expectations of female body size in a heteropatriarchal culture. These wasting bodies were topped with very intelligent heads: what had gone so terribly wrong? Some were daughters of very famous men. Had they found power in self-denial, in corporeal vanishing? Furthermore, outside the clinic doors in those mid-1980s days, there was a far more politicized wasting illness devastating the gay community, the AIDS epidemic. Extreme thinness in young men was already assumed to be a marker of full-blown AIDS, no longer the more prestigious male-pattern anorexia of ballet dancers and jockeys. How did the NIH patients feel about the gendered competition, then, for AIDS research money versus funds for women's breast cancer, eating disorders, and pelvic inflammatory disease from poorly designed contraceptive devices? But the more I initiated dialogues in the dayroom, the more the clinic staff chafed and glowered and complained about my outsider/feminist "influence." My presence on the ward became an internal problem for NIH; one nurse accused me of trying to seduce a patient, easily the farthest thing from my mind. What NIH wanted was my body fat index and muscle mass and "good" cholesterol numbers, my willing and joyful digestion of dairy products, my routine and regular output of excreta. My historical analogies, my feminist analysis of the beauty myth which sends many young women into diet pathology, were not welcome. So it was that after my last week of hospital tests, I came home to find a phone message from the director of the eating disorders clinic, kindly requesting that I and my copy of *Our Bodies, Ourselves* never return. In fact, I did return for a few more summers – these studies were longitudinal, and they needed normal volunteers.

But what was normal for a lesbian in the mid-1980s? When I wasn't giving blood or eating measured fats and proteins for science, I was dating women. There were two different factions in the lesbian community: the vegans and vegetarians who criticized meat and dairy eaters as pawns of corporate agribusinesses and animal abuse, and the political activists who, while certainly willing to boycott Nestlé, were also invested in ensuring Black, Latina, Arab, Asian, Pacific Islander, Indigenous, and Jewish dykes had something to eat at a feminist table including them. Whose animals were sacred? Kosher? Ritually slaughtered and eaten on feast days, at luaus, after sweat lodges? Whose foods were served at international conferences, at block parties, at what served as the social event of the season in lesbian culture: the women's music festivals?

During my dates with other Jewish lesbian foodies, romantic, candlelit scenarios permitted sensuous taste. We went to the movies first, and the distasteful chow of my recent hospital tests receded into memory, replaced by the oozing oils of Junior Mints. We feasted on a Jewish menu of challah and rugelach, latkes and sour cream, and chilled vodka, talking about the food-based Yiddish we knew, the crass kitchen-garden insults for women of the *shtetl* to shout at men: You should grow like an onion with your head in the ground! Beets should sprout from your belly! This reminder of the role root vegetables played in my own heritage was something I vowed to bring up as soon as I returned to the eating disorders clinic at NIH. God damn it, why wasn't Jewish cuisine part of any food study? Could we talk about the way dieting had the effect of eliminating ethnicity? As I had been the *only* "normal" volunteer that summer, would it have cost so much to have my binge study include bagels and cream cheese? Even one rugelach?

"Rugelach," my girlfriend and I whispered, our tongues lingering over the word's prolonged throatiness. "Challah." If eating a loaf of challah, pulling its softness apart, rolling it into a damp and airy mouthful, can be construed as foreplay, then we were already in trouble over the hors d'oeuvres.

Bread. Jews were by now a tiny minority hanging onto planet Earth. Yet everybody liked bagels. I was finding that although generic Jewish food trickled down into American cuisine, in most parts of the country it wasn't how people ate every day.

Having saved up the money I needed for another year of graduate school expenses, I considered the additional economizing and sisterhood that might come with living in a lesbian collective. There were many such group houses forming, and I pored over the wanted ads until I found what seemed like a good match. The women of this household had a clever and creative outgoing message on their answering machine when I immediately made an appointment to be interviewed as a potential housemate. But here's where everything fell apart. Operating as a collective, they explained, each woman would take her turn grocery shopping for the entire household – using a set list of basic staples. Every month, each housemate contributed an agreed-upon amount of dollars to the food budget, and the grocery list ensured that the kitchen was always full of food. No one was unduly burdened with running to the store all the time, and the budget plan for each month of nutritious, home-cooked meals was consistent and fair.

It all sounded great in principle, until I saw their list of what counted as "staples." It was, like so many white dyke food plans at that time, the least ethnically comprehensive pantry grid in America. This was a self-righteous era of no butter, no salt, no dairy, no sugar, no chocolate, and wheat-free everything. The ultimate indulgence permitted and sanctioned might be powdered yeast and tamari sprinkled on one's organic popcorn. I was fine with living without meat. It was the lack of soul that troubled me.

Nervously, I enquired: what if the housemate sent to go get the regular groceries wanted something a little different, for herself? Say, kosher pickles? Or, even – sour cream? Well, but that came out of *her* pocket. Such radical foods were *extra*. What counted as a staple was not negotiable; anything "other" was a luxury. In other words, as usual, it cost to be a Jew, colouring outside the culinary lines. Of course, in this group house, it would also have cost to be Italian, Arab, Asian, Black, Latina, Greek, Armenian …

And yet, these very kind and wholesome women were outspoken defenders of diversity, openly lamenting that they couldn't seem to attract more women of colour to their events. We were all reading Audre Lorde's popular memoir *Zami*, in which Lorde wrote nostalgically about gay-girl house parties of the 1950s, noting that the more affluent white women never served enough food, in contrast to the generous spread offered at Black women's homes. As much as I supported collective housing, I just didn't see myself living on a mandated diet of bran, molasses, navy beans, yeast powder, tapioca, tempe, granola, plain yogurt, and carob chips. I would never have fit in. So I went back to renting a one-room studio, where I could chew my way through a robust snack of hummus and Greek olives on an onion bialy, with lumpy kosher chocolate spread. My cupboards overflowed with regional and personal tastes, groceries selected from the Amish market (red velvet whoopee pies, pickled beets), the Vietnamese market (avocado bubble shake, "Aroma" coffee, coconut rice, mangoes), and North African and Central American fare (ful medames, horchata, cinnamon sticks).

Of course, ethnic grandstanding also allows one to claim a high-salt, high-fat cuisine regimen as part of one's identity, as something that should not be taken away. Moderation is key. Laurie Colwin's essay "Friday Night Supper" warns that "The traditional Friday night fare – pot roast and potato pancakes – is not something you would want to make a steady diet of, nor would you be comfortable serving it to your cardiologist." But by the 1980s, ethnic pride and identity politics helped make us aware that in America, women were routinely expected to lose weight (or modify their cholesterol and carbs) by abandoning the in-group soul food of their childhoods for "lite" cling peaches on cottage cheese with iceberg lettuce. I felt that reaching for *non-fat sour cream* in the dairy section was a betrayal of righteous living. Any mainstream diet would rapidly de-Judaicize a person.

At the end of that odd year of hospital tests and food politics and time spent reflecting on feminist appetites, it was Yom Kippur. Now I was fasting; a fasting process of renewal and redemption that had not been on the long-form NIH questionnaire. After a year of writing about food and Jewish women's relationship to food, I stood waiting for sunset and the soft scraping of a purple carrot, the peelings of my old sins down the drain. In my refrigerator, a jar of gefilte fish, and a little tub of whitefish from *So's Your Momeli*, and a bottle of Gold's beet horseradish. These were secret Jewish treats which I saved for after the fast; often I chose to feed my Jewish soul alone. I'd break the fast with couscous, wine, and fishes, mixing Sephardi and Ashkenazi tastes. I'd be entered in the book of life again, as life re-entered me, deliciousness in forkfuls. Tomorrow, I'd lightly brown my blintzes in olive oil from Palestine, consuming my peace politics, the olive branch itself.

This act of keeping faith alive, not by scrupulous observance of kosher laws, but through pleasantly gastronomic Judaism is, of course, the sort of cop-out that drives more Orthodox Jews wild. It's Moses, Pharoah, the Red Sea, and the Torah words at Sinai reduced to an onion bagel. Elizabeth Ehrlich writes in *Miriam's Kitchen*, "With freedom and opportunity came new undreamed-of choices – to believe in your grandparents' religion, or to believe in nothing, or to believe but eschew the trappings, or to embrace the trappings with all your heart, and make a corned beef sandwich on "Jewish" rye the only religion you need." She explores the concept of "kosher-style" as "the taste without the blessing." Yet when my friend Lauren Heller peeled the lid off a tub of whitefish and sighed erotically, "Ah, the taste of Judaism!" – I knew exactly how she felt.

Eating, security, staying alive, observing tribal rituals – they're all interconnected, and I was invested in making a place for talking about all of this in lesbian culture. Though she acknowledges the heaviness of the Shabbat evening meal, Laurie Colwin goes to bat for the home team: "For those who have let it lapse, Friday night supper is a tradition worth reviving. It is a night when the heart of even the most assimilated Jew cries out for something more substantial than one skinless chicken breast." Our ancestors might have come to America to get ahead, to offer their kids better opportunities, even to assimilate willingly in most ways, but there would always be that jar of gefilte fish (or Filipino bagoong sauce, or Mexican dulce de leche, or Lebanese kibbeh) in the fridge. Where we came from was part of our palates, shaping how we chose to live now. The test for the LGBTQ+ community, in all its magnificent intersectionality, would be learning to accept without judgment the intimate hungers and appetites of all our differences; to feed one another's survival in ways no test, so far, had measured.

References

American Psychiatric Association. (1973). *Diagnostic and statistical manual of mental disorders II.*
Beck, E. T. (Ed.). (1982). *Jewish girls: A lesbian anthology.* Persephone Press.
Ehrlich, E. (1997). *Miriam's kitchen.* Penguin.
Lorde, A. (1982). *Zami: A new spelling of my name.* Persephone Press.
Newman, L. (1986). *Good enough to eat.* Firebrand.

16 Breaking Out of the Pack

Roller Derby and the Journey to Self-Discovery

Kaitrin Doll

It's been 14 months, two days, 12 hours, and 13 minutes since the world shut down, and we were all forced to let go of the lives we once knew. Now we all exist in this new reality of isolation, physical distance, and the unknown; for the greater good, we let go of people, plans, dreams, and expectations. Possibly the scariest part of the pandemic for someone like me is the loss of control, not knowing. While many people perfected their sourdough recipes, for those of us who navigate issues with food, body image, and exercise, the pandemic brought on new challenges; being home with food and mirrors, staring at ourselves on zoom, then of course being disconnected from physical support systems and coping mechanisms. My whole life has been a battle with food, exercise, and a general disdain for my body. Even a few stints at treatment weren't enough to "fix" me, and I was resigned that I would move through my life with this shameful secret. It's been 14 months, two days, 12 hours, and 14 minutes since we lost derby. A sport, community, and lifestyle that deeply altered the trajectory of my life. I mourn the loss of roller derby more than you probably should for a recreational sport, but this wacky sport repaired my relationship with food, my body, and my identity in ways that years of mainstream therapy couldn't.

Cereal and Running

Since I was a kid, I've had a complicated relationship with food. I recall never quite feeling full and even after eating three bowls of cereal, always reaching for another. This would have been chalked up to me going through growth spurts but as a chubby awkward child, there was always a feeling that I shouldn't be having more even though I may want it. Despite being active, involved with dance and various sports, I was always aware of my body and how it wasn't quite right. When I was a kid, I couldn't identify that I was pressured by the heteropatriarchal ideals around femininity and what was considered an acceptable assigned female at birth (AFAB) body, but now I recognize that even at age ten these suffocating social and cultural norms infiltrated my psyche, made me feel unworthy and left me with baggage that I still carry to this day. Back to my childhood. I'm not sure why or how, but at age 13 I decided to start running and I ran a couple of times a week. I could still eat three bowls of cereal, but now my body started to feel

DOI: 10.4324/9781003217121-18

different. As soon as I started to take up less physical space in the world, I got positive reinforcement. Patriarchal societal discourses cause AFAB people to hate our bodies so much that the only way we're acceptable is to take up as little space as possible, especially with our bodies; big bodies are offensive and presumptuous while small bodies are desirable, correct, controlled, and reinforced.

Back to the running, positive reinforcement felt good, and like cereal, I always wanted more. So, running a couple of times a week turned into every day and I started to shrink, and the reinforcement got louder, now with an added layer of envy. I was hooked and wanted more; I desperately clung to this attention, the affirmation that I was now finally worthy. One day, just a flicker of a thought barged into my mind and was too persuasive and tempting to ignore; *what if I stopped eating the three bowls of cereal and kept running?* It was like a light switch; it unlocked a powerful force inside me that embedded into my consciousness and is with me even today. Without the cereal (or any food for that matter) and the daily running, I was shrinking at an incredible rate; I had almost totally disappeared, and the positive reinforcement was now concern but it didn't matter anymore. I didn't need the positive reinforcement because I had a new fix, a new voice that drowned out any positive reinforcement or concern. I had a voice inside me fuelled by social and cultural discourses around the acceptable body that kept pushing me forward, *"harder, faster"* and was never satisfied despite how I rose to the challenge. This is how I ended up in an eating disorder treatment programme shortly after my 14th birthday.

Roller Derby: The Awakening

Even after a few stints in treatment, I still carried that voice like a presence inside me. As the years drew on, I coexisted with this unwanted tenant; sometimes they were very loud and kept me up all night, reminding me I didn't measure up, and other times they settled down and I could recognize the absurdity and intrusiveness of their accusations.

In 2007, I moved reluctantly to a new city and province with my partner at the time. I didn't know anyone in the city; I was out of my comfort zone which fuelled old insecurities. Feeling vulnerable and left to my own devices, the inner voice emerged with a vengeance, and although I knew better, it felt comforting to let the voice lead me down the path of restriction, exercise, and hypercontrol. I controlled my body because I felt out of control in my life, hyperfocusing on what I ate and how much I exercised was my harm reduction strategy to cope with my insecurities, which meant walking a fine line between being ok and totally spiralling. What felt like serendipitous timing, one day at work I got a flyer in my mailbox from a colleague for a local derby bout. Like many others, I had seen the movie *Whip It* and not only developed a huge crush on Elliot Page but was also completely fascinated with the sport and culture of derby. I went to the bout and was in awe; I saw strong, aggressive bodies wearing tights and booty shorts, smashing into each other as they skated around an oval track. I had no idea what was going on, but I was hooked immediately; I had found my people and I needed to play derby. After the bout, I went online and found the first learn to skate pro-gramme I could and signed up. I had two weeks before the learn to skate started and I wasn't very comfortable on quad skates, so I would bike around the city and find any parking lot, school playground, or smooth surface I could skate on to practice. As my excitement for roller derby grew something else started to happen, that inner voice was being stifled by my new fixation and instead of spending all my time at the gym or obsessing about food, I was trying to get comfortable on my skates. The goal wasn't to disappear, it was to be seen and I wanted to be spectacular!

Every Body Is a Derby Body

At the first session I did well, my two weeks of practice made me stand out from the other new skaters and I quickly graduated from the learn to skate programme to all-league practices. Going to all-league practices was a totally different scene. At all-league practice, there were skaters from the competitive team who were happy to put you in your place as a new skater. Lots of new skaters were intimidated by this, and of course, so was I but I had years of the inner voice bullying me, so I knew how to handle intimidation. In the same way that I would rise to the occasion with my inner voice, I rose to the occasion with derby, pushing as hard as I could, getting up after every big hit, skating one more lap than what I was asked to do. My goal was to make the travel team in my first season, and I was determined to get there. Derby was the first full-contact sport I ever played, and I learned very quickly that being frail and going into practice having not eaten wasn't going to get me on the travel team and it wasn't safe. The best skaters had strong bodies, and there were all types and sizes of bodies in derby and every body had its strengths. The best hitters had big booties that were celebrated for sending people flying off the track, tiny jammers twisted, juked, and jumped around blockers, and bigger bodies became impenetrable walls. There was also a positive culture around food; I have fond memories of team bonding at the many potlucks and post-game dinners. Derby's culture of all bodies being good bodies and eating food because it tasted good was a shift for me. It wasn't always easy but being part of a culture that actively resisted the stereotypes that dictated how bodies "should" be was incredibly empowering and helped me to question my inner discourses around why I hated my body. I came to recognize that eating food made me stronger. I remember the first time I shoulder-punched a blocker in the chest, sending them flying onto their ass and feeling so powerful that I could do anything! For as long as I can remember exercise was an obligation, a punishment. Derby shifted that as well; I started to focus on what my body could do so I could be better at my sport and not what it looked like. I needed to be able to hold my ground so I could make the travel team so instead of torturing myself on the treadmill for hours, I started to train for the sport. I finally had a positive outlet, one where I was literally smashing the patriarchy by smashing myself into other badass folks on the track. Solidifying my love and obsession with derby, I did make the travel team that first year. More importantly, I entered a new phase of my life where I finally started to love my body for what it could do not for how it met the standards.

Roller Derby Can't Make You Gay But …

Derby didn't just transform my relationship with food and my body, it also helped me actualize my sexuality and gave me space to explore my gender identity. Derby is known for fostering an environment and community where queer athletes are celebrated and affirmed. Many of the sport's top athletes are unapologetically queer and it's common to see roller derby names like: Alien InvadeHer, Vagetarian, or Queerella D'evil. Growing up in a small rural town, there were few positive representations of queer people. I'm sure queer people were around but queerness wasn't celebrated and if people were queer others accepted them despite this and as long as their existence didn't collide or call into question heterosexual norms and discourses.

I found my big gay self in roller derby. At this point, I'd been playing for a few years, immersed in a space with queer folks and part of a larger roller derby community where queerness was celebrated. This gave me the space and freedom to start deconstructing my subconscious obligatory straightness. A turning point was going to watch the roller derby championship playoffs in Portland and being enveloped in a mass of queer bodies. At this event most of the top players were out, proud, and celebrated and the spectators were queers and allies. Standing in the crowd, cheering my face off, I felt euphoria like I'd never experienced; something finally aligned, and I knew I was never going to stifle my queerness again. I wanted to be out and proud like those skaters on the track, and after that tournament I rejected heteronormativity and all its pressures and constraints and finally started to be who I really was. The more I started to reject the suffocating heteropatriarchal social and cultural expectations the less that inner voice nagged at me to disappear; I no longer believed that I had to be feminine or that I had to marry a man and have kids. I started to realize all the ways that the social expectations had fed that inner voice and led me down a path of self-loathing and destruction, blocking me from actualizing my queerness. I decided to stand up for myself, and I had a derby family with open arms ready to support me on my new journey.

Beyond the Binary

In 2016, the Women's Flat Track Derby Association (WFTDA) introduced a new gender policy, effectively removing any requirements for gender-affirming hormones or gender-affirming surgery as a qualification for trans and gender-diverse athletes to participate in the sport. The policy meant that anyone who felt that women's derby was the version and composition of the sport that they most closely identified with could now participate. This policy is one of the more progressive gender policies for a sporting organization, and it means that gender-diverse and trans athletes can continue to participate or can join roller derby without having to conform to strict gender categorization that misaligns with their gender identity. This expansive definition of women's derby has meant that gender-diverse and trans athletes are also affirmed and protected in the sport; it's common practice at all roller derby bouts to have all-gender washrooms and changing rooms and game rosters now include players pronouns. These policies and practices are yet another way that derby is radically redefining sports environments so that all athletes are welcomed and affirmed to participate in sport and where people have the space to be dynamic, fluid, and expansive in their gender presentation and identity.

In the same way that I was also never exposed to sexual diversity, gender diversity was not really on my radar until my immersion in roller derby. Particularly after the WFTDA gender policy, it seemed like more people felt comfortable coming out and in my most recent league, there were many trans and gender-diverse players, refs, and volunteers. Anytime our league had a new or visiting skater everyone formed a circle and names and pronouns were shared. Having the privilege of being in this space, I got those same feelings of freedom and solidarity I felt giving space to my queerness. With the support of my league mates, a self-proclaimed group of queerdos, I started using different pronouns and finally feel like I have the space to breathe and be on my own gender journey. I don't really know what that means for me other than my gender identity is broader, bolder, more fluid and complex than can be captured by a binary category. Being surrounded by a community of people that reject social norms and happily exist outside of hetero/cisgender societal pressures has helped me to see another way that I can live my life. By recognizing and unpacking these influences I feel empowered to push back and resist toxic discourses that contributed to my contemptuous relationship with my body. The more I deconstruct and problematize gender categorization I have come to realize that femininity never felt completely genuine for me; I felt pressured to perform femininity, this felt non-consensual, and I was consistently shoved into a box that didn't quite fit.

I'm not a derby girl; I'm an athlete and as I expand my understanding of my own gender identity the more that inner voice becomes muffled and often, I don't hear it at all. Derby made me realize that I don't need to subscribe to strict social and cultural rules around the body, gender, and sexuality; this radical resistance has shaped my journey of actualizing my identity, healing my relationship with food and my body, and empowering me to live my life authentically.

Waiting for the Return

As we enter the third wave of COVID-19, with new lockdown restrictions, I sit here with a freshly broken ankle that happened while park skating (something I took up in the pandemic to keep skating and feel connected to derby and my teammates). I can't use movement to cope and distract me from my feelings. I now must sit uncomfortably with the immense grief and loss for the sport that's helped me to redefine my identity in a way that aligns with my authentic self and helped me repair a lifelong relationship with food and my body. I grieve for myself, as I feel that inner critic starting to voice its opinion again, I grieve for my roller derby community, who need the sport as much as I do, I also grieve for all those people who haven't discovered roller derby yet and may not have the chance to be part of a community and culture that would support them on their own queer journeys. I hope that roller derby can survive the pandemic because so many of us need this sport, community, and culture to have a space where we can truly discover our authentic selves.

17 Social Failure and Personal Best

An Autoethnography of Food and Gender in the Life of a Queer Youth Who Cooks with Vermouth

Edward Chamberlain

Culinary Beginnings: From Cooking in Popular Culture to the Cult of Popularity

On the popular television programme, *The French Chef*, the American culinary icon Julia Child once explained that numerous Americans have a fear of failing in the kitchen (Child et al., 1970). In an effort to teach viewers how to cook, Child draws upon her personal experience and reflects on the process of learning. Instead of saying that cooking comes naturally from within, Child highlights how the art of cooking commonly involves the process of trial and error. In an earlier episode, Child allows herself to be filmed as *failing* to achieve the desired result – the perfect flip of a pancake – and in the process, she endears herself to viewers by showing herself to be a chef who is imperfect (Child et al., 1963). Despite the television industry's aim of showcasing a professional demonstration, Child reveals a process that looks *less than perfect* at times. Her embrace of this error – or what would commonly be viewed as *failure* – exhibits some parallels with viewpoints in the academic field of Queer Studies, where the scholars Jack Halberstam and Alpesh Kantilal Patel illuminate the generative powers of *failing* in several contexts. Halberstam and Patel offer an alternative set of viewpoints that lead readers to rethink the public discourse associated with failure, including the pejorative label of ineptitude and the shaming that often is placed upon people who fail.

As these thinkers show us, the experience of failure can function as a means to social and intellectual development. In many cases, failing can foster positive forms of "transformation" including adaptation and learning new ideas (Halberstam, 2011; Patel, 2017). Taking a cue from these perspectives, this chapter uses the critical and reflective tools of autoethnography, such as introspection, for the sake of explaining how a queer youth took to the culinary arts as he navigated moments of social failure shaped by societal structures of normativity including the cultural ideals of the 1980s and 1990s. Historically, much of the normative thought about the culinary arts has been predicated upon patriarchal ideologies and capitalistic visions of family, in which a father is perceived as the breadwinner who works in the public sphere, while a mother is the domestic sphere's cook. Amid these roles,

DOI: 10.4324/9781003217121-19

the figure of the *queer child who cooks* was never a variable in the equation of US familial life. Histories of young queer cooks in America remain largely silenced and untold. To break the silence, I study personal experiences as evidence and cast a critical eye upon them, using the intellectual lenses of scholars in the fields of Cultural Studies and Food Studies. This approach allows me to analyze how my culinary experiences happened in tandem with moments of failure and feelings of powerlessness in my youth. Early in elementary school, I experienced distressing feelings of failure in my maths class, sports, and related social contexts – the sites where boys are expected to succeed and gain the respect of peers. In examining these moments, I evaluate how my life as a young queer cook in a largely white suburb is legible as a challenge to dominant expectations, which define boyhood in terms of certain knowledges, popularity, and sport. Far from being successful in those areas, I found a meaningful sense of solidarity among community members, teachers, and relatives who similarly possessed a passion for discussing and sharing knowledge about the culinary arts.

The Cultivation of a Queer Sense of Self and Intimacy through Culinary Arts

Looking back to my time in fifth grade, I recall pursuing a modicum of talents, which included one of my personal best: the preparation of more elaborate dinners. Reflecting on this time, I see the queerness of being an artsy boy who talked recipes with teachers outside of class. As I talked with my English teacher about cooking, I felt a connection – as though I had gained entrance to a secret adult league of chefs. My teacher gave me a recipe for Chicken Vermouth, and though I was too young to purchase the vermouth myself, my parents supported my culinary endeavours, enabling me to embrace my precocious talents. In time, I came to accept my more feminine form of "gender performance" as well as my own budding queerness (Butler, 1990). These personal characteristics are likely what caused my classmates to label me – *Martha Stewart* – another popular version of the "good woman" that the scholar Katie Hogan theorizes about in her study of American women caretakers and mothers (Hogan, 2001). Being labelled in this way made me feel *different* and contributed to an emerging set of anxieties that I came to understand later in life. Some of these same phenomena are explained by the researchers Stephen T. Russell and Jessica N. Fish, who have stated, "sexual minorities experience distinct, chronic stressors related to their stigmatized identities, including victimization, prejudice, and discrimination. These distinct experiences, in addition to everyday or universal stressors, disproportionately compromise the mental health and well-being of LGBT people" (Russell & Fish, 2016). Like many young LGBTQ+ people, at first, I denied my sexual identity, and as a result, I dealt with several kinds of troubling states: a sense of self-loathing, social anxiety, and bouts of depression. To counter these experiences and the stressors of *difference*, I explored the culinary arts, which allowed me to find an alternative pathway through negativities I encountered, thus leading me to align myself with creative thinkers. I connected with TV personalities like the Chinese American chef Martin Yan and the white New Yorker Dom Deluise, who evinced a great love of food and sometimes departed from strict gender norms of the time. As a result, I felt a little comfort in knowing that there were some artistic, sensitive, and tender-hearted men existing in the world.

In recent decades, the study of personal narratives has evolved considerably, and writers such as Stacy Holman Jones and Anne Harris have developed a *queer approach* to such self-study. They evince a common cause with early researchers such as Carolyn Ellis and Tony E. Adams. They speak to the belief that studying one's personal experiences can enable a writer and their readers to understand our process of self-development and relationality. In a collaborative essay, they explain, "autoethnography is a method that allows us to reconsider how we think, how we do research and maintain relationships, and how we live" (Adams et al., 2015). To enact this method, I began by reflecting on my relationships in school and at home. From a young age, I learnt about culinary diversity through the various foods enjoyed at my family's table. Although my father's family has lived in the United States for generations, he is descended from German and English immigrants. Similarly, my mother immigrated to the US from Australia, having ancestral origins among Welsh people. As a youth, my mother's immigration to the US granted me a rather unique way of viewing the world and its food. She introduced our family to foods from *down under* such as queen pudding, which is a creamy custard topped with a sweet fluffy meringue. This recipe and several more favourites were printed in my mother's trusty *Commonsense Cookery Book* (1970), a key text that guided my early cooking and played a role in my sense of self (and my difference). While our food created a *different* sense of home, I appreciated these differences too. This difference became visible as I noted my school's homogenous population, which primarily consisted of middle- and working-class white students for whom activities like sports were major guideposts.

My small town's shared interest in sports was a site of social bonding and personal development for classmates who conformed to social standards of gender. Thankfully, my schools kept *alive* a lifeline for unconventional youths like myself. Our school's extracurricular activities – the yearbook group and the music programme – granted me creative opportunities. In the chorus, the more artsy and unconventional youths could find a place to express their non-athletic talents. I pursued these because I found little success on the playing field. During one autumn, I had tried to play football with the boys during the lunch hour when I was 11 years old. On that day, amazingly I caught the ball, but I failed to make the play properly, which caused some boys to laugh at me. In particular, I remember having a crush on one of the boys who laughed, and his laughter caused me pain that led me to avoid football games thereafter. At that time, I was fearful of failing and lacked the resilience to counter it. Consequently, I decided to avoid sports that usually happened during the lunch hour and rode my bike home to make my own lunch. While I wanted to connect with classmates, I also wanted to live as my non-conforming self – beyond the norms we see in football and lunchrooms, where athletic skill and popularity give one power.

As some boys were learning about professional athletes, I connected more with people – both real and imagined – who showed an interest in new and diverse forms of eating. For instance, I was intrigued by the literary character of Sam Gribley in Jean Craighead George's youth novel *My Side of The Mountain* (George, 1959). Sam was a young outsider who made food for himself on the wild terrain of his grandfather's homestead in the Catskill mountains of New York. Living a life of self-exile, Sam's consumption of acorn flour, wild bulbs, and cattail tubers resonated with my younger self, who was intrigued by adventurous eating. Although I never followed Sam's move to the mountains, I enjoyed experimenting with food at home, where my family had managed to assemble a respectably diverse pantry of foods. During this time, a classmate and I decided to mix an odd selection of ingredients in a blender – elements infrequently used together. Mixing milk with more savoury ingredients created a peculiar milkshake, yet it also made me wonder about *what else could be created* when we step outside the sanctioned activities and social boundaries. These culinary experiences allowed me to think in new ways and see myself as an inventor instead of simply a failure and outsider. In reflecting, I had experienced a sense of anguish as well as shame for not succeeding in traditional male arenas, yet intellectuals such as Carolyn Ellis have shed light on what these moments of struggle can mean. Ellis envisions such reflection as not simply one's own "victim tale" but rather autoethnographies like this one actually can be "survivor tales for the writer and for those who read them" (Ellis, 2009).

In taking this introspective approach, I have realized I was trying to find my place in the world, searching for a place to belong. For young people in the United States, developing a sense of belonging is a part of one's social development, yet for many queer youths, unfortunately there are many roadblocks obstructing the common pathways *through culture*. As the writers Stacy Holman Jones and Anne M. Harris explain, the act of writing autoethnography can be a means to "write-the-self-in-culture" and thus (re)situate ourselves in existing heteronormative narratives (Holman Jones & Harris, 2019). In writing this autoethnography, I re-situated my sense of failure in several contexts, observing I had found success at times. Through doing so, I observed a community that enabled my younger queer self to find an *alternative* social membership in cooking, thereby empowering me to survive the daily challenges and social exclusions that often prevented me from connecting with young people. Despite the successes of feminists and the sexual revolution in the 1960s and 1970s, there have remained many young people who were subject to a set of cultural ideals that delineated a reductive notion of social propriety as well as paradigms like *the normal citizen*. Through my recollecting, I see how *the political* intersected with *the personal* to create a certain ideal of boyhood, which was a normative performance of gender that was held in place by a slew of social phenomena, including acts of silencing and traumas caused by instances of bullying, harassment, intersectional bias, abusive relationships, and similar violence. This qualitative research illuminates the benefits of questioning how a developed society seldom creates a place for LGBTQ+ youths beyond that of marginality.

Concluding and Moving Forward: Young Queer Homebodies and Their Sustenance

In connecting my reflections, it dawned on me that my youthful acts of culinary creativity are more than simple expressiveness. Cooking opened doorways that I have come to see as being a means of creating connectivity, exploration, and sustaining oneself. These reflections yield a critical remembrance constituted in justice, in which achieving a sense of fairness remains a significant goal. Relatedly, later in life I would read the writing of the Black poet Audre Lorde, who offers a telling perspective, in which she makes a comment on the way that conventional learning often leaves many youths yearning for something more. *In Zami: A New Spelling of My Name*, Lorde writes, "How meager the sustenance was I gained from the four years I spent in high school; yet how important that sustenance was to my survival" (Lorde, 1982). Lorde's words inspired me to reflect on the fact that my early cooking experiences indeed were a productive form of education and daily living. Even though I failed to master the lessons in maths class, the culinary arts created a key space for survival. Such experiences point to the fact that a pluralistic set of learning options can be beneficial to youth who find themselves feeling like a failure in pre-established modes of learning. In this way, *rethinking the systems* in which we live – and not the youth's identity – exhibits a notable potential for ensuring a higher quality of life.

Reflecting on these moments has led me to see how it wasn't *my own* failure but actually the failure of existing systems that glorify success and define certain gender roles. Although I can see how the idea of a young person cooking with vermouth may bring to mind oddity or risk, we benefit by recontextualizing such notions. Instead of a simple oddity, I observe how our prevailing systems of gender and sexuality have involved a dynamic where our patriarchal cultures have required boys to attain a gendered ideal, which is like that of adult males, who frequently reap the benefits of making *Others* cook for them. In contrast, learning the culinary arts can enable young LGBTQ+ people to build allyship amid the web of normativity perpetuated by powerful figures like teachers, school systems, and the state. Of course, the culinary arts are by no means free of inequity and struggle. Indeed, as activists such as Ron Finley have shown, eating and growing food are interwoven with bias and privilege (Finley, 2013). Nonetheless, in a time where many LGBTQ+ people commonly express feeling unsatisfied in several contexts – the family sphere, school, work, politics, and community – there remains the social realm of the culinary arts, which offers some opportunities for satisfaction – even if it is only a fleeting moment in one's daily life. Such moments – like exchanging a memorable recipe – can make a positive difference in a queer youth's early development, inspiring greater perseverance.

References

Adams, T., Jones, S. H., & Ellis, C. (2015). *Autoethnography: Understanding qualitative research.* Oxford University Press.

Butler, J. (1990). *Gender trouble: Feminism and the subversion of identity.* Routledge.

Child, J. (writer) & Atwood, D. (Director), "Gâteau in a Cage". (1970). *The French Chef.* Season 7, Episode 9. WGBH-TV, December 23. https://vimeo.com/6202899.

Child, J. (writer) & Morash, R. (Director), "The Potato Show". (1963). *The French Chef,* Season 1, Episode 22. WGBH-TV, June 29. https://www.dailymotion.com/video/x2gtq66.

Craighead George, J. (1959). *My side of the mountain.* Dutton Books.

Ellis, C. (2009). *Revision: Autoethnographic reflections on life and work.* Left Coast Press.

Finley, R. (2013). A Guerrilla gardener in LA. TEDTalk. Youtube. https://www.ted.com/talks/ron_finley_a_guerrilla_gardener_in_south_central_la

Halberstam, J. (2011). *The queer art of failure.* Duke University Press.

Hogan, K. (2001). *Women who care: Gender, race, and the culture of AIDS.* Cornel University Press.

Holman Jones, S., & Harris, A. (2019). *Queering autoethnography.* Routledge Press.

Lorde, A. (1982). *Zami: A new spelling of my name.* Crossing Press.

NSW Cookery Teachers Association. (1970). *Queen pudding: The commonsense cookery book.* HarperCollins.

Patel, A. (2017). *Productive failure: Writing queer transnational South Asian art histories.* Manchester Press.

Russell, S., & Fish, J. (2016). Mental health in lesbian, gay, bisexual, and transgender (LGBT) youth. *Annual Review of Clinical Psychology, 12*(1), 465–487.

18 Recipe for a Queer Cookbook

Alex Ketchum

Recipe for a Queer Cookbook

So you want to cook up a queer cookbook? Here's a recipe that you can customize to your tastes. Begin by assembling your ingredients.

Required ingredients:

(1) An author or authors who self-identify as LGBTQ+, ideally in the cookbook itself.
(2) A discussion of LGBTQ+ community, culture, or issues in the front matter, introduction, surrounding recipes, and/or in section headers.
(3) Instructions for preparing food or drink (it is possible to have metaphorical recipes, yet most of the cookbook should centre on creating food or drink).

Additional ingredients that you can mix and match. Choose your *toppings* based on your aesthetics:

(1) **Photographs of the dishes, authors, or other content related to the cookbook.**
     You might want to go high gloss like *Drag Queen Brunch* (2020), *Antoni in the Kitchen* (2019), *Big Gay Ice Cream* (2015), Lagusta Yearwood's *Sweet and Salty* (2020), and *Tasty Pride: 75 Recipes and Stories from the Queer Food Community* (2020). You can keep production costs down by printing the photographs on uncoated book paper stock such as *Cookin' with Honey: What Literary Lesbians Eat* (1996) and Jenice R. Armstead's *Lesbians Have to Eat, Too!* (2011). You can combine both techniques and print only some of your photos on glossy paper such as the Bloodroot Collective's *The Perennial Political Palate* (1993).
(2) **Illustrations to accompany the dishes – expressive and campy cartoons are highly encouraged!**
     Whimsical illustrations such as the joyful fairies in *The Gay of Cooking* (1982), the "campy cartoon" line drawings of Lou Rand Hogan's chef swimming in fruit salad by David Costain (1965, p. 30), David Shenton's stylized cartoons of people cooking in *The Queer Cookbook* (1997), and the loose-lined

DOI: 10.4324/9781003217121-20

portraits in *The Art of Gay Cooking: A Culinary Memoir* (2019) adorn many of the cookbooks.

(3) **Erotic content and/or nudity.**

The Lesbian Erotic Cookbook by Ffiona Morgan Genre (1998) has erotic and nude photographs, but many queer cookbooks that do not have naked photos still utilize sexual innuendo and word play.

(4) **Purple ink.**

The use of purple ink and a purple colour scheme is common in many queer cookbooks such as *Cooking with Pride* (1989), the Kitchen Fairy's *The Gay of Cooking* (1982), and *The Lesbian Erotic Cookbook* (1998).

There are vegetarian, vegan, and meat versions of this recipe. Cookbooks written by and for lesbian and queer women are more likely to be vegan or vegetarian. There are queer cookbooks that address a wide variety of dietary needs, including gluten free, kosher, and more! There are cookbooks, such as *Out of Our Kitchen Closets: San Francisco Gay Jewish Cooking* (1987) that address religious dietary needs. You can customize your cookbook to meet these requirements.

Instructions:

(1) **Place the recipe in a story** like the authors of *Cookin' with Honey: What Literary Lesbians Eat* (1996) and *Lesbians Have to Eat, Too!* (2011). Or better yet – **write the whole recipe in a memoir format** like *The Alice B. Toklas Cookbook* (1954) and *The Art of Gay Cooking: A Culinary Memoir* (2019).

(2) **Reference other queer cookbooks within your own.** Make clear that you see your cookbook in relation with other queer cookbooks. In *The Butch Cook Book* (2008), the authors Lee Lynch, Nel Ward, and Sue Hardesty write explicitly about how they see their cookbook as a part of the butch lesbian community and part of a longer lineage. Isengardt models *The Art of Gay Cooking* (2019) on Toklas's cookbook. Skyler Blue's *The Gay Man's Cookbook* (2011) references Lou Rand Hogan's *The Gay Cookbook* (1965).

(3) **Salt with camp and humour to taste.** Consider puns and sexual innuendos in recipe titles. The titles can be explicit such as the ones in *The Gay Man's Cookbook* (2011) or playful puns. In the Kitchen Fairy's *The Gay of Cooking* (1982), the word play begins in the table of contents. Each section has a whimsical title, and a translation "straight talk" is below it. For example, "A little starch will keep it stiff" is for "Pasta, Rice, and Potatoes." Titles should reflect your personal preferences. There are so many ways to be LGBTQIA+ and your cookbook should reflect your or your community's wide variety of experiences.

(4) **Optional Step: make your cookbook a fundraiser for a LGBTQ+ organization or cause.**

For example, *Cooking with Pride* (1989) is a queer community cookbook that fundraised for Pride and PFLAG committees.

Want to add the special sauce? Add more recipes from friends (Figure 18.1).

Figure 18.1 A digital collage of queer cookbooks stacked on top of each other. The titles and illustrations on the cookbook covers glow and the image is saturated in purple. Alex Ketchum.

What is a queer cookbook? Is there a set recipe for what makes a cookbook queer? Is it that the author is queer? Or is there something inherently queer about the cookbook itself? What do Lou Rand Hogan's *The Gay Cookbook* of 1965, the Bloodroot Collective's *Political Palate* of 1980, the Cincinnati Lesbian Activist Bureau's 1983 cookbook *Whoever Said Dykes Can't Cook? The Lesbian Erotic Cookbook* by Ffiona Morgan Genre (1998), and *Lesbians Have to Eat, Too!* by Jenice R. Armstead (2011) have in common? Does a cookbook published by a global media company and marketed as "queer," such as Buzzfeed's *Tasty Pride: 75 Recipes and Stories from the Queer Food Community* (2020) count as a queer cookbook? In the summer of 2021, I curated an exhibit on American and Canadian queer cookbooks and zines which sought to answer these questions. The physical exhibit was at McGill University from August 18 until December 20 and showcased 17 queer cookbooks from my personal collection, three publications on loan from Les Archives Gaies du Québec, and three zines from Les Archives

Lesbiennes du Québec. The digital exhibit lives on The Historical Cooking Project website and includes more cookbooks. I drew on the scholarship of Stephen Vider "'Oh Hell, May, Why Don't You People Have a Cookbook?': Camp Humor and Gay Domesticity" (2013), sociologist Stacey Williams's "A Feminist Guide to Cooking" (2014), historian Katharina Vester's *Taste of Power: Food and American Identities* (2015), and social anthropologist Rachael Scicluna's *Home and Sexuality: The "Other" Side of the Kitchen* (2017) who explore lesbian and gay cookbooks.

This chapter includes a literal recipe for creating a queer cookbook based on the commonalities of 42 Canadian and American LGBTQ+ cookbooks published between 1954 and 2021. As the recipe demonstrates, there are some key features of queer cookbooks. Authorship, connection to the queer community, and the use of aesthetic choices to emphasize the cookbook's relationship to queer cultures are necessary. The use of humour, puns, sexual innuendo, erotic content is prevalent, but not required. Recipes from friends or other community members appear in community cookbooks and single-authored texts.

The Alice B. Toklas Cookbook (1954) and *The Gay Cookbook* by Chef Lou Rand Hogan (1966) set important precedents for what makes a cookbook "queer." Toklas's genre blending of memoir and recipe work has inspired numerous queer cookbook authors. Hogan's use of illustrations and playful tone (including numerous innuendos and puns) is echoed in later cookbooks. In these two cookbooks, we already see that the author's identity, the formatting of the cookbook, the relationship to community, the use of images, and the recipes are all part of what makes a cookbook queer. The later-published queer cookbooks build on this legacy and continuously reference the queer cookbooks that came before.

Queer cookbooks have changed in some significant ways since the mid-20th century. The production value has generally increased. There tend to be more glossy images. Recipes tend to be written by authors under their actual names as more LGBTQIA+ people are out. This shift is noteworthy because Hogan was a pen name for Louis Randall, and in *Cooking with Pride*, Leatherella O. Parsons writes in the introduction that

> we are gaining ground daily, but the number of recipes which came unsigned or signed with an obvious alias, let us know how many, for one reason or another, are still in the closet. Let's hope this book gives us all a bit of courage
> (Parsons, 1989, p. 1).

However, the legacies of humour, community sourced recipes, and queer authors endure.

While the cookbooks may include metaphorical recipes, to be a queer cookbook the book must include actual recipes for food and drink. The formatting can vary, and recipes range from opening a pack of kraft dinner mac and cheese, as joked about by the authors of *The Butch Cook Book* (2008), to multi-course meals. There can be drink-centred cookbooks such as *Queer Cocktails: 50 Cocktail Recipes Celebrating Gay Icons and Queer Culture* (2021) and tips for party planning in *The Queer*

Cookbook: A Fully Guided Tour to the Secrets of Success in the Homosexual Kitchen! (1997). However, all these books are part of the cookbook genre.

A cookbook's author or authors must also self-identify as LGBTQIA+ for the cookbook to be queer. In *Cookin' with Honey: What Literary Lesbians Eat* (1996) and *Lesbians Have to Eat, Too!* (2011), the recipes' authors make clear that they identify as lesbians. While quoting his husband Filip Noterdaeme, Daniel Isengart reflected his cookbook *The Art of Gay Cooking: A Culinary Memoir* (2019), "You are gay, your approach to cooking is gay, why bother trying to write a conventional cookbook?" (p. ii). For a cookbook to be queer, the authors must utilize their experiences as LGBTQ+ individuals to shape the cookbook that they create. However, if a cookbook's authors are queer, is their cookbook necessarily queer?

A recurring article is the yearly LGBTQ+ cookbook list of the year. Examples include Buzzfeed's *16 LGBTQ-Authored Cookbooks To Feast From During Pride Month* (Szewczyk, 2018), Tasty's: *18 LGBTQ-Penned Cookbooks To Cook From During Pride Month* (Szewczyk, 2019), Chowhound's *14 Must-Have Cookbooks by LGBTQ+ Cooks* (Paget, 2020), Food and Wine's *13 Cookbooks by LGBTQ+ Authors of Color to Buy Right Now* (Chapple, 2020), and Autostraddle's *7 Super Queer Cookbooks For Your Super Queer Kitchen!* (Charles, 2018). These lists share cookbooks by LGBTQ+ authors, yet the cookbooks are not always explicitly queer in their content; they do not make connections to other queer cookbooks; and the authors do not always connect their recipes or content with the LGBTQ+ community. Therefore, while representation and authorship are important components for making a cookbook queer, they are not the only factor.

The third necessary requirement for being a queer cookbook is that the cookbook makes connections to LGBTQ+ community. Authors can make these connections by utilizing memoir and story to link their recipes to their experiences as LGBTQ+ individuals. Photographs, illustrations, and graphic design can emphasize the authors' queer aesthetics. Some authors discuss their cookbook's connection to LGBTQ+ organizations and may donate a percentage of the profits to queer causes. Other authors include recipes from the larger LGBTQIA+ community/communities. While that inclusion is beneficial in representing more queer perspectives in a single cookbook, this is not the same as a queer community cookbook.

As cookbook historian and antiquarian bookseller Don Lindgren writes in *UNXLD: American Cookbooks of Community and Place* (2018), community cookbooks tell stories of community and place. The recipes that they contain are "mementos of shared experience, of friendship" and they are "preserved records of collective effort in service to a cause" (2018, p. 5). While Lindgren primarily collects women's community cookbooks, queer community cookbooks share the similar features of publication on a shoestring budget, recipes coming from local sources, created to generate revenue for a charitable cause, often spiral-bound (2018, p. 7). While the cookbooks by Toklas (1954), Scholder (1996), Isengart (2019), and Armstead (2011) bring recipes from friends, lovers, and community members, queer community cookbooks, such as *Cooking with Pride* (1989), compiled by Leatherella O. Parsons, show these roots more explicitly.

Cooking with Pride (1989) is a queer community cookbook that fundraised for the International Association of Lesbian and Gay Pride Coordinators (IAL/GPC), as well as the various Pride Committees and PFLAGs (founded in 197, the first and largest organization in the United States uniting parents, families, and allies with people who are lesbian, gay, bisexual, transgender, and queer) who submitted recipes. The cookbook is a compilation of nearly 300 recipes representing entries from 30 cities in 20 states or provinces, in three countries on two continents. It is spiral-bound and printed in black, white, and purple. The formatting of the cookbook emphasizes the importance of every member of the community by reminding readers about shared pride conference experiences. The appetizer section includes a story about the first Pride Coordinators Conference in Boston in 1982. The beverage section begins with a story about the pride conference in St Louis. As a community cookbook, *Cooking with Pride* declares that this cookbook exists to build and serve the queer community.

The three features of queer cookbooks: authorship, connection to the queer community, and being an actual cookbook with recipes, are required. Within these parameters, the cookbooks range widely in production value, costs, aesthetics, and publishing. As LGBTQ+ people have gained more acceptance; larger publishers and digital media companies such as Clarkson Potter of Penguin Random House and Tasty of Buzzfeed have partnered to publish cookbooks targeted towards queer audiences. The publication of *Tasty Pride* (2020) raises questions for the future of queer cookbooks.

Does *Tasty Pride* still count as a queer cookbook? The editor Jesse Szewczyk identifies as queer. The collectively sourced recipes come from 75 queer cooks and celebrities. A story accompanies each recipe and authors make the connections between their identities and the dish they have prepared. The introduction explains that the publisher donated US$50,000 to GLAAD, an organization that works towards LGBTQ+ acceptance. Does Buzzfeed's involvement in the cookbook's publication undermine the community aspect of the cookbook? Did Buzzfeed work to publish the cookbook because the company actually cares about queer representation? Was the decision to publish this text just to capitalize on the LGBTQIA+ market? Or does a major media company wanting to publish a pride cookbook indicate mainstream acceptance and evolving cultural views of the LGBTQ+ community?

Queer cookbooks continue to have value. Inside the cover of *Tasty Pride*, large font declares:

> To all the queer cooks who have longed to see themselves represented in mainstream food media. We are in every restaurant, test kitchen, hotel, catering company, studio, and publication. This book and the stories within it prove that there is a seat at the table for all of us.
>
> (*Tasty Pride*)

Later in the introduction, Szewczyk discusses wishing that he had seen himself represented in kitchens and cookbooks. He writes that the impetus of editing this cookbook was "to pass on the gift of finding joy in each other's successes" (2020, p. 12). Queer cookbooks offer more than representation. They serve to preserve and share LGBTQ+ cultures and socializing. That sounds like a recipe for success!

References

Armstead, J. (2011a). *Lesbians have to eat, too!* Self-Published, CreateSpace.

Armstead, J. (2011b). *Lesbians have to eat, 2!: More stories, memories & thoughts in food.* Self-Published, CreateSpace.

The Bloodroot Collective. (1980). *The political palate.* Sanguinaria Publishing.

The Bloodroot Collective. (1984). *The second seasonal political palate.* Sanguinaria Publishing.

The Bloodroot Collective. (1993). *The perennial political palate: The third feminist vegetarian cookbook.* Sanguinaria Publishing.

Blue, S. (2011). *The gay man's cookbook: It's a way of life!!!* Self-Published, CreateSpace.

Brown, S. E. (2013). *The queer vegan cookbook.* Self-Published.

Chapple, J. (2020). *13 cookbooks by LGBTQ+ authors of color to buy right now.* Food & Wine. https://www.foodandwine.com/lifestyle/books/13-cookbooks-by-lgbtq-people-of-color

Charles, R. (2018). *7 super queer cookbooks for your super queer kitchen.* Autostraddle. https://www.autostraddle.com/7-super-queer-cookbooks-for-your-super-queer-kitchen-419408/

Clark, D., & Shenton, D. (1997). *The queer cookbook.* Bloomsbury Publishing.

Cooking with trans people of colour. (2021). Self-Published. https://www.the519.org/programs/tpoc

Doroshow, C. (2012). *Cooking in heels: A memoir cookbook.* Self-Published, Red Umbrella Project.

The Gay Gardeners Garden Club. (1962). *Bouquet of recipes.* Self-Published.

Hardesty, S., Ward, N., & Lynch, L. (2008). *The butch cook book.* TRP Cookbooks.

Hogan, L. R. (1965). *The gay cookbook.* Shelburne Press.

Isengart, D. (2018). *The art of gay cooking: A culinary memoir.* Outpost19.

The Kitchen Fairy. (1982). *Be gay! Eat gay!: The gay of cooking.* Fairy Publications.

Laney, L. (Ed.). (2021). *Queer cocktails: 50 cocktail recipes celebrating gay icons and queer culture.* Ryland Peters & Small.

Lindgren, D. (2018). *UNXLD: American cookbooks of community and place.* Rabelais Books.

Merrin, A., & Alvarez, R. (2019). *Husbands that cook.* St. Martin's Press.

Moskowitz, R. (1987). *Out of our kitchen closets: San Francisco gay jewish cooking.* Self-Published.

Miriam, S., & Furie, N. (2007). *The best of bloodroot, volume one: Vegetarian recipes.* Anomaly Press.

Miriam, S., & Furie, N. (2008). *The best of bloodroot volume two: Vegan recipes.* Anomaly Press.

Miriam, S., & Furie, N. (2018). *The bloodroot calendar cookbook.* Anomaly Press.

Morgan, F. (1998). *The lesbian erotic cookbook.* Daughters of the Moon Publishing.

Mueller, C. (1983). *Le gay gourmet.* Data-Boy Instant Press.

North, C. (1993). *But can she cook?* Bittersweet Press.

Paget, S. (June 1, 2020). 14 Must-Have Cookbooks. LGBTQ+ Cooks. URL: http://www.chowhound.com/food-news/230270/best-lgbtq-chef-cookbooks/ (from the wayback machine: https://web.archive.org/web/20200620051220/http://www.chowhound.com/food-news/230270/best-lgbtq-chef-cookbooks/)

Parsons, L. O. (1989). *Cooking with pride.* Act One.

Petroff, B., & Quint, D. (2015). *Big gay ice cream: Saucy stories & frozen treats: Going all the way with ice cream*. Clarkson Potter.

Porowski, A. (2019). *Antoni in the kitchen*. Houghton Mifflin Harcourt.

Ramstetter, V., & Contenta, M. (1983). *Whoever said dykes can't cook?* Dinah.

Scicluna, M. R. (2017). *Home and sexuality: The 'other' side of the kitchen*. Palgrave Macmillan.

Scholder, A. (1996). *Cookin' with honey, what literary lesbians eat*. Firebrand Books.

Sindaco, A. (2014). *Cooking with the bears*. Drago International Publishing House.

Szewczyk, J. (2018). 16 LGBTQ-authored cookbooks to feast from during pride month. *BuzzFeed*. https://www.buzzfeed.com/jesseszewczyk/lgbtq-cookbooks

Szewczyk, J. (2019). 18 LGBTQ-penned cookbooks to cook from during pride month. *Tasty*. https://tasty.co/article/jesseszewczyk/queer-authored-cookbook-roundup

Szewczyk, J. (2020). *Tasty pride: 75 recipes and stories from the queer food community*. Clarkson Potter.

Toklas, A. B. (1954). *The Alice B. Toklas cook book*. Harper & Brothers.

Tooker, P. (2019). *Drag queen brunch*. Pelican Publishing Company.

Williams, J. S. (2014). A feminist guide to cooking. *Sage Journals*, *13*(3), 59–61.

Vider, S. (2013). "Oh hell, may, why don't you people have a cookbook?": Camp humor and gay domesticity. *American Quarterly*, *65*(4), 877–904.

Vester, K. (2015). *A taste of power: Food and American identities*. University of California Press.

19 Girlfriends

A Culinary (Re)collection

Gunita Gupta

I don't always recall the specifics. Names elude me, lost almost
as soon as they are uttered.
Time passes people pass through my focal point,
into the periphery and beyond.
But the food – the flavours, sensations, smells, textures – all we shared is
always there, it seems, just on the tip of my tongue.
I suppose one can't constrain (re)collection –
this is what I remember.

Clementine

Best friends hidden by spindly fir trees and our own invisibility, dripping with sap, a carpet of brown needles below us releases the fragrance of indifference. What do you think it means to neck? She asks and I pause a segment halfway to my mouth – chance a glance at her tanned skin and wonder what it might be like to lick it. The thick heat of boredom and late summer encourage this conspiracy my eyes say silently, *"Could it be this?"* I lean over and place my sticky lips below her ear, sucking slightly. Explosions on my tongue – acid, salt, sunshine, sweat. Sweet juices dribble down my chin. We sat on the low retaining wall and kissed and ate and laughed. Suddenly September and summer's fleshy fruits quietly grew dry and bland.

Teen Burger

At the mall after school, a riot of shiny surfaces and the ubiquitous smell of adolescence. We made our way to the food court and ordered. We both knew it was a ruse, like the way I doubled her home on her bike, heedless of stop signs, her hands at my hips. Tempting fate. At the tables with the chairs attached I strain against the urge to get closer, content to brush hands as we share fries and onion rings. Stare as her delicate fingers deftly remove the pickles. Every time. I never think about why she won't just ask for exactly what she wants. I never think about why I don't. On the bus ride home, we held hands hidden under her jean jacket. The smell of vinegar lingered long after we parted.

DOI: 10.4324/9781003217121-21

Vegan Pizza

The end of that summer snuck up on me and she crossed my path like a mirage. Wonder and magic, wavy lines in the distance, the hot sun beating down on our backs and heads. Dykes on Bikes. PFLAG. The roar in my ears resolved to find out if her skin was as soft as I remembered. As we slow-danced in the basement bar and finally kissed after all those days holding hands in junior high, I thought, with a sigh. Finally. The next morning awoke in my double bed in the den of my mom's one-bedroom apartment, our mouths full of garlic from the falafels. Our lunch on the Drive. She was vegan and I was determined to like – no, love – the pizza we got from the place in the old square. But the "cheese" gave me a stomach ache like swallowing bad news or the culmination of a fantasy. The first time she cheated on me. The second time I cheated on her. Past promise notwithstanding, I was never sure whether I could reconcile ideology with pizza. I liked it simple and traditional. I didn't know that yet.

Butter Chicken

By this time, I was grown up, at least by my own account. Having moved on, moved out, moved down the street after parental cohabitation got in the way of our sex life. Late fall or early winter – who could tell it was all so cold, wet, and dark. She called the room the melon for its hot pink walls; it felt like a womb and steamed up her dark-framed glasses. She was so much cooler than I was. So much more worldly. Cumin, cayenne, turmeric, and coriander – this was not the familiar food of my childhood. Sweet creamy butter sauce hiding charred chicken conspicuous with their pierced centres. Later, in the back seat of her shitty little car, her fingers/tongue pressing my sweet flesh piercing *my* centre culminates in searing heat as I gasp, and she laughs into my throat. I smell myself on her lips. She tastes of rose-scented saccharine endings.

Pancakes

As far as hovels go, this one was the best of the pathetic lot. The long space like a torso, the rooms like haphazard limbs. At least it was above ground and had a full-size stove. We spent barely any time in the living room; the living was in the kitchen. The IKEA table I fancied covering with pen and ink scrolling patterns but only ever managed to complete the corner: it was my first grown-up purchase. I was vegan then because of some other girl, and as I taught myself to make pancakes without butter, eggs, or milk we sat there, late at night, Pat Metheny on the CD player perched atop the fridge, and chatted. My love for her was unlike all the others. Poetic, calm, sweet, like the scent of vanilla, syrup, warm coffee with cream.

Vegetarian Chili

I guess, in a way, she was my first straight girl. I was scared of her at first: she was "that" girl sitting at the desk in the womyn's centre, long hair and Converse, perpetually pissed-off in a way I could never be. I came to the door that January and it was her. I moved in the following week. My room was off the kitchen, which somehow seemed fitting. Exercising my culinary prowess with bulgur wheat and a copious – if unceremonious – dumping of store-brand spice powder. The smell of cumin lingered in the air as we played the guitar in her room and composed songs about the incomprehensibility of Judith Butler. And then that one time, as she lay on the bed, beckoned me over, kissed me. Soft and sweet. I would have done anything for her. I don't know if she knew that. Maybe she did, which is why it never happened again – neither kiss nor chili.

Gin

She brought the squat brown bottle over that night and took it when she left. Barely touched.

Tofu and Rice Samosa

This is what I remember: I had heard about her, the tales were wild, my mind's eye had conjured a picture of her well before we met, so then, when we finally did, I knew (I knew!) it was her. It wasn't anything but magic, and I wanted her in a way I have never wanted anyone before. I made it my mission to insinuate myself into her space. I didn't give a shit about her girlfriend. Purchasing envelopes. And chit books. Innocuous conversation about paper permeated my day until one day we made a lunch date. Down the street to the vegetarian eatery for a tofu and rice samosa – fried not baked. (To be perfectly honest I was too nervous to eat.) We sat at the base of the statue in the park, homeless people and drug addicts and mothers and children. It was summer, I think. As I ran my hand down her arm and admired her tattoos I knew that she was it for me. She. Was. It. But … we didn't become until much later, in another summer whirlwind, fuelled by my unsuspecting bravado. That afternoon, I crawled home on my knees and tucked up into my bed, numb. And later, when the rains came, and over mediocre sushi, she apologized. Even now when we meet, I still have trouble eating.

Bran Muffin

My existence with her was punctuated by discomfort: the burn of smoke in my lungs peaking on the warm concrete, a deep smoulder of jealously – self-loathing and her icy gaze turning away and back and away – the anger that unfolded within. Once (only once) at the westernmost edge of the island, gazing out at an endless roiling ocean, I glimpsed softer edges. The imprint still visible beneath the sediment. Then it was only peanut butter pie and seemingly endless cheesecake martinis. It was all a game. Culminating in a visit home – a bran muffin and a late-night trip to the ER. The brochures said six hours: you must wait six hours. Go immediately if you throw up, but … I never threw up. I just suffered. Always alone even when she was with me.

BLT

She was different. My age almost exactly and a relief. Walking up the stairs to the queer film fest, smelling slightly of demi-glace reduction and sweat. Her head, then glasses, then face coming slowly into view – a revelation. Then that first meal at the Cat's Meow. Maybe it was just drinks. Later at her place cooking dinner on her tiny, retro kitchen counter trying not to bump my head on the overhead cabinets. I was in cooking school and wanted to impress her. Italian of some variety which prompted mention of an Italian "girlfriend" causing me to falter – I think it was a test. White wine at mine, trips to her mother's place on the ferry. We garnished the plate with foraged rosehips, breaking my rule never to decorate with anything inedible. She broke all my rules. The summer before the dog we took a road trip to her childhood home. At the highway diner she ordered a bacon, lettuce, and tomato sandwich. A sworn vegetarian once again undone by salted and cured meats.

Cosmopolitans

Food was always our connection. Late night meals out: I smoked then, just to get away and that is precisely when we met again. We were always eating together. Her brothers and their girlfriends and their pretty, straight girl and boy friends. Our parties were well attended, infused with booze because in those days it was just so easy to be special if you had lychee liqueur and imported European beer. She liked cosmopolitans. Such lofty aspiration with a tall, thin stem. After years watching her fall asleep on the couch at 8 p.m., gently removing the glass from her hand, I had had enough light pink drinks to last me a lifetime.

Mojitos

That summer was her mouth, rum-soaked mint-tinged cigarette smoke-filled. Kisses in the alley behind my best friend's apartment. Kisses while my real girlfriend sat inside.

Veal Parmesan

She was a series of misadventures which fed the excuses I made to myself and the dogs. I used to love to listen to her speak Italian on the phone to her family. The most interesting thing about her. Often returning with a surly expression and plates warm with loosely covered foil: moist pork loin, bites of pasta, veal parmesan with homemade marinara. My father never puts garlic in his sauce, she told me. I believed everything she said – that I was special and deserved more. I ate it all. She was older, straight with queer-leaning tendencies, but she would never call it that. Of course, we were drunk. We were always drunk. Or I was alone. First the nights then the mornings blinded me with shame and pathos. She was a tornado and yet. The scent of perfume, booze, cigarettes still stirs something in me.

Niçoise Salad

I would procure the albacore loin from the Korean guy who ran the sushi place up the street from our apartment. He worked with his mom. Eight dollars for 48 dollars-worth of fish. I would poach it in olive oil, lay it on mesclun greens tossed with pitted Kalamata olives, room temperature roasted potatoes, thinly sliced peppers, and blanched *haricots verts*. It was the only thing she wanted. Not traditional but close enough. We lived on someone else's property, buying eggs from coolers at the ends of driveways with jars for bills and coins. I loved the speckled blue ones the most: their delicate shells contrasting with the deep yellow yolk within. Our end came like the rich soil emerging from compost and horse manure: slowly, deliberately, steaming with secret heat from somewhere deep within. Or just not here anymore.

Assorted Meats

The first time we met she turned around, looked me up and down. Decided that today, despite hunger and a tired face and early allergies, she would grant me – small, brown, tattooed, pierced, lesbian – the honour of her company. Chatting her up in line for the shittiest food-truck food either of us have ever eaten. Neither of us cared. Which is what happens when two carnivorous souls finally meet in the line-up to a gluten-free, vegan food truck. We were at the wrong truck and made a sharp turn right to the other. Still not very good. The cheese wasn't melted on my sad little chicken wrap, the meat dry as I wolfed it down in the car. She brought me sausages the next first time. Smoky with a slight heat, garlicky. The first time we fought she called me fractious and combative as she abandoned her plate and fled. Eight years later she eschews flesh in all its forms but takes bites here and there. She trusts me. At last, I am full.

20 Gender-Reveal Cakes and Transphobia

L.M. Zoller

In 2018, I started decorating "Gender-Reveal Disaster Cakes" to mock increasingly bizarre and violent "gender-reveal" celebrations. In a "gender reveal," medical staff give the (genital) "results" of the foetal ultrasound to the parent to be. The parent can give that sealed information to a bakery or friend to conceal pink or blue items to be "revealed" inside a cake or other item, which the parent/s cut open to reveal pink for vulva or blue for penis. However, genitals and chromosomes do not determine gender; the practice of "gender reveals" and gendering infants is reductive and transphobic. Only the child can determine their gender or lack thereof when they are able to communicate.

I collect examples of gender-reveal party mishaps and memorialize them in cake. Past pieces included "Fight at Applebee's" and "47,000 Acre Wildfire." Unable to bake large cakes during the pandemic, I created artistic prototypes of my cake designs instead. These designs are based on actual gender-reveal "fails," including a black balloon full of pink or blue glitter that escaped before the parents could pop it; parents who fed a watermelon dyed with pink or blue food colouring to an alligator; and a box of balloons opened, not to reveal pink or blue balloons, but a rainbow of colours. Through this series, I hope to draw attention to both the trans joy of watching gender reveals fail, as well as to the hypocrisy of cisgender "allies" who continue this harmful practice.

Balloon Escape

Collage prototype of a three-tiered layer cake depicting two partygoers chasing after an gender-reveal black balloon, which escaped while the expectant parents were attempting to pop the balloon to reveal pink or blue glitter. The bottom layer, the largest, is frosted in white buttercream with the text "Do Not Perceive Me" piped on in cursive. The middle layer is frosted in green buttercream, using the grass frosting tip to create a grassy texture. White frosting is piped on to depict a fence. Fondant sculptures of two partygoers, one in blue and one in pink, are climbing up the second layer's fence. A spring of candied rosemary represents backyard foliage/trees. The top layer is the smallest tier, frosted in sky blue buttercream. At the very top of the cake is a cake pop coated in black candy melts to represent the black balloon flying away (Figure 20.1).

DOI: 10.4324/9781003217121-22

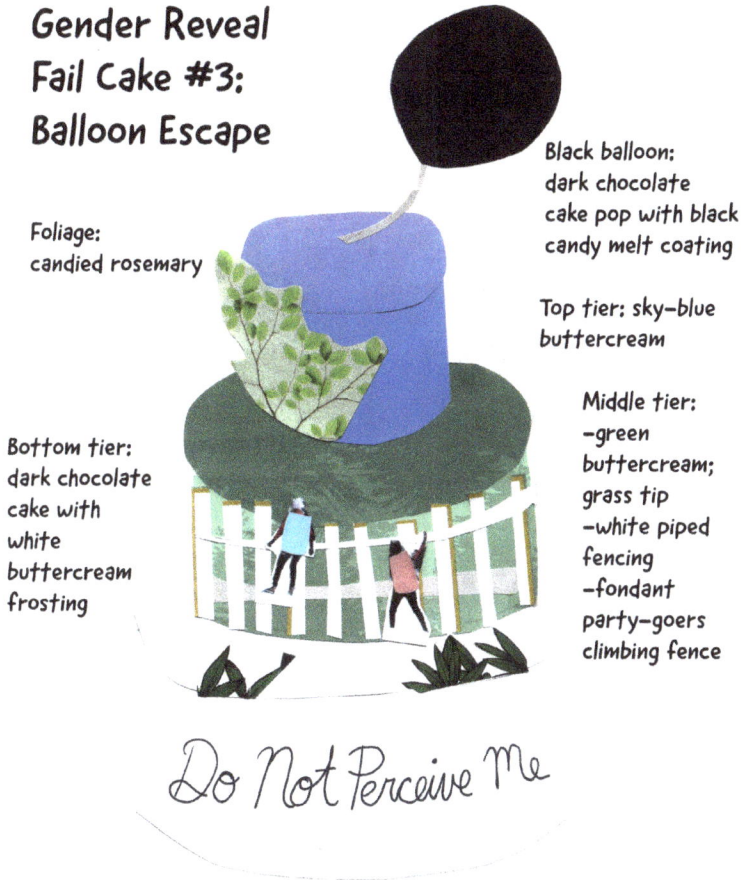

Gender Reveal Fail Cake #3: Balloon Escape

Black balloon: dark chocolate cake pop with black candy melt coating

Top tier: sky-blue buttercream

Foliage: candied rosemary

Middle tier:
-green buttercream; grass tip
-white piped fencing
-fondant party-goers climbing fence

Bottom tier: dark chocolate cake with white buttercream frosting

Do Not Perceive Me

Figure 20.1 Gender-Reveal Cake Fail: "Balloon Escape," collage (analogue and digital), L.M. Zoller. L.M. Zoller.

Rainbow Balloons Surprise

Collage art prototype of a square layer cake frosted in chocolate to look like a box that has been opened with balloons flying out. Based on a real incident in which expectant parents opened a box of party balloons to "reveal" the "gender" of their unborn baby, expecting the balloons to be pink or blue, but six balloons in rainbow colours came out. The cake is cut open to reveal six layers in the colours of the rainbow: red, orange, yellow, green, blue, and purple. The top of the cake has a square cut out to look like an empty box. The top is a dark brown for the chocolate ganache filling. Out of the "hole" in the box are six balloon-shaped cake pops on sticks. The side of the box has light pink and light blue polka dots on it

Gender Reveal Fail Cake 5
Rainbow Balloons
Surprise

Square 6–layer vanilla
cake; each layer is
a different color of
the rainbow

Balloons:
balloon–shaped sandwich
cookies or macarons
on sticks

Frosting: chocolate

The top of the
"box" is carved
out and filled with
chocolate ganache

Decorations: frosting or
fondant dots in
baby blue and baby pink

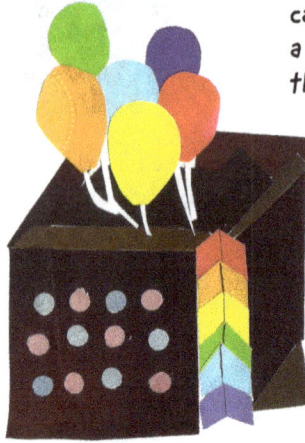

Not pictured:
cis–tears martini

Figure 20.2 Gender-Reveal Cake Fail: "Rainbow Balloons Surprise," collage (analogue and digital), L.M. Zoller. L.M. Zoller.

Gender Reveal Fail Cake #6
Alligator with Watermelon

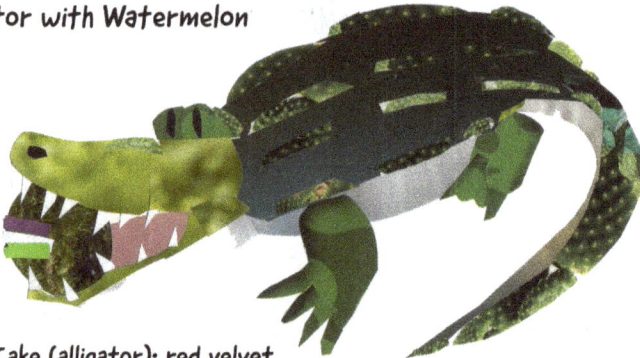

Cake (alligator): red velvet
Frosting: matcha buttercream
Watermelon: watermelon–flavored cupcake covered in fondant
partially crushed to reveal genderqueer–flag colors

Figure 20.3 Gender-Reveal Cake Fail: "Alligator with Watermelon," collage (analogue and digital), L.M. Zoller. L.M. Zoller.

to represent the "expected" foetal genitals to be revealed by the balloons (pink for vagina, blue for penis) (Figure 20.2).

Alligator with Watermelon

Collage art of a cake that is shaped like an alligator. The alligator is holding a watermelon in its mouth, which has been partially crushed in its jaws to reveal the interior is genderqueer pride colours: purple, white, and green. This cake is based on an incident in which expectant parents put a watermelon in an alligator's mouth. The intent was for the alligator to crush the watermelon in its powerful jaws to reveal the interior to be pink or blue (Figure 20.3).

21 Meat Cute

Mikhail Collins

I have never eaten meat.

This sentence causes outrage, shock, bewilderment. I answer to a never-ending chorus of haughty one-liners such as "what do you even eat?", overly concerned queries of "aren't you starving?" or "how have you survived this long?", and presumptuous investigations like "is this for a medical reason? You must be unwell." This statement involuntarily invites strangers to comment on my body with "that's why you're so tiny" and uncomfortably flirtatious, "I hear that's beneficial in the bedroom." It is always an interview process, nothing is off limits, and I am to answer all questions willingly and readily. My "meatless-ness" is an aberration, a shame and a pity, something to be challenged, and something to be feared.

In reality, my vegetarianism stems from my parents, who ceased their meat consumption before I was born, at first abstaining from red meats for health reasons and then all meats for ethical ones. Growing up I was given the option to try meat but by grade school the pinkish substance looked so foreign and unappealing I could not understand why anyone else would willingly, enthusiastically eat it. I recall finding the pepperoni – then called "red circles" – on top of pizza at a friend's birthday party strange and grotesque, telling my mother in a bewildered tone that the other children kept pressuring me to eat it. I can remember other children learning that their burgers were once cows with horror, some crying and others quickly coming to terms with the fact their food was once very much alive. I had known this for far longer than they had and had quickly accepted the fact that it was not a "food" that I wanted anything to do with. Coming across an old magazine on my parents' bookshelf that featured prominently "the inside scoop: hidden cameras expose torturous slaughterhouse conditions" was more than enough to instil in me that meat and the meat industry is not something I could morally condone, even as a child.

When I disclose that my meatless-ness is from my parents I am met with a mixture of sympathy and disregard. I am told tragically "it is a shame that your parents decided that for you" or snidely with a laugh, "you must be very obedient to still listen to them even as an adult." My choices around my food consumption then, are negated because this was not my choice but another's choice *for* me: I am made both a victim and a coward. Ultimately, the belief is that no one would willing choose to abstain from meat, because there must be some medical condition,

DOI: 10.4324/9781003217121-23

perhaps a forced diet exclusion, a concerning obsession with body image, or simply my own ignorance.

I recall my parents teasing me when I was younger, "what if your future partner eats meat?" Impossible, I had thought then. Of course, my partner would not eat meat. I can show them the slaughterhouse magazine and that is all it would take. Why would I be involved with someone who thought it was right to kill and consume another?

My partner does eat meat. My partner, at times in his youth, ate almost only meat. My partner was awarded high honours in culinary school. He has medals, certificates, and letters of recommendation on how incredible his culinary skills and butchering techniques are. I find some of these facts quite revolting, and he finds these facts to be quite a proud accomplishment.

My partner, Logan, hates strawberries, hates Brussels sprouts. He finds asparagus disgusting and refuses to eat cherries because of the texture. Bananas give him heartburn. Apples are too sweet. The smell of pumpkin makes him nauseous, and he especially hates artichokes. Cauliflower, black beans, grapes, peas, lemons, avocados, eggplant, squash, cucumbers, sweet potatoes, oranges not in juice form, all vary in degrees of dislike. He somehow, miraculously, also received perfect scores on his tasting exams. He likes to tell me that he has a "perfect palate" and brags about his willingness to try anything once. He just happens to not like much. In terms of food preferences, I would say we could not be further apart from one another.

--

He describes to me in great, agonizing detail how to debone a chicken while we are waiting for our food in a restaurant. The noise of the other patrons is so loud I can barely hear him. He does not seem to notice as my eyes wander to the hand-drawn poster of a bright purple gorilla drinking a strawberry milkshake. I'd sure like a strawberry milkshake right now.

I glance back at him occasionally and nod. I wonder if he will realize his error and change the subject, but he goes on, gesticulating something crude and speaking about the importance of flexible boning knifes. I raise my eyebrows at him, perplexed, and he motions as though he's slicing the air. I make eye contact with the purple gorilla instead.

He finishes his explanation, looking proud.

I feel ill.

--

Meat makes me sick. I'm not used to how it looks, how it smells. I see commercials, advertisements, billboards for meat products and it takes a conscious effort to recognize this as a much-treasured food. When it's wrapped up in a burrito across the table or a distant order of chicken strips I can manage. It's when it's pink and red I feel the heaviest unease. A slice of ham. A sizzling, bleeding steak. A rare burger. Raw chicken posed strangely the in deli aisle. I have seen my insides before and they too, are pink and red. I can't grasp the difference. Eating it is like eating me.

I have been told stories of Americans who go abroad only to see whole animal carcasses hung from meat hooks and recoil in horror, as though they did not know the pre-packaged, pre-sliced, pre-cooked bacon they had been eating for decades was once a living, breathing, fleshy creature. And there is much truth to this, the way we deal with meat makes it easier to detach it from the living being it once was. Adams (2010) refers to this concept as the "absent referent."

The language surrounding "meat" recalls dishes of holiday ham, fragrant beef, and freshly cooked turkey as food instead of the immediate death of an animal. This "mystifying" of meat pushes the idea of the killing of animals for consumption further from our consciousness, and allows meat to exist solely as a food, as devoid of animal despite being wholly animal. Meat cannot be meat without first killing an animal. "The absent referent functions to cloak the violence inherent in meat eating, to protect the conscience of the meat eater and the render the idea of the individual animals as immaterial to anyone's selfish desires" (p. 304).

--

"Wait, what's that?" I lean over him, peering intensely at something odd in his refrigerator. There's a sealed plastic bag on the bottom shelf full of something pale pink. In response he gently turns my head the other way with a few fingers.

"It's chicken," he holds his hand in front of my eyes like a shield, "you don't want to see that."

"Oh," I pause, wait a moment, then two. "Why does it look like that?"

"It's boiled, for the cats. Chicken is a little pink or white. It's called a 'white meat'."

I frown. "Well, what are other kinds of meats called?"

"Red. Or white."

"Oh."

I study the wrinkles on his palm.

"What's a red meat?"

"Steak."

"Steak is?"

"Cow."

"Cow is?"

"Beef."

"Beef is cow. Cow is steak," I repeat. He doesn't lower his hand. We stand in silence. He moves to close the refrigerator door, but I stop him.

"Uhm," I pause again, "can I see it?"

He places the sealed bag of chicken on the counter, steps back for me to examine it. It's odd. Very odd. The chicken looks as though it's been bleached, shredded into chunks for an easier cat dinner. It is also unbelievably stringy. It was alive once, and now it's here in a bag, in a fridge.

"Why does it look like the bristles on a broom?"

He laughs suddenly, "is that what it looks like to you?"

I make a morbid realization and clutch at my fingers anxiously. "No," I feel deeply unsettled, I look away quickly, "it looks like tendons."

--

I feel about meat the way I feel about gender: by the age I was supposed to "get it" I most certainly did not "get it." What is there to "get?" A lot, apparently.

Gender is just as ingrained as meat, with food itself assigned gendered roles as masculine or feminine. Adams describes how meat serves as a tool for male bonding, "bestow[ing] an idea of masculinity on the individual consumer" (p. 303). Masculinity is linked to the domination, killing, and consumption of another living being, and to take great pride in these actions.

I feel wrong as a woman. I feel wrong as a man. I feel a distinct repulsion to both man and woman, and I feel a distinct repulsion to meat. Not eating meat is just as confusing as rejecting the gender binary to a bystander. Those refusals carry weight, the non-doing of a thing is often more upsetting, more menacing than the doing of one. Thus, rejecting the consumption of meat is just as integral to my identity as rejecting the construction of gender.

--

Logan casually orders a burger when we go out to eat.

I find it repulsive. It's dead flesh and muscle. It bleeds. It was alive once but all that is left is flesh, a corpse. I watch him eat with a growing horror. Dead. Alive. Dead. Alive. It's on the brink of food and rot. Death and life. A reminder of once what was here but now is gone. He notices me watching and smiles, tries to kiss me. I gag.

When he gets a burger next time, he doesn't try to kiss me after.

We establish a strict no-contact rule when meat is consumed: he brushes his teeth immediately afterwards.

--

I've been handed pieces of bacon with pleading eyes; told I would like it if only I tried it; told that I'm desperately missing out; told that if I don't try it once, how will I ever really know what I like? My choices surrounding what I eat are invalidated, as I am not an individual who can pick and choose what I enjoy because I cannot even tell what it is that I do enjoy. I am rendered helpless, and my self-autonomy is ultimately undermined, if not thoroughly destroyed. My "lack of" meat is a threat, and the threat is in the refusal to partake.

There are heterosexist parallels to my meatless-ness and to queer sexualities. The "try it and you'll like it" argument that so many queer people – particularly queer women – hear in regard to their sexuality is a noteworthy parallel. The prominent link between meat and masculinity is not lost on me, as though the rejection of meat is simultaneously the rejection of men. Queer people are seen oftentimes as confused and uncertain of what they truly want and, of course, the heterosexual is here to help them in their time of deep, prolonged disorientation – a saviour in a dark tunnel. This is coupled with an overarching infantilization of those who are not straight. My queerness paired with my vegetarianism doubles this sentiment of "lost child needing help," where the meat eater – nearly always a man – lends me his hand triumphantly and reassures me that he can help me, he can fix me, he can make me never look back.

--

Logan is cooking a vegetarian meal for me. He admits that he spent several days combing over recipes online in hopes of finding something good enough, easy enough, to prepare together. We are at his house, the counters are covered in red cabbage, garlic skins, and juice from tofu. He's mincing garlic with a confidence that I rarely see him with, shoulders back and hands moving swiftly with the knife. I watch as he adds garlic to the pan, moves it with a wooden spoon, and turns to me smiling and focused.

"The recipe says to cook sesame oil with the garlic, but I've always considered that more of a finisher," he points to the cabbage, "we can top everything with the cabbage last."

"This would have been really good with broccoli," I say wiping dry the wet counters.

He laughs lightly, makes a face. The face of a guilty broccoli hater.

We cook in silence for a while before he realizes the tofu is sweating, unattended in the corner.

"Oh, uh," he stammers, chuckles, looks away, "we have to press that."

He lifts the tofu like it's a small living creature, cups it in both hands tenderly before wrapping it in a multitude of paper towels. I watch transfixed, his motions clumsy and obviously foreign.

That's a lot of paper towels.

"That should be good!" He delicately places an unused frying pan on top of the damp towels with wet hands.

He's mummified the tofu.

Logan catches me eyeing the tofu suspiciously. Embarrassed he tells me, "I've never cooked tofu before."

"Never would have guessed. They didn't teach you about tofu in chef school?" I break my gaze with the Halloween tofu as he tosses some cabbage in the pan with some seasonings, oil, brown sugar, scallions, more garlic.

"Nope."

"That's sad. You can do a lot with tofu. It's like a sponge."

He makes an unpleasant noise, "sponge, huh?"

The unused frying pan is supplying an unimpressive amount of force to the tofu. The wetness continues to slowly seep out from underneath its tomb.

We eat together perched on his bed, the cabbage has a definite raw crunch, and the tofu is still slightly wet, slightly oily from lack of a proper pressing and being placed in oil without marinating.

"You know," he begins, collecting tofu and scallions on his fork, "I cook because I just like to make people smile. Eating is when people have some of the best memories. Food brings people together and being together is good. I really like cooking for you." He looks over at me fondly, "do you like the tofu? I think it's a little bland, actually."

Suddenly it's the best tofu I've ever eaten.

--

I am told if I really cared about the environment, I would buy only local foods, use only public transport. I am told that vegetarianism does more harm to my health than good, that meat is required to live, to be human. I am told that I do eat meat and just haven't realized it yet, I am pelted with questions of if I eat gelatine or marshmallows, as though I can be caught in a trap. I am told that eating meat doesn't matter anyway, that there are more important things than animals, that I should focus on something of actual significance. I am told that when you are raised with meat is it harder to stop, nearly impossible to give it up.

Logan brings me to vegan restaurants I have never heard of before, tries the food excitedly, tells me confidently we can cook this at home, whispers tips on how to improve the texture, the taste. He sends me recipes and outlines how we can substitute the meat: we use mushrooms in his family's chicken croissant recipe, garbanzo beans in veggie burgers, plant-based sausage for breakfast. I ask him, apprehensive and sceptical, if this is genuinely something he enjoys or if meat consumption is as integral to his identity as its absence is to mine. He tells me softly, "what a unique opportunity. I get to serve a devout vegetarian and learn about a world of cooking I never would have entered on my own. Think of all the fun dishes we can come up with."

I will never eat meat. I avoid it whenever possible, and I will continue to do so. Nothing will change how I feel, and as I age, I find my revulsion growing stronger. My partner understands and accepts this, and despite his lack of vegetarian/vegan culinary experiences, purposely seeks to appreciate and recognize my beliefs, thoughts, and limitations on food. He teaches me that my vegetarianism is something that can be admired and learned from, instead of something that should be feared and mocked. In return I teach him new recipes, give new perspectives, offer new foods. I feel truly included within food by another for the first time outside of my parents and it feels indescribably tender, thoughtful, and kind. Together we have learned to bond intimately over food instead of being drawn apart by it.

Reference

Adams, C. J. (2010). Why feminist-vegan now? *Feminism & Psychology, 20*(3), 302–317.

22 Achāri Anecdotes

Exploring Queer Food Cultures in Indian Kitchens

Anil Pradhan and Andronicus Aden

With the advancement of cultural studies, one can discern that "home" has come to symbolize more than just a space, either shared or not, for emotions and ideals to be celebrated, where one's personality and sexuality thrives in a safe space marked by recuperation, protection, nourishment, and intimacy. It serves as a platform to represent and uphold social norms and idealized heteropatriarchal systems which require investment, continual labour, and repetitive actions in order to assert its hegemonic legitimacy (Butler, 1990). Thus, "home" also signifies a confluence of gender inequality and a "space of negotiation and resistance as well as oppression" (Cox & Buchli, 2017, p. 15). Conventional heteronormativity often divides home into gendered spaces, restricting movement both within as well as outside, with the dialectics of the inside/outside delegating gendered roles at the threshold, between the realm of the domestic/feminine/unremunerated labour and the world/masculine/employed respectively (Szabo, 2017, p. 17). Contemporary studies have now focused on the need to deconstruct the preconceived standards of the domestic space as a cisgendered heteropatriarchal construct, to acknowledge the bias and privilege granted to heterosexual couples as the ideal model for all things domiciliary, and to explore alternative, non-normative versions of domesticities vis-à-vis sexualities. Within the complex politics of gendered domesticity, the kitchen not just emerges as a space assigned for food preparation and consumption but also as a place of friction vis-à-vis gender, class, race, and economy.

Studies on food and its relation to gender have explored the invariable relationship between masculinities and domesticity, where heterosexual men's connection with food and cooking occur within the static boundaries of leisured, segregated spaces such as backyards and professional kitchen and food items such as meat and game (Julier & Linderfeld, 2005). The traditionally stigmatized space of the kitchen is now being occupied by single men, single fathers, and gay/queer couples/individuals, claiming the kitchen as a space for meal preparation and nutrition either out of volition or necessity (Szabo, 2017, p. 19). Within this existing gendered deviation in terms of masculine domesticity, Szabo (2017) points out the emergence of "gay domesticity" as an alternative construct, where non-heteronormative ideas of "home" and domestic comfort and care are inculcated (p. 23). Furthermore, Cook (2014) asserts a need to view and study queer histories and

DOI: 10.4324/9781003217121-24

domesticities by accepting the presence of gay individuals in spaces that are more private. After all, the heteronormative home has mostly excluded queer individuals, who then create alternative versions of it, contesting against the norms and their previous familial spaces and creating a niche for acceptance, expression, and belonging. The queering of the kitchen vis-à-vis the home can be interpreted as not just a transgressive act but also an everyday political assertion of one's identity and a reimagination of non-normative domesticities (Campkin & Pilkey, 2017, p. 85). Although existing research has explored queer food cultures through ethnographic studies in Australia, Israel, Guyana, Singapore, the United Kingdom, and the United States (Pilkey et al., 2017), there remains a glaring gap in terms of exploring the narratives of those marginalized within the marginalized groups in the Global South, when it comes to the queering of domesticities.

In the Indian context, queer food culture studies is a *terra incognita*; existing research has focused mostly on literary texts and criticism (Menon, 2018; Pradhan, 2020; Sareen, 2021; Vanita, 2014). However, food culture studies with Indian context have recently made an entry towards a multidisciplinary study on food: preparation, consumption, and dynamic, multifaceted relationships between the establishment of power structures and their subversions. *Food Culture Studies in India* (2021), with articles focusing on literary criticism, visual cultures, popular media, and identity politics, is a major addition to this specific field and has explored how food becomes "a source of contestation, coercion, resistance, subversion and negotiation" (Malhotra et al., 2021, p. vii), but it is clearly lacking in terms of focus on food vis-à-vis non-heteronormative sexualities. Since no proper ethnographic study has been conducted on gay individuals and their domestic negotiations in the kitchen spaces of India, within the larger framework of food cultures in an economically and culturally diverse India, where does one situate queer food cultures and their dynamic narratives? Specifically, what are the relationships between queerness, food, and cooking when it comes to focusing on the domestic space of the Indian home? Our ethnographic study (perhaps the first of its kind in India) attempts to explore these non-normative narratives of the queering of the Indian kitchen and the multiple subjectivities that negotiate and emerge from the varied processes and negotiations. We are not making an argument that Indian queer men (and LGBTQ+ individuals) have a special, experiential relationship with food and cooking by virtue of their sexual identities, but, through this chapter, we are attempting at unearthing the intimate ways in which interactions and contestations have shaped relationships between queer men and the way they consider, cook, and consume food.

Method

The study deals with queer men in India as participants via prior contacts, using the snowballing technique. The ethnographic discussions presented in this chapter are part of an independent study undertaken by the authors, and the data are drawn from interviews conducted in the month of November 2021. All participants (n = 13) self-identify as queer men and were aged between 23 and 54.

Most of them belong to the socioeconomic middle-class (ranging between lower and upper middle-class) and were educated in English-medium schools. The ethnic diversity in our sample was as such: Bengali (n = 6), Indian, Nepali, Gorkha (n = 5), and Punjabi (n = 2). Most of them were located in East India, in the state of West Bengal (in the cities of Kolkata and Siliguri, the towns of Kurseong and Kalimpong, and rural areas of Darjeeling), with two participants based in North India (Sonipat and Chandigarh) and one in South India (Bengaluru). The interviews were conducted primarily in English with occasional digressions into Nepali, Bangla, and Hindi. Rather than adopting structured questionnaire schedules, we chose to let informal conversations and semi-structured interviews be the mainstay of our method. Eight participants have been referred to using their real names, following their signed consent, whereas five participants have been provided pseudonyms upon their explicit, verbal request.

Discussion and Analysis

Queer Men, Kitchen, and Homemaking

In the context of the liberative and transformative politics of food and cooking among queer Indian men included in this study, the construct of the domestic space of the kitchen and the idea of queer homemaking feature as important aspects of negotiating with the heteronormative and patriarchal space of the gendered home/domestic. It helps them in laying claim to an alternative form of belonging in the family and refashioning romantic relationships in shared domestic spaces and the notion of queer homemaking that is both non-normative and unconventional. Several participants commented that the act of reclaiming the kitchen space in order to assert a certain degree of agency is often met by surprise, from figures who support a heteropatriarchal idea of the domestic space, especially when the everyday-ness of the activity presents itself as an unconventional reality in the Indian household. The responses to such acts, even if accepted and encouraged, were often veiled in heteronormative inflections. For example, Dawa (name changed) recollected how, while cooking in his Tibetan household in the Darjeeling Hills, his mother had once commented, "buhāri chāhindaina" (Nepali: "There is no need for a daughter-in-law"), revealing how such instances reinforce the heteropatriarchal norm as the invariable scenario. However, another aspect of reclaiming the kitchen space was highlighted by Patrick (name changed), who informed how his foray into the domestic space of the kitchen at home, located in a Christian family in the Kalimpong Hills, helped him access an alternative sense of belonging in the family. He made use of cooking as a medium of gaining acceptance and approval from his father, who, he informs, respected men who were self-dependent in matters of the kitchen. For him, entering the kitchen space altered the domestic dynamics of the Indian household, especially in terms of the gendered notions of cooking in the kitchen.

Furthermore, cooking as an artistic medium also seems to have helped queer men find solace and positive reinforcement when it comes to socially inflicted trauma related to non-normative sexuality. For example, Avro Basu mentioned that cooking at home and the organic movement in the kitchen space has been a detoxifying experience and has helped him explore his imagination; for him, the kitchen acts as a space for seeking and finding solace, transforming it into a "sacred space." In this context, Avro highlighted how his cooking food in the familial domain on a daily basis challenges notions and stereotypes of the normative, societal idea of men not generally cooking in the middle-class Bengali household in Kolkata. On similar lines, Sunny (name changed) stated that cooking has been a form of refuge for him, citing incidents of abuse and bullying in school, along with his introversion and closeted-ness that propelled him towards the kitchen as a space of restoration. The narrative of exposure and trauma in the "outside"/world got contested through the "inside"/home where he could find protection and resistance through food and cooking, i.e., the kitchen, which Sunny describes as his "saviour." Also, since childhood, he stated that he had a proclivity for the arts, and through cooking, he could express a different perspective of art. Since he was not only preparing ordinary dishes but also experimenting and innovating new garnishes, he described it as his "artistic approach towards food." As such, queer men's self-expressions through the food they create are not only an essential part of their subjectivity but also their artistic claims on queering food cultures.

For the participants, food and cooking also feature as an inextricable part of projecting queer subjectivity and in sustaining relationships with romantic partners, wherein queer men's refashioning and reclaiming of the domestic sphere and homemaking envisages queering the dynamics of the Indian home. For example, Phurba Sangay Sherpa's reclaiming of domesticity is visible in his rented house in Bengaluru, especially in his fully stocked kitchen, and the assertion of domesticity that is reflected through his association of "home" with the smell of his kitchen. When guests (queer or otherwise) enter his home, he wants them to smell the aroma of *sabji* (cooked vegetables) or *dāl* (cooked lentils) wafting from his kitchen, showcasing how the construction of a functioning kitchen vis-à-vis gay domesticity can reclaim the domestic space as an inclusive, comforting space. In the context of relationships with same-sex partners, the responses were further interesting. Patrick quoted the oft-repeated saying, "If you want to get to a man's heart, it's through his stomach" while confessing that he had often made good use of his cooking skills toward both impressing his romantic partners and expressing his affection and love for them. Similarly, Vivek (name changed) mentioned that he has had prepared "better" food (varied, special dishes from other regions of India that are generally not prepared at home in the Nepali-dominated hills in North Bengal) for men he has had a liking for, putting in more labour into the process of cooking and the presentation of food. Avro also spoke of instances when the familial and the romantic merged in the dining space and mentioned that food has often acted as a gelling agent between his parents and his same-sex partners. However, the act of cooking in the queer domestic space, for almost all of the participants, entails a need to de-heteronormativize labour and involvement in the kitchen in a manner that does not replicate heteropatriarchal structures of gendered divisions and stereotypes. When it comes to sustaining a domestic and romantic relationship with another man, for example, Patrick revealed how he has had negotiated power politics and exercised caution through division of labour and duties when cooking with someone else as a gay couple. Kaustav Bakshi also remarked that gendered notions of men cooking and considered as housewives should be challenged by queer folx so as not to reimpose heteropatriarchal notions of domesticity when it comes to the kitchen. Suraj (name changed) goes so far as to equate one-sided cooking for a partner to be akin to "pampering" them. Such comments by participants highlight how an idea of similarity/equitability in sharing domestic responsibilities and labour, including cooking, for queer couples is essential in refashioning the liberating and democratic agency of non-heteronormative relationships and coupledom.

Men Queering Food and Recipes

One aspect that the study also focuses on is an idea of queering food and culinary practices by queer men. Elsewhere, I have discussed how "queering culinary practices and food items entails projection and presentation of food as something 'different' from the 'normal' and/or the 'normative,' while making it acceptable in the popular imagination of its consumers, admirers, and critics" (Pradhan, 2020, para. 5). For Doonan (2012), the queering of food entails two elements of the appropriation of culinary practices: firstly, the process and the art of creating something edible and simultaneously different that symbolizes a response to hegemonic homophobia; and secondly, the idea of transferring the culinary art of one culture into the culinary parlance of another and producing a consumable piece of novelty that denotes hybridity, symbolizing the pride of being variedly queer in a polarized hetero-normative society. Similarly, this study tries to elicit and explicate how connotations of sexual politics and culinary experimentation might collude to present "queer-ious" results in the food–sexuality dynamics and praxes. Patrick, who is aware of the ideas of certain food items connoting queer politics, provided a relevant example in this context. He recalled preparing vibrant, rainbow-coloured trifles for visitors at a church-organized event, that, though as a private joke, made him feel personally happy upon seeing them gorge on it, given the generally negative stance of the Church on queerness and non-normative sexuality. Patrick also highlighted how if one is to queer food and cooking, experimentation and refashioning would be involved in creating something that is at once different but also unique, that, for him, has often provided the upper hand at the dining table. He provided examples of certain dishes he has tried refashioning that include Indian-style baked chicken and capers with local fishes. As such, assertions vis-à-vis food and cooking by queer men, like Patrick's, show how, often, experimenting with food through new forms of refashioning can become an important part of claiming agency through acceptance, applause, and even awe.

A few participants also talked about queering the menu at home in multifarious manners, entailing various intersections, especially when cooking involves gay romantic partners. For example, Parjanya Sen opined that queer identity entails different vectors and registers which include class dimensions and sexuality, as well as caste positions and, thus, one must look at various vectors to understand a certain notion of the "queer." One way in which he has attempted to recognize this diversity within the domestic space is through the act of cooking different ethnic cuisines for the same meal. For example, Parjanya and his partner were able to bring together dishes such as *Emā Dātshi* (a traditional Bhutanese dish) and *Ilish Māch* with *Shorshé* (a typical Bengali dish) on the same day, hinting at how such mix and matches on a daily basis in their house cut across various gender-queer boundaries including race, ethnicity, and sexualities through food. Kaustav provided another interesting commentary on how recipes can be queered and new queer food items can be created out of non-normative friendship and kinship. He recalled how he had once recreated a specific dish for his close friend Rituparno Ghosh (the deceased Bengali film director) that he wished to be cooked. The unique, unnamed *paneer* dish entailed dipping the *paneer* (a form of semi-firm, fresh cottage cheese) in egg and frying it in a curry containing mustard seeds. In recreating this "queer" dish (that blurs, transcends, and even blasphemes the boundaries between the strict "vegetarian" and the "non-vegetarian" categories in India) that he named "Paneer Rituparno," and through cooking it again and again for other queer friends, Kaustav's example pointed out how food can be queered in an imaginative and empowering manner through memory, intimacy, and camaraderie among queer folx.

In relation to sexual expression through food, a few participants also commented on the aesthetic contexts entailed in the queering of food by queer men and how their relationship with queer aesthetics cannot be neglected. For example, Samudranil Gupta opined that queer people come up with their own forms of queer aesthetics as he has observed that most queer individuals are concerned with presentation; he clarifies that this is a general idea because a lot depends on how one appears. This idea/question of appearance is intricately linked with the question of expression, visibility, acceptance, and assertion within the queer community which consequently gets reflected in their sense of aesthetics-via-food. Presenting a dish is not just for himself but is a complete process of becoming and, as a result, Samudranil claimed that his presentation of the food that he creates sustains and reflects his queerness. On a similar note, Sunny stated that the designs of his cakes and pastries come out as "different" compared to mainstream bakers; he claimed that they come across as more artistic since he uses a lot of floral motifs. In this context, he commented that belonging to the queer community creates a different mindset, especially in terms of aesthetics. He recalled how he has always been interested in colourful preparations and pink being his favourite colour, he would incorporate it into his cakes. He would also incorporate floral flavours in his dishes, such as infusing jasmine essence in his *pulāo* (a form of fried Indian rice prepared with fresh vegetables). Sunny's utilization of floral motifs to express his queerness in terms of flavour, visuals, as well as olfactorily experiences resonate the ways in which queer men can and have queered food and cooking in an agential manner.

Queering Masculinity through Food

While foraying into the contexts of the constructions of masculinity in India, cooking and its attendant politics featured as a potential challenge to heteropatriarchal hegemony. Pawan Dhall asserted that an act of consciously staying away from cooking is "a form of toxic masculinity," where, within a heteropatriarchal system, some men are unwilling to literally enter the kitchen space. Similarly, Sandip Roy commented on how some heterosexual men in India "take pride in the fact that they cannot cook food," hinting at a problematic relationship between masculinity and cooking when it comes to a gendered and patriarchal notion of cooking and the kitchen space in India, especially with respect to the "taken-for-granted" aspect of cooking being a woman's business. Therefore, men cooking in general, and queer men cooking in particular, can act as a medium of challenging heteronormativity. In this context, Pawan highlighted the dialectics between the segregation of gendered spaces between the outside/occupation (male-centric) and the inside/home (female-centric) spaces. For example, a male chef is not viewed as something unnatural or feminine; here, cooking doesn't really challenge heteronormativity because it is often excused by the society as a professional, monetary requirement. However, the moment men start cooking for their families, or their wives/sisters, cooking as an everyday activity gains a queer, political valency.

For queer men, the way food is cooked and presented often becomes a medium of not only challenging discriminatory distinctions in the societal constructs of masculinity but also asserting their queerness through liberative forms of expressing femininity and/or blurring the lines of the binary. For example, Patrick talked about a gendered division of labour when it comes to the responsibilities in the kitchen at home where men tend to dwell in the realm of meat-based food items that symbolize masculinity through the process of killing, skinning, chopping, and cooking chicken or beef for curries at home; as opposed to the dishes relegated to a more feminine context, such as preparing *rotis* and *chutneys*. In this context, his dealing with all forms of food items and dishes challenges the gendered, normative notions of what a man should cook in the household. Specifically, Patrick asserts pride in shouldering the responsibility of the entire process and by not adhering to the gendered division of labour in the heteropatriarchal sense (when it comes to the outside-male roles of buying/marketing and collecting vs the inside-female roles of preparing, cooking, serving, and cleaning). Further examples from other participants highlighted how when it comes to cooking and its processes, for queer men, the performative aspects themselves challenge presumptions of masculinity. For example, Sahil Sood provided a narrative of gendered behaviours where he equated patience and gentleness with femininity, a trait, which he opines, is useful in the kitchen while preparing custards, oven-based dishes, or dishes that require gentle hand movements. Avro also highlighted how, in the larger Bengali society, where men cooking is often relegated to the category of *shokher rānnā* (Bangla: cooking as hobby), the regular-ness of men cooking could be subversive in the context of challenging heteropatriarchy. Such relationships of queer men with food and cooking not only challenges the heteropatriarchal constructs of masculinity but also colours the challenge through queer self-dependence in executing the process of cooking.

Apart from the process of queer cooking, several participants drew attention to the queer relationship between certain flavours and food items and the societal constructions of masculinity (and femininity). In terms of the connection with food and sexuality, Dawa argued that a lot of people categorize spicy and sour food with femininity and womanhood. He mentions how he loves the Nepali recipe of *Karji Marji* (an appetiser made with the innards of chicken or mutton), in which he incorporates a lot of chillies along with butter and oregano. Given his affection towards such "feminized" flavours, he has often received comments like "kasto keti jastai amilo ra piro khāko?" (Nepali: "Why do you eat sour and spicy things like a girl?"). Furthermore, Dawa noted how rigid such gendering of food is when his heterosexual male friends "don't even look at such dishes, let alone taste/eat them." Similarly, Samudranil also shared an anecdote where while eating *fuchkās* (a sour-spicy street food famous in East India, also known as *pāni puri* and *golgappā*), how, in a group of customers, when a wife asked her husband to join in, he retorted that "*fuchkās* were meant for girls." Given that such associations with certain flavours unsettle notions of the heteropatriarchal norm, Kaustav also pointed out how the obsession for sour food among queer men, especially the fascination for *achār* (pickles – either preserved or freshly prepared), could reveal how notions of hegemonic masculinity can get challenged and subverted through queer men's preference for food that is traditionally associated with women. One example he provided is *kotbel achār* (fresh pickle of wood apple with green chili, mustard oil, and coriander leaves) – a favourite among his queer friends. Kaustav goes so far as to claim that the process of *achār*-making by men could be considered as expressing androgyny through the bottled and picked *achār* – preparing and persevering *achār* – which has traditionally been considered a woman's job, entailing a non-normative boundary crossing in the context of food and sexuality, and revealing how notions of hegemonic masculinity are both fragile and malleable. Such pickled anecdotes provided by the participants of this study showcase how queer men's relations with food, cooking, and kitchens can be both personal and political when it comes to the ways in which food is envisioned, prepared, consumed, and relished in colloquial contexts in India.

Conclusion

The claiming of a queer subjectivity within the strictures of domestic, heteropatriarchal spaces allows a degree of agency for non-heteronormative men in India. However, we had not contemplated the melange of narratives, like the depth of flavours and spices in Indian cuisine, that would emerge out of our research. Our ethnographic study has merely scratched the surface, and already issues such as the invariably gendered Indian kitchen, agential access to such spaces, queering of food and sustaining queer relations through food, differences in terms of "gay domesticities," the need to de-gender the kitchen space, and gendering and queering of flavours vis-à-vis masculinity have emerged from our findings. As complex and multifarious as the term "queer" is, so is the kitchen space and its dynamics; the everyday politics of negotiation vis-à-vis lesbian consumption, transgender foods, caste-based queer cooking, and queer diasporic food cultures are just some of the areas that are yet to be explored within the field of queer food culture studies in India. One thing remains clear: such negotiations and reclamations not just assist in queer visibility within the framework of heteropatriarchal hegemony but also represent the intense longing and effort to establish, fashion, and sustain queer homes in India, marked by a sense of refashioning, resistance, and reclamation through one of the most basic aspects of life: food.

References

Butler, J. (1990). *Gender trouble: Feminism and the subversion of identity*. Routledge.

Campkin, B., & Pilkey, B. (2017). Introduction: Queering home. In B. Pilkey, R. M. Sciluna, B. Campkin, & B. Penner (Eds.), *Sexuality and gender at home: Experience, politics, transgression* (pp. 83–87). Bloomsbury.

Cook, M. (2014). *Queer domesticities: Homosexuality and home life in twentieth-century London*. Palgrave Macmillan.

Cox, R., & Buchli, V. (2017). Series preface: Why home? In M. Szabo & S. L. Koch (Eds.), *Food, masculinities, and home: Interdisciplinary perspectives* (pp. 15–16). Bloomsbury.

Doonan, S. (2012). *Gay men don't get fat*. Penguin.

Julier, A. & Lindenfeld, L. (2005). Mapping men onto the menu: Masculinities and food. *Food and Foodways, 13*(1–2): 1–16. https://doi.org/10.1080/07409710590915346

Malhotra, S., Sharma, K., & Dogra, S. (2021). Introduction. In S. Malhotra, K. Sharma, & S. Dogra (Eds.), *Food culture studies in India: Consumption, representation and mediation* (pp. vii–xvii). Springer.

Menon, M. (2018). *Infinite variety: A history of desire in India*. Speaking Tiger.

Pilkey, B., Sciluna, R. M., Campkin, B., & Penner, B. (2017). Introduction. In B. Pilkey, R. M. Sciluna, B. Campkin, & B. Penner (Eds.), *Sexuality and gender at home: Experience, politics, transgression* (pp. 1–11). Bloomsbury.

Pradhan, A. (2020, January 28). Too gay an oreo!: The cultural connotations of queer(ing) food. *Café Dissensus, 52*. https://cafedissensus.com/2020/01/28/too-gay-an-oreo-the-cultural-connotations-of-queering-food/

Sareen, S. (2021). Food, love and the self in Indian women's poetry in English. In S. Malhotra, K. Sharma, & S. Dogra (Eds.), *Food culture studies in India: Consumption, representation and mediation* (pp. 49–58). Springer.

Szabo, M. (2017). Introduction. In M. Szabo & S. Koch (Eds.), *Food, masculinities, and home: Interdisciplinary perspectives* (pp. 17–51). Bloomsbury.

Vanita, R. (2014). Chaini, chocolate and pan: Food and homoerotic fiction. In S. Singh (Ed.), *Gay subcultures and literatures: The Indian projections* (pp. 153–164). Indian Institute of Advanced Study.

23 Not Ready Yet

Laura Bockus-Thorne

Artist Statement

"Not Ready Yet" is a mixed-medium art piece constructed from polymer clay, paint, wire, string, glue, and saran wrap. The artist chose these mediums to make the piece more vibrant and realistic through the use of a 3D format (Figure 23.1).

The fruit and vegetables arranged in a rainbow are the artist's expression of the intersection of LGBTQ+ and the field of dietetics. The butterflies whose wings represent different LGBTQ+ groups, signify how many LGBTQ+ people in the field of dietetics the author has met. At the bottom of the art piece is a chrysalis, still in its cocoon hanging below the fruits, vegetables, and butterflies. Even though the butterfly has not yet emerged to show its wings, through the cocoon we can see a swirl of colours.

The artist created this artwork as an expression of self; her own experiences with the intersection of LGBTQ+ and the field of dietetics. The scarcity of people being out about their identities, the prejudice she has seen in a typically conservative field (healthcare), have helped to contribute to a sense of "Not [being] Ready Yet," to be out about her own identification(s). Beyond this is an understanding towards others, who may not feel ready yet either.

DOI: 10.4324/9781003217121-25

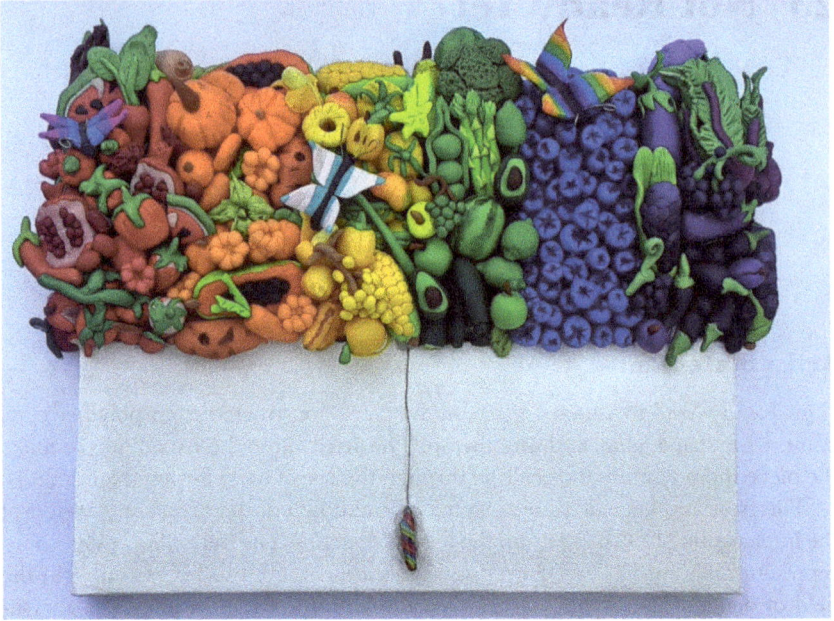

Figure 23.1 Not Ready Yet. Laura Bockus-Thorne.

24 Food, Consumption, and Queer Subjectivity in Contemporary American Cinema

Megan L. Wilson

The 21st century has seen unprecedented visibility for LGBTQ+ (lesbian, gay, bisexual, transgender, and queer) people in American cinema and television, proliferating discourse on the construction of sexual subjectivity on screen. The popularity of several widely released and critically acclaimed gay films in the last decade points to a growing cultural and economic value in LGBTQ+ identities and narratives. As such, same-sex desire and intimacy have become sutured to certain cultural markers in order to be made legible to mainstream audiences. This chapter examines how such desires and intimacies might surface on the screen through images of food and its consumption. As powerful cultural signifiers and sensuous objects, images of food solicit a range of senses from the observer beyond sight and sound, with sense memory opening up a two-way carnal dialogue between cinematic text and spectator. Whilst ostensibly very different narratives of gay male coming-of-age, two recent critically acclaimed films, *Moonlight* (Jenkins, 2016) and *Call Me by Your Name* (Guadagnino, 2017), share a similar access point to queer subjectivity: food. The infamy of the peach scene notwithstanding, both films offer a mode of textual address founded in the phenomenological capacity of food and eating scenes to communicate queer pleasure, community, and intimacy.

British baker and author Ruby Tandoh (2018) wrote an article, entitled "A Feast for the Eyes," on the vital role of food in LGBTQ film. Tandoh suggests that food can be representative of intimacy and nourishment that is desired by queer people, yet often forbidden or withheld due to their marginalized social status. Acts of cooking, sharing, and feeding have the potential to bring people together but can be a difficult matrix to navigate for those who do not find themselves welcome at every table. Tandoh's article makes way for a compelling study which suggests that the use of food as a sensory device in film can be traced as a paradigm within a larger range of contemporary queer films. Beyond acting as a prop, food in film takes on a phenomenological capacity, engaging our hungry, feeling bodies. In academia, critics have also written on the role of food and consumption in the formation of subjectivity, largely through lenses of culture, race, and sexuality. This area of study can be neatly summed up by the term "foodways," that is, "a critical lens that enhances the analysis of the personal and political dimensions of food," stressing its significance beyond mere sustenance (Baron et al., 2014, p. 16). The foodways lens puts

DOI: 10.4324/9781003217121-26

into more concrete theoretical terms what Tandoh began to explore in her article, that "eating might nourish us – that mashing of food in teeth and gums – but it's in feeding that we get a taste of the relationship we have with the world and with the people around us," (Tandoh, 2018). For queer people, such relationships are inherently challenged by heteronormative and homophobic societies, which exclude and even outlaw non-normative social and sexual practices. Even the title of Tandoh's article lends itself to a more phenomenological reading of the films therein, suggesting that our eyes may feast upon an image, and perhaps even taste it.

Laura Marks, writing on "The Memory of the Senses" in intercultural cinema in her book *The Skin of Film*, states that

> I will argue that the senses are a source of social knowledge [...] I will point out that the organisation of the senses, that is, the sensorium, varies culturally as well as individually; thus we would expect cinema to represent the sensorial organisation of a given culture
>
> (Marks, 2000, p. 195).

In this way, the senses become indicative of both a personal and collective experience of the culture and ideology which has informed them. This demonstrates that though senses like touch and taste are embodied and considered primal, the experience of and response to our senses are equally learned, as "sense organs are the sites where culture crosses the body," (Marks, 2000, p. 201). At this juncture we can see where food and consumption in film come into play, as food as an object and eating as an activity comes into direct contact with bodily senses such as taste, touch, and smell. Phenomenology has a largely feminist tendency in its understanding of embodiment, as "feminist phenomenological film theory turns to the bodily sensations we experience in responses to cinema, arguing that these have the potential to destabilize dominant ways of understanding cinema's cultural and subjective effects," (Stephens, 2012, p. 530). Indeed, traditional scholarship on spectatorship in film has suggested that the act of looking is imbued with an irrevocable heteropatriarchal subjectivity, a theory first suggested by Laura Mulvey (1975). Therefore, we might look to other senses and ways of experiencing film in order to explore queer subjectivities as subordinate to these traditional concepts of spectatorship. Marks emphasized the importance of sense memory in the representation of minority subjectivity, as "these memories are especially crucial as repositories of knowledge for people whose experience is not represented in the dominant society," (Marks, 2000, p. 199). From this, we might consider that when the experiences of a certain social or cultural group have not been privileged by society to be preserved in text, other means of recording and communication must pass on these experiences.

Communal Eating and Queer Kinship in *Moonlight*

In *Moonlight*, a 2016 American drama film, protagonist Chiron's relationship to his queer desire is copulated with his relationship to eating and those who nourish him throughout his life. The film focuses on the coming-of-age of the young Black boy, who realizes during adolescence that he is gay. The narrative is divided into thirds, chronologically depicting Chiron as a child, teenager, and then young adult living in Miami, Florida. Chiron's gay identity is a continual source of tension throughout the narrative, as he struggles to find healthy ways to communicate his desires in a repressive home environment which does not nurture him physically or emotionally. An intrinsic focus in the film is Chiron's bond with his non-biological father figure, a drug dealer named Juan, who takes Chiron under his wing, and later, his romantic relationship with his childhood friend, Kevin. An essential foundation of these relationships is feeding, and the associated sensations of physical nourishment that formulate "a gateway to trust and familiarity" (Leszkiewicz, 2018). The film's climactic love scene is not a sexual one, but an intimate meal prepared by one man for another. *Moonlight*'s narrative resolution rests on the assurance that Chiron is not only sexually fulfilled, but tenderly nourished by another man.

The first scene in which Chiron appears is a great example of the importance of eating and nutrition in the child's experience of found family and acceptance. The scene begins with Chiron being chased by other children, who force him to hide in an abandoned apartment littered with drug paraphernalia whilst they beat on the door. A terrified Chiron is discovered there by a strange man, who introduced himself as Juan. Chiron does not reply verbally but leaves with Juan when invited to get something to eat. We transition from drug den to diner, where Juan and Chiron sit opposite one another. Juan has bought the boy a meal, placed in front of him on a tray. The spatial evolution from the bare, dingy drug den to the bright, spacious restaurant represents a shift from a space of drug consumption to one of food consumption. The colour palette of the diner scene is drastically different; high-key lighting and soft reds dominate the frame as the camera slowly tracks forwards into a two-shot, framing Juan and Chiron at the table (Figure 24.1).

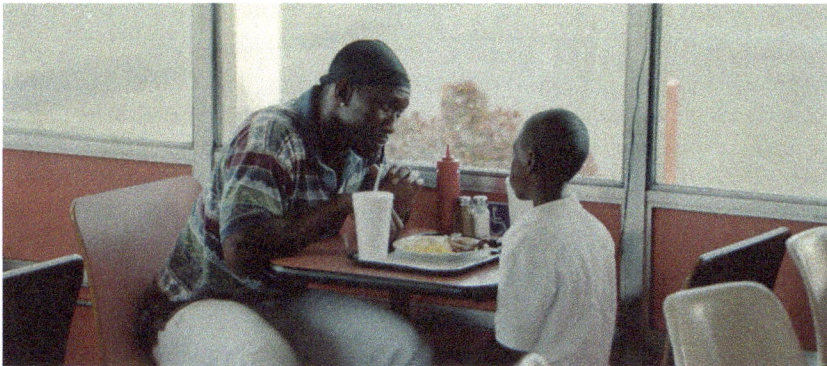

Figure 24.1 Juan and Chiron at the diner. Source: Jenkins, B. (Director). (2016). *Moonlight* [Film]. A24; Pastel Productions; Plan B Entertainment. Format: Prime Video (streaming online video).

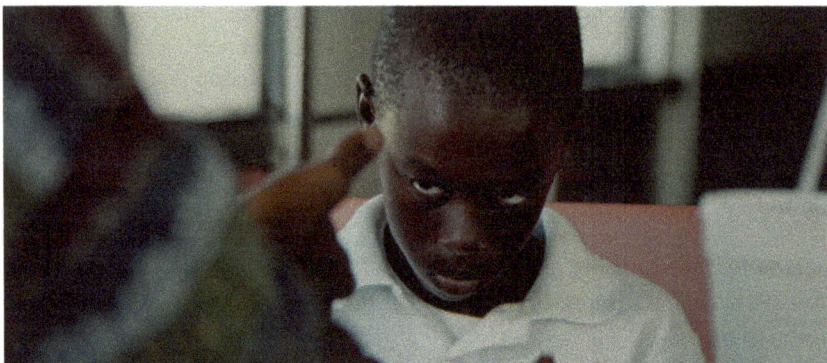

Figure 24.2 Close-up of Chiron at the diner. Source: Jenkins, B. (Director). (2016). *Moonlight* [Film]. A24; Pastel Productions; Plan B Entertainment. Format: Prime Video (streaming online video).

The warmth of the colouring emphasizes the homey atmosphere of the restaurant and evokes the flavour of the hearty meal that Chiron so fervently shovels into his mouth. The frenzied action suggests Chiron's vulnerability, as if he is afraid that the meal will be taken from him. Thus, when Juan pulls the plate away from Chiron to coax him into conversation, the shot cuts to a close-up of Chiron (Figure 24.2), the editing implying a severance in their potential connection. The boy looks down with a dejected expression, clearly betrayed. Juan realizes his mistake, returning the plate and joking "you know I wouldn't do you like that," realizing the significance of the meal in gaining the boy's trust.

Chiron learns through this encounter that Juan is not going to punish him but is in fact trying to take care of him. Writing on food and the body, theorist Carole M. Counihan suggests that "precisely because eating and intercourse involve intimacy, they can be dangerous or threatening when carried out under adverse conditions or with untrustworthy people" (Counihan, 1999, p. 10). As such, it is revealing that the film uses this eating scene as a narrative device to indicate a change in Chiron's psyche; in accepting the meal from Juan, Chiron opens himself up to vulnerability. We do not see Chiron eating with his biological mother at any point in the film; the only thing that she alludes to consuming is drugs, which is one of the reasons for the breakdown in her relationship with her son. Instead, the dinner table at Juan's house becomes a space around which Juan and his girlfriend Teresa establish an alternative, nurturing family model for Chiron. This example of kinship is formative in Chiron's coming-of-age, as Juan and Teresa offer an accepting, loving father and mother figure who provide him with not only food, but emotional support. It is no coincidence, then, that the dinner table is the first place where Chiron vocalizes an awareness of his otherness to Juan and Teresa, having been called a "faggot" by another child. Chiron's queer subjectivity is anchored by the table and the queer family model he has established around it, giving him access to love and sustenance from his nurturing parental figures.

Food consumption takes on a more significant phenomenological capacity by the third act of the film, when Chiron is a grown man. After some years in prison, he returns to Miami to visit the man with whom he had his first sexual encounter as a teenager. Kevin now works in a restaurant, and Chiron visits him whilst he works an evening shift. The fact that the men's reunion takes place in a dining space is suggestive of the nurturing and nourishing nature of Chiron and Kevin's relationship – something that the spectator only sees replicated by Juan during Chiron's childhood. Upon their reunion, Kevin offers Chiron a meal – either from the menu, or the "chef's special." There is an implicit understanding that by choosing the special, Chiron is accepting a far more intimate gesture. The scene transitions to the kitchen as Kevin prepares the meal, and the cinematic rendering of the space is deeply romantic. In contrast to the bright, clinical space expected of a commercial kitchen, Kevin's workspace is dark and intimate; warm light bathes the countertops and casts Kevin in a silhouette as he handles the food slowly and carefully (Figure 24.3). The hand-held camera travels across the workspace like a wandering eye, closely framing Kevin's hands as he makes steady movements (Figure 24.4). The squeezing of a lemon and chopping of coriander have an aromatic sensuality to them; though the dish is simple, it incorporates strong, traditional flavours. The combination of soft focus and the rousing, deep string score emphasize slowness and the importance of preparation that make this meal so significant.

Gaye Poole suggests in *Reel Meals* that "because the preparation of food requires thought, labour, time, and in some cases love, it is an ideal conduit for emotional language. It is possible to 'say' things with food – resentment, love, compensation, anger, rebellion, withdrawal." (Poole, 1999, p. 3). Given that this is the only scene of detailed food preparation in the film, it solicits a sensual, fulfilling effect from the spectator, as the narrative has so far lacked this nourishing attention to detail. The spectator is able to feel, through their phenomenological realization, not only the emotional impact of Kevin's cooking for Chiron but its significance in the re-establishment of their kinship. As such, *Moonlight* demonstrates how Chiron's

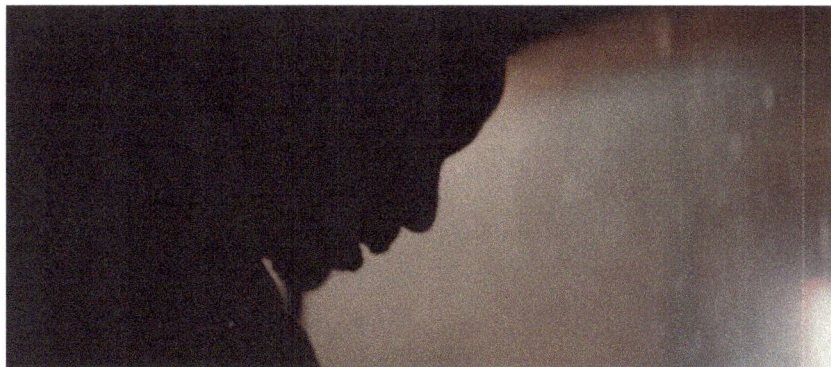

Figure 24.3 Kevin's silhouette in the kitchen. Source: Jenkins, B. (Director). (2016). *Moonlight* [Film]. A24; Pastel Productions; Plan B Entertainment. Format: Prime Video (streaming online video).

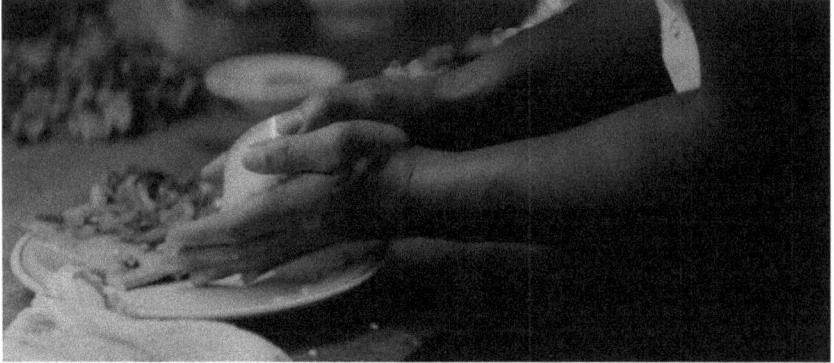

Figure 24.4 Kevin prepares the "chef's special." Source: Jenkins, B. (Director). (2016). *Moonlight* [Film]. A24; Pastel Productions; Plan B Entertainment. Format: Prime Video (streaming online video).

subjectivity as a gay man is structured by the nourishment he receives (or does not receive) from other people. Where he begins as a frightened, lonely child unsure of his place in a hypermasculine, heteronormative society, Chiron learns to accept love and sustenance from those outside of his biological family, communicated sensually through his relationship to food. The preparation and serving of a meal show Chiron how to accept affection from other men, something he admits he has never done since he and Kevin had their only sexual encounter. The intimate shared meal represents a form of love and betterment that can be explored in a safer and more protected environment than sex, allowing Chiron to confront his insecurities and reveal himself as vulnerable to Kevin.

Moonlight offers just one example of how communal eating plays a crucial part in contemporary queer subjectivity. Aside from the brief sexual encounter between Kevin and Chiron in their youth, *Moonlight* does not feature explicit gay sex, nor is this necessarily the main concern of the characters. As such, the film lends itself to Elspeth Probyn's argument that "queer theory needs to relinquish its dependence on sexuality as the sole optic of analysis," and instead examines how queerness inflects subjectivity beyond sex, particularly with regards to kinship (Probyn, 1999, p. 423). As I have argued in the case of Jenkins's film, foodways and sense memory form a subtle but integral part of the queer narrative, allowing for a more embodied experience of queer subjectivity as a continuum for the spectator, regardless of their own sexual identity.

Food, Desire, and Queer Sexual Fantasy in *Call Me by Your Name*

Another, more recent, example of popular American cinema that shows an explicit gay relationship is *Call Me by Your Name* (2017). The film's subject is the 17-year-old Elio Perlman, an American living in Italy with his parents. During the summer, an older man named Oliver comes to stay at the house as an intern, assisting Elio's father, a professor. After initial hostility and a clashing of personalities, Elio and Oliver embark on a secret sexual relationship that catalyzes Elio's coming-of-age. Although the film explores same-sex desire more explicitly than *Moonlight*, Elio's subjectivity as the protagonist is still impacted by his somewhat troubled relationship to his sexuality, compounded by shame and secrecy despite his liberal upbringing. This can be identified through the use of eating and the associated sensations that suggests fundamental differences in Elio and Oliver's subjective experiences as queer men. As in *Moonlight*, communal eating is a significant occurrence throughout the narrative in *Call Me by Your Name*. As well as contributing to the idyllic atmosphere of the rural Italian home, it establishes the close bond of the Perlman family, and the shift that Oliver's arrival triggers. During Oliver's first breakfast with the family, he clumsily smashes a boiled egg when trying to remove the delicate shell and proceeds to eat it sloppily, oozing yolk. Oliver is established as having a great appetite, which translates to eagerness and an unselfconscious disposition that, at first, irks Elio. It is also suggestive of the concept of the sexual appetite; indeed, it is Oliver that takes on the more dominant, assertive role in the men's subsequent relationship, whilst Elio's position as an emerging queer subject is much more uncertain.

Later in the narrative, after the eventual consummation of Elio and Oliver's relationship, Elio is lying alone on a mattress in a secret hideout which he earlier used to have sex with his girlfriend, Marzia. He is eating peaches, picked from the trees on the Perlman's land, which are ripe and juicy. After a moment of contemplation, Elio hollows out the peach with his finger, spilling juice all over himself (Figure 24.5). He then uses it to masturbate. This action occurs in a long take,

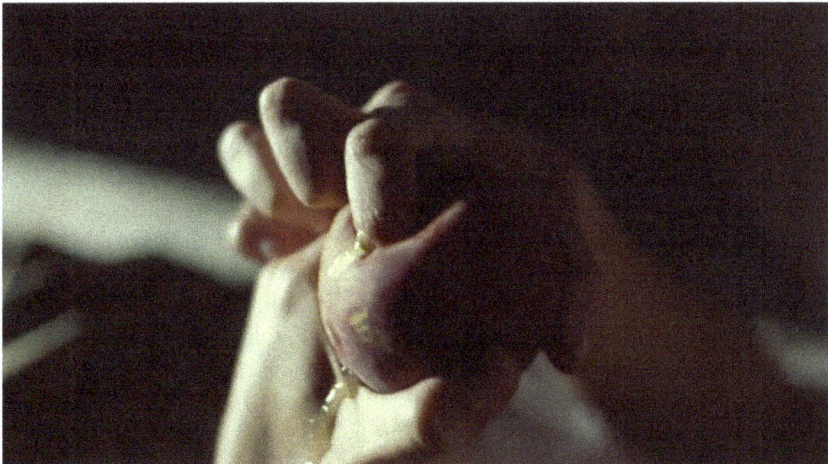

Figure 24.5 Elio punctures the peach. Source: Guadagnino, L. (Director). (2017). *Call Me by Your Name* [Film]. Lá Cinefracture; Frenesy Film Company; RT Features. Format: Prime Video (streaming online video).

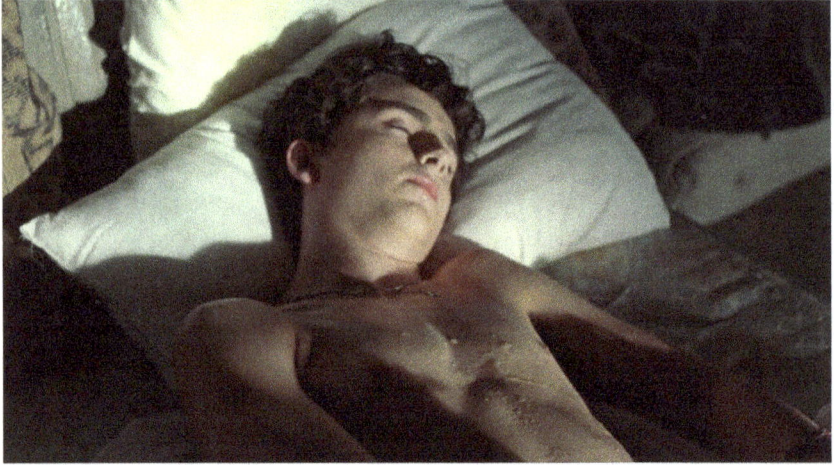

Figure 24.6 Elio masturbates with the peach. Source: Guadagnino, L. (Director). (2017). *Call Me by Your Name* [Film]. Lá Cinefracture; Frenesy Film Company; RT Features. Format: Prime Video (streaming online video).

emphasizing the sensual intensity of the moment as Elio reaches climax, filling the peach with semen (Figure 24.6). There is also a lack of non-diegetic score, which intensifies the sounds of the sticky fruit and Elio's heavy breathing. The sensuality is intensified by the summer heat and Elio's bare, juice-drenched chest, regarded in close-up by the camera's gaze. Elio's sexual exploration with the peach extends his bodily experience outwards, engaging with multiple senses and encouraging the spectator to dually experience the tactile pleasure. In terms of phenomenology, Marks suggests that "fetish objects are used to extend bodily experience into memory," and in this way, the peach acts as a "prosthesis for memory," (Marks, 2000, p. 201). As such, Elio is able to fantasize about his sexual encounters with Oliver and use the similar sensations to explore and physicalize his queer sexuality in private.

A similar effect is also elicited earlier in the film when Elio trespasses in Oliver's bedroom, and puts Oliver's worn swimming shorts over his head, breathing in his scent. Through these fetish objects, Elio's queer desire for Oliver is accentuated by his experiences of smell and taste, which is then communicated to the audience via sense memory. After Elio finishes with the peach, Oliver enters the room and begins to pleasure Elio with his mouth, where he inevitably tastes the residue of the peach. Realizing what Elio has done, Oliver takes the peach and attempts to eat it, but Elio is embarrassed, thinking he is "sick." By contrast, Oliver is amused by Elio's actions, and is clearly aroused by the idea. Here, the difference in queer subjectivity between Elio and Oliver is apparent, as Elio begins to cry, betraying his shame. This exchange is similarly framed in a particularly long take, and the continuing lack of score emphasizes the intense bodily focus of the scene. For Oliver, the peach is a part of sexual play, but Elio evidently harbours anxiety regarding his queer sexuality, which he has realized through his defilement of the fruit. This scene is an example of how a phenomenological foodways lens in particular can be a window into a queer character's interior feelings and sexual desires, as "the links between food taboos and sexual taboos make foodways analysis a useful means for exploring representations of sexual identities." (Baron et al., 2014, p. 239). As such, it can be seen how the foodways lens particularly lends itself to subversive readings of gay and lesbian films, where any romantic or sexual activity is already more charged with tension and illicitness due to the persistence of homophobia. *Call Me by Your Name* explores the interior anxiety of the queer subject, whilst also externalizing this through explicit sexual encounters, which demonstrates a shift in attitudes in mainstream filmmaking. For a gay and lesbian audience, it provides a more complex and full-bodied exploration of queer subjectivity which allows for the experience of a multiple interplaying senses. Meanwhile, the film also provides an access point for heterosexual audiences in that the sensory associations made by the peach scene are such that in theory, any person, regardless of sexual orientation, can experience similar sensations and find themselves engaging (if not quite identifying) with the queer subject.

Final Thoughts

Throughout this chapter, I have aimed to construct a theoretical and analytical model that allows us to explore contemporary films in a way that transfers and displaces same-sex desire and intimacy from the body as the sole basis of sexual figuration on screen. *Moonlight* and *Call Me by Your Name* both make compelling case studies in the advancement of queer foodways, respectively demonstrating how both positive and negative queer effects can be produced from image sequences centred on communal eating and food-centred sexual play. The result of this study has been rewarding in exploring new ideas about meaning-making and subjectivity in LGBTQ+ films, electing to distance these ideas from the physical body and instead externalize them through food as object and consumption as activity. Though this is not unique to gay and lesbian films – heterosexual desire may be similarly represented – I maintain that the consumptive embodiment of desire speaks to queerness in a way that captures both the abjection and illicit indulgence that many queer people face when realizing their sexuality.

I intend my analysis to lend itself to further potential research to expand the scope of this paradigm beyond Hollywood, perhaps by looking further back into cinema's history to locate the possible origins. One way to do this would be to examine other contemporary national cinemas and identify how LGBTQ+ narratives entwine with foodways and phenomenology, particularly when food and consumption are inevitably entrenched in different economic and cultural value systems. A recent example that engages with queer kinship through food production and consumption is the German Israeli film *The Cakemaker* (Grazier, 2017). A German baker, Thomas, has an affair with a married Israeli man, Oren, which ends abruptly when Oren is killed in an accident. Thomas travels to Jerusalem and finds Oren's wife, Anat, in the café she runs, where he secures a job in the kitchen. Thomas grows closer to Anat and her son, without revealing that he was Oren's lover. A strange kinship is formed between the three, with Anat unaware that she and Thomas are grieving the loss of the same man. Thomas and Anat make cultural exchanges through food preparation, as Thomas must learn the regulations of a kosher kitchen, and Anat grows fonder of Thomas after noticing his gift as a baker. In one scene, Thomas shows Oren and Anat's son, Itai, how to ice cookies. Close up, long takes of the boy's hands being guided by Thomas' as he draws with the icing bag convey the tenderness of the activity, emphasized by the soft focus of the camera. Within *The Cakemaker*, this sequence functions as an indication of the building emotional closeness of Thomas and Oren's son. Though Thomas is initially a stranger to Anat, their shared appreciation for food catalyzes their kinship, queered by their shared desire for Oren. This brief example demonstrates the potential of my theoretical approach to reach beyond popular cinema in the US, and to illuminate many cultural influences which contour queer desire and intimacy.

To return to Probyn's discussion of queer appetites, she asks: "Beyond sex, is there anything else that might differentiate a queer assembling of bodies, that recreates relationships to others, to selves, to the world differently?" (Probyn, 1999, p. 422). This chapter argues that yes, indeed, there are multiple affective and erotic registers through which same-sex desire and intimacy can be read in contemporary cinema. I argue for the usefulness of foodways in combination with feminist phenomenology as a framework for reading gay and lesbian films as they engage the spectator's senses to generate queer eroticism and bodily effects. Under this lens, *Moonlight* and *Call Me by Your Name* become much more nuanced figurations of homosexuality whereby the act of sex itself is not the sole visual register of sexual subjectivity.

References

Baron, C., Carson, D., & Bernard, M. (2014). *Appetites and anxieties: Food, film, and the politics of representation*. Wayne State University Press.

Counihan, C. M. (1999). *The anthropology of food and body: Gender, meaning, and power*. Routledge.

Graizer, O. R. (Director). (2017). *The cakemaker* [Film]. Film Base Berlin; Laila Films.

Guadagnino, L. (Director). (2017). *Call me by your name* [Film]. Lá Cinefracture; Frenesy Film Company; RT Features.

Jenkins, B. (Director). (2016). *Moonlight* [Film]. A24; Pastel Productions; Plan B Entertainment.

Leszkiewicz, A. (2018, April 20). The hand that feeds: How food scenes became the home of intimacy, sex and power in film. *New Statesman*, Culture. https://www.newstatesman.com/culture/film/2018/04/hand-feeds-how-food-scenes-became-home-intimacy-sex-and-power-film

Marks, L. U. (2000). *The skin of film: Intercultural cinema, embodiment, and the senses*. Duke University Press.

Mulvey, L. (1975). Visual pleasure and narrative cinema. *Screen, 16*(3), 6–18. https://doi.org/10.1093/screen/16.3.6

Poole, G. (1999). *Reel meals, set meals: Food in film and theatre*. Currency Press.

Probyn, E. (1999). An ethos with a bite: Queer appetites from sex to food. *Sexualities*, 2(4), 421–431.

Stephens, E. (2012). Sensation machine: Film, phenomenology, and the training of the senses. *Continuum*, *26*(4), 529–539. https://doi.org/10.1080/10304312.2012.698033

Tandoh, R. (2018, March 18). A feast for the eyes: Ruby Tandoh on food and film. *The Guardian*, Food. https://www.theguardian.com/lifeandstyle/2018/mar/18/food-and-film-ruby-tandoh-call-me-by-your-name-moonlight-tampopo

25 Have You Eaten Today?

David Ng and Jen Sungshine

The phrase "Have You Eaten Today?" is shared amongst many racialized communities, as a language-signifier of familial love and nourishment. As a group of queer artists of colour, Vancouver-based collective Love Intersections has employed this theme of diasporic food culture as a medium to explore intersectional and intergenerational stories of queer, trans, intersex, Black, and Indigenous people of colour (QTIBIPOC). Food-sharing and food cultures have been a medium for our approach as "social practice" artists – artists who use social exchange as the primary medium for art creation. We, as Co-Artistic Directors of Love Intersections' and artists of Chinese and Taiwanese descent who use arts for social change, were drawn to this theme. We were interested in thinking about the significance and role of food and food culture as a facilitator of social relations (Motta & Martín, 2021, p. 514), and as a medium to evoke the senses towards social change. In both our respective cultures and languages – 你食咗飯未呀 (Cantonese) and 你今天吃了嗎? (Mandarin) – this phrase, "Have You Eaten Today?", is often the first thing that our friends and family will say when they greet us, or when they pick up the phone. While the phrase is a common greeting, the semantic implications and cultural significance of food within our culture – as well as many other Black, Indigenous, people of colour (BIPOC) communities – resonated deeply with us, and we employed this theme throughout several of our projects as a metaphor for community nourishment and love. In this chapter, we explore the possibilities of food-based social arts practices, as a strategy of community care, and the implications of these gestures as a form of artistic resistance and resilience for queer people of colour who navigate white-centric systems in their communities.

The ways in which food is signified is entangled amongst broader systems of socio-political, cultural, and economic dynamics (Motta & Martín, 2021, p. 504). For example, access to food security is imbricated with experience of race, class, and gender. The food from racialized communities is often appropriated as markers of difference – for example, both of us share experiences of receiving xenophobic comments about "smelly" Chinese food. The role of food in racialized communities has deep implications towards identity, and for people with a diasporic experience, histories of movement of bodies is discursively entangled with the movement of food and language (Mintz, 2008).

DOI: 10.4324/9781003217121-27

The act of doing, replicating, and sharing of "traditional" food cultures has different meanings and significance for communities of colour in white-dominant societies. Werbner and Fumanti (2013) explore the notion of "mimesis" performed by people of colour, and the transformative power that practising and replicating traditions has for people with diasporic experiences: "what appears on the surface to be derivative and imitative, taken from elsewhere, engenders authentically felt cultural competences and a sense of ontological presence" (p. 149). The engendering of belonging, being, and identity that becomes heightened during the practice of traditions from people with a diasporic experience, has affirmative and transformative potential regarding cultural identity, in societies where racialized people are situated outside of the norm.

As (queer of colour) artists, we employed these themes of food-sharing amongst racially marginalized communities as a form of dialogical relational aesthetic, to intervene on dominant discourses of white supremacy within the queer community, through our art practice. Inspired by Tao Leigh Goffe's theorizing on "gastropoetics" vis-à-vis "the materiality of food as a sensorium to open alternative forms of knowledge production from the colonial archive" (Goffe, 2019, p. 31), this chapter explores a "queer of colour gastropoetics" of food-based practices that Love Intersections has utilized to cultivate community anti-racist transformation in Vancouver's queer landscape. In particular, we will reflect on our projects, *Diverse Appetites* (2015) and *Hot Pot Talks* (2021) that produced cultural dialogues on the intersections of food and diaspora, race, gender, and sexuality.

As a collective of queers of colour who use art for social change, we draw on "mimesis" (Werbner & Fumanti, 2013) as a strategy of community care, and also resistance and survival. In "Feeling Queer, Feeling Asian, Feeling Canadian," Kojima, Catungal, and Diaz (2017) argue that queer Asians face erasure on multiple fronts, existing on the periphery from white-dominant queer communities, while simultaneously occluded by heteronormativity within diasporic communities (p. 70). They argue that this convergence of marginalization, requires that we explore creative strategies of resisting formations of normativity, and that the operationalization of "queer," and what it "does," offers an array of possibilities in transforming systemic power (p. 70). These themes of mimesis, the role of "queering" in our arts practice, identity affirmation, and employing arts to foment social dialogues is an approach that stretches across many of our food-based projects, including the marketing and design work that we curate. For example, in Figure 25.1, the graphic for "Hot Pot Talks! Season 2" (by Annie Canto) includes food elements from our culture(s): napa cabbage, rice bowls, and ginger, and the Chinese calligraphy that reads "Have You Eaten Today?" was written by Jen's father. Infusing these cultural elements into our communications strategy allows us to triangulate our intention of queering dialogues on issues related to identity, ancestry, and family.

As artists that straddle social and community-based practices, the modality of the facilitation, and how our arts practice can engage the public, informs how we employ queer of colour food practices as a form of relational aesthetic. Bishop describes the complexity of the history of artists that fuse art and pedagogy, "while

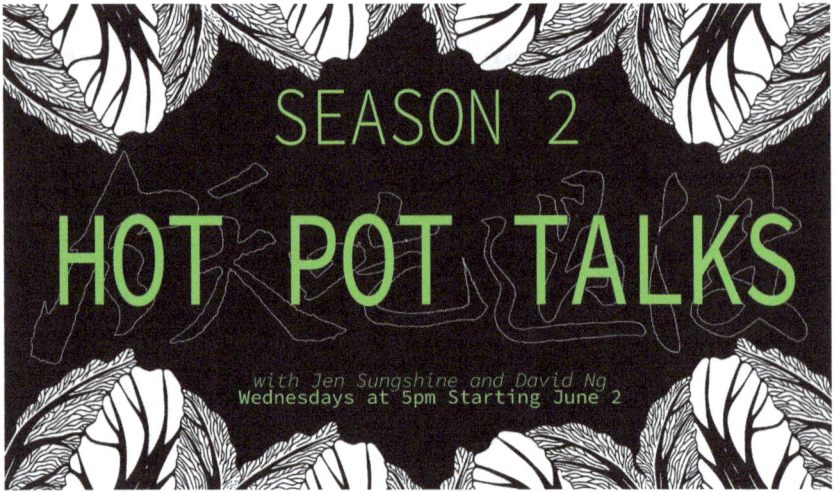

Figure 25.1 Hot Pot Talks Season 2. Annie Canto.

attempting to augment the intellectual content of relational conviviality" (Bishop, 2004, p. 241). Love Intersections' artistic practice is situated within this genealogy, where our pedagogical practice overlaps with our aesthetic inquiries. Drawing from popular education theory (Friere, Boal), and the approach of using publics as the form for cultural production, Love Intersections' food-as-art-practice approach has also adhered to this interrogation and the collapsing of the boundaries between arts practice/process and the public. Bishop's inquiry "How do you bring a classroom to life as if it were a work of art?" resonates with our own food-based arts practice; how can we bring to life the dialogical aesthetic of *Diverse Appetites* and *Hot Pot Talks*, as if it were a work of art? This interrogation of form, reflects some of the conflations of art, pedagogy, and performativity that our food practice falls into, contending with the possibilities of performing and making public diasporic food cultural traditions, as a conduit for community dialogue.

Diverse Appetites

After forming Love Intersections in 2014 on the premise of transforming systemic racism, one of the earliest debates about race and culture that we encountered was on the topic of cultural appropriation. Heightened conversations about cultural appropriation in and around Vancouver's queer and BIPOC communities became ever more present in online spaces where mainstream and subcultural practices in food, fashion, and even language were called into question. We witnessed arguments on social media erupting around different instances of cultural appropriation, with the rhetoric against cultural appropriation becoming a symbol of continued racial inequity. We found ourselves at the centre of these polarizing conversations while pulled into simplified definitions of cultural appropriation, delimited by the technology of social media platforms. Online conversations became just that, limiting and simplified: your "exhibition" of culture is either appropriation or not. Of course, real life and deep, relational understandings of food and "our" culture exist in between a layered continuum that is elastic through time and history, and undeniably messy.

Through a series of video work produced under the title, *Diverse Appetites* (2015), we began seeking what decolonial artists and art practitioners call "ways of doing otherwise," for example, evoking the senses: the visual, the smell, sound, feeling, as a way of gesturing towards transformative possibilities (Rojas-Sotelo, 2014). Thinking through a decolonial aesthetics lens, we embarked upon a six-month project timeline eating, filming, talking, and diving into the ethics of food-based cultural exchange at the dinner table. We filmed participants preparing food, while they talked through their familial and cultural histories that turned single ingredients into multiple, storied dishes. Together we began theorizing on, and employing food, as a medium to *think, feel,* and *digest,* about cultural appropriation outside of dialogue or debate.

In "What is (the Wrong of) Cultural Appropriation?" Lenard and Balint (2020) discuss the complexities of discourse on cultural appropriation, and the forms of cultural misrepresentation and offence that are often confused with it (p. 346). By unpacking different formations of "cultural appropriation," they suggest that contextual conditions can amplify the harm caused by cultural appropriation, including power imbalances, absence of consent, and profit that the appropriator accrues (p. 331). They argue that while social media debates and "call-outs" of cultural appropriation reflect persisting historical (racial) injustices, there is a gap in public discussions on the topic regarding the role of cultural interaction and exchange when communities of different cultures encounter each other. As an organization founded upon a mandate to do anti-racist work through building communities instead of building barriers, we were drawn to the complexity of the cultural appropriation debates – as a formation that emerged due to conditions of racial inequality. We had many conversations about what accounted for "cultural appropriation;" from the most egregious forms, such as selling (and wearing) Indigenous warbonnets as music festival attire, wearing Black face as a Halloween costume, to The Mahjong Line – where a group of white women redesigned the traditional Chinese game Mahjong, and marketed their product based on critiques of the Chinese symbols and characters that appear on the original game tiles; to the debates around appropriating food – such as Lucky Lee's restaurant in New York, where a white Jewish woman marketed her Chinese restaurant as a health alternative to (what was implied as unhealthy) Chinese food. While cultural exchanges happen in communities all the time and are documented throughout history – from the Chinese influence of noodles, to Indian spices, to cocoa, coffee; the question of when one culture encounters a dominant culture, and when "appropriation" debates emerge, is rooted in the power dynamics that underpin systems of racial dominance and asymmetry.

As a collective, we were curious as to the possibilities of cultural exchange: what constitutes cultural appropriation, and when is cultural exchange ethical? After a conversation about food and the historical exchanges that have allowed for the fusing of different cultures and cuisines that have produced hybrid – and delicious – foods, we also wanted to explore the potential that the act of food making, food-sharing, eating, and digesting food could have on this conversation on cultural appropriation. We wanted to incorporate our shared love for experiencing food cultures through the senses within this exploration on the complexity of the cultural appropriation debates. What potential does food have in infusing, fermenting, and facilitating a form of "digesting" of these conversations on cultural appropriation and cultural exchange? Working with the tangible materiality of ingredients creating an opening to talk about the intangible, the very *values* that underpin each dish. It is the exchange of *values* through the act of sharing: "In the [cultural] exchange, it's not just about the superficial, tangible thing. One thing Canada is pretty good at is exchanging the tangible: food, outfits, music. We can talk about that. But what we're not very good at [talking about] is the values underneath. So it's not just, when you go for dim sum, you knock your hand. It's "you knock your hand *because*, and so we're sharing the values, the *why*" (Shopland in Love Intersections, 2016). "Knocking your hand" on the table is a common gesture that represents "Thank you" when someone pours you tea. The legend is that a Chinese emperor wanted to go out to visit his subjects in disguise, and so when he went to eat with his bodyguards, in order to maintain discretion, the "knocking on the table" was devised by the bodyguards to thank the emperor whenever he poured tea for them, as a symbol of bowing or kneeling in gratitude.

In one *Diverse Appetites* video, Jane recreated her mom's Ghanian plantain and beans recipe, and describes the dish as "home" and coming to home:

> This is something that is like a home to you almost, food is like where you find comfort like your home. I like that kind of exchange, so when you're dealing with food there's way more opportunity to do that - so I like starting with food, and then bringing people in understanding. (Love Intersections, 2016)

The dialogue in the clip reflects notions of mimesis, and sensorial identity experience, that through the medium of the food-sharing, and the dialogical process, the video offers an insight into discursive nuances that are embedded in a cross-cultural encounter. In another video, David talks about his passion for sharing the ceremonial aspects of Chinese food culture, and the underpinning ethico-ontological layers of his Chinese heritage, that is an important cultural value in his life. In both videos, food practices are deployed to elicit embodied and sensorial aspects of food practices – to ferment a dialogical aesthetic that queers polarizing debates on the identity politics of cultural appropriation.

The nexus of the complexities in debates around cultural appropriation – cultural values, racial power, colonialism – inspired our journey in grappling with the nuances and the discomforts of the cultural exchange vs appropriation debates, while contending with our own discursive instability regarding what we did not know (regarding the ethical parameters of cultural encounters), and what we were trying to make knowable. The notion of eating and digestion argued by Hrorch (in Loveless, 2020), offer several tools to analyze the discursive possibilities offered by food practices in *Diverse Appetites*. Hrorch suggests that the process of digestion occurs at multiple scales; when we attend to the biological transformations that happen while we "digest," we are digested as we digest (p. 34). Metabolization, decay, and flow occur simultaneously on multiple scales, suggesting that the transformations of materiality into energy are intertwined through the process of digestion (p. 34). In their racial analyses of the colonial archive, Tompkins contends with the notion of "eating" in historical texts, where the act of eating produces political subjects through the process of fusing the social with the biological (p. 1). Hrorch and Tompkins's notions of digestion and eating illuminate the discursive possibilities of food practices as a political act; as a mode of interrogating the colonial archive, and an instrument to contend with emergent modes of knowing and unknowing (Hrorch in Loveless, 2020).

If the production of a narrative of who is eating and who is being eaten can foment and reinforce racial hierarchy (Tompkins, 2012), what opportunities does the act of food sharing and eating offer as a practice, regarding intervening in systems of oppressive power? *Diverse Appetites* became a conduit for us to employ this literal and metaphoric act of digesting, as a process to grapple with our own discursive instability regarding the debates on cultural appropriation and cultural exchange, while practicing acts of embodying "digestion" and "sharing" of discourse. As discussed previously, the social practice of eating is loaded with the practice of delineating difference and distinguishing between social group formations – the practice of eating has political and material implications (p. 4). Drawing from Judith Butler in *Bodies That Matter*, Tompkins explores "how the act of eating dissolves the boundary between self and other, between subject and object" (p. 4), contending that the process of materialization of the body is a discursive process, entangled within systems of power.

Diverse Appetites was a medium for us to journey through these aforementioned themes, starting with mimesis, and the act of replicating and practicing our own diasporic cultures, creating a space where we could engage with our own cultural identities. The dialogical process of food sharing, coupled with convivial conversation, allowed us to have a conversation on the nuances of cultural exchange and appropriation. Through the project, we recognized how the cultivation of care, and the nurturing of relationships and trust, plays a role in the possibilities of cultural exchange. This concept is not new – "breaking bread together" and "family style" eating, for example, are other formations in which "food-sharing" is a symbol of communing together, or an invitation to a deeper, embodied engagement. While the act of sharing food on its own does not necessarily transform systemic inequity, the act of sharing food can be a conduit for building relationships that open up safer spaces for cross-cultural exchange – which offers a foundation for building community instead of building barriers.

Hot Pot Talks

What started out as a response to the social and community isolation brought upon by a global pandemic, *Hot Pot Talks* (2021) became more than a virtual talk show series and conversational hot spot. Within the free-flowing conversations with artists, activists, chefs, performers, poets, intellectuals, and community organizers, we met each guest at the philosophical nexus between art, activism, and cultural production. *Hot Pot Talks* employed the image of the "hot pot" – a style of meal sharing that involves a simmering pot of soup stock that sits in the middle of the table where the raw ingredients are cooked throughout the duration of the meal – as a metaphor for community dialogue, nourishment, and cultural sharing. The aesthetic of *Hot Pot Talks* employs notions of "queer sensibility," referencing Isherwood, Greene, and Munoz's theorizing on the possibilities of envisioning and imagining, versus conforming and homogeneity – which are core strategies for survival for queer and other marginalized communities (Isherwood, 2020, p. 230). *Hot Pot Talks* attempts "to queer" normative systems and categories – of art, theory, activism, grassroots, academia, performance – through conflating and interrogating these boundaries through the virtual metaphor of the hot pot. Governed by this queer sensibility, our conversations stayed and strayed on topics ranging from anti-Asian racism, BIPOC futurity, Chinatown solidarity, diasporic food cultures, and interrogating the boundaries between everyday activism, "fine art," and cultural work.

Notions of intimacy and pleasure as a strategy of relationship-building for queers of colour, were also themes that underpinned *Hot Pot Talks* and *Diverse Appetites*. This intimate notion of *feeling queer* in Kojima, Catungal, and Diaz's introduction chapter in *QUEER/ASIAN/CANADIAN*, offer generative tools for us to examine and explore queerness. They argue for the political potential of "seeking pleasure" as a form of queer of colour (and in particular, queer Asian Canadian) critique. They suggest that the possibilities of pleasure as queer of colour resistance and critique can stem "from the pursuit of intimate relations, from the performance of multiple acts of resistance, or from animating diverse creative practices" (p. 76), the latter forming the intimate basis of *Hot Pot Talks*. The lure of *Hot Pot Talks* stems from turning the lens on ourselves as we "perform" conversations with guests that draw viewers into the intimacy of our living rooms and minds. Employing this notion of "pleasure," the hosting of *Hot Pot Talks* was predicated on a relational conviviality, with the food practice of the hot pot operating as a facilitation tool to invoke taste-pleasures, while cultivating a friendly/convivial conversation with our guests.

We witness these intimate moments across multiple episodes of *Hot Pot Talks* as we serve each guest with one consistent question throughout the series: "what is your favourite hot pot ingredient or experience?" A simple question on the virtual platter unlocked the sensorium of memory, nostalgia, family tradition, and cultural practices, and anchored each episode around the guests' own unique story. From Kai Cheng Thom's description of napa cabbage and its texture and versatility in kimchi, slaw, stews, and soups, to Chiyi Tam's father eating hot pot in

×30°C weather with open doors and windows in Winnipeg, to Tao Leigh Goffe describing her inaugural hot pot experience:

> I was there with my mother and sister. It was my first time visiting Asia … I just remember that first hot pot experience … These two older women, we didn't know what we were doing [but] they set it up for us. We didn't speak the language of course and I think food is just this language where you're able to learn and also have this kind of acrobatics of dancing with the noodles. Just incredible.
>
> Goffe

The images conjured by each guest were steeped in history, story, relationality – oscillating between personal, political, and theoretical.

For Love Intersections, employing food practices has been a tool to tap into multiscalar, embodied dialogues of identity, culture, politics, and social justice. Thinking about and employing food as an arts practice, food as a medium for brewing social bonds, food as a dialogical aesthetic, and food as ceremony, has been a vessel in which Love Intersections has cultivated difficult, nuanced, pleasurable, convivial conversations. As artists, utilizing diasporic food discourse as a queer practice, and reflecting on the significance of food practices in communities of colour has been a method of facilitating relational dialogues towards envisioning just futures. This dialogical and literal act of "sharing" nutrition, warmth, and care is a practice that is not only our activist ethos but is also our philosophical approach to artmaking: relationships, collaboration, and building communities instead of building barriers, preferably on a full stomach. And so, we end this chapter with the question that started it all, *Have you eaten today?*

References

Bishop, C. (2004). Antagonism and relational aesthetics. *October, 110*, 51–79.

Goffe, T. L. (2019). Sugarwork: The gastropoetics of Afro-Asia after the plantation. *Asian Diasporic Visual Cultures and the Americas, 5*(1–2), 31–56.

Isherwood, M. (2020). Toward a queer aesthetic sensibility: Orientation, disposition, and desire. *Studies in Art Education, 61*(3), 230–239.

Kojima, D., Catungal, J. P., & Diaz, R. (2017). Introduction: Feeling queer, feeling asian, feeling Canadian. *Topia (Montreal), 38*, 69–80.

Lenard, P. T., & Balint, P. (2020). What is (the wrong of) cultural appropriation? *Ethnicities, 20*(2), 331–352.

Love Intersections. (2016, July 15). *Diverse appetites: Andrew and Jen* https://www.youtube.com/watch?v=o0hGK1IRSfk

Loveless, L. (2020). *Knowings & knots: Methodologies and ecologies in research-creation.* (1st ed.). Canadian Electronic Library, University of Alberta Press.

Mintz, S. (2008). Food and diaspora. *Food, Culture & Society, 11*(4), 509–523.

Motta, R., & Martín, E. (2021). Food and social change: Culinary elites, contested technologies, food movements and embodied social change in food practices. *The Sociological Review, 69*(3), 503–519.

Rojas-Sotelo, M. (2014). Decolonizing aesthetics. *Encyclopedia of Aesthetics*, *2*, 300–304.

Tompkins, K. W. (2012). *Racial indigestion: Eating bodies in the 19th century*. New York University Press.

Werbner, P. and Fumanti, M. (2013). The aesthetics of diaspora: Ownership and appropriation. *Ethnos*, *78*(2), 149–174.

26 Food as Cultural and Body Shame

Experiences of an Ethnic Sexual Minority Emerging Adult

Enoch Leung

Though food choices are thought of primarily through health or taste, food is also related with the social context in which the food is connected with the individual's social identity (Higgs & Thomas, 2016). Through the lens of social identity, food choice can be understood as a social construct and central to our identities. Social identity theory posits how individuals come to develop a sense of self based on features of the social groups that are salient to them (Stets & Burke, 2000). One aspect relevant to social identity in schools is food choices. Food can be an approach where adolescents can express their belonging to their social group. Grounded in social identity theory places food choice and practice as an artifact to an individual's social identity. In schools where adolescents can be stigmatized for being outside of the socially created school norms, adolescents can be marked as different or similar via their food choices.

Food choices are also influenced by pressure on physical appearances, particularly for adolescents who are increasingly aware of such sociocultural pressures making this developmental period at risk for body dissatisfaction and disordered eating (Romito et al., 2021). Both sexual- and gender-minority adolescents were found to have a higher prevalence of unhealthy eating practices to control their weight (McClain & Peebles, 2016). As there are limited studies looking at the food eating practices and experiences for lesbian, gay, bisexual, transgender, and queer-youth of colour (LGBTQ+-YOC), this chapter draws upon an autoethnographic perspective (O'Hara, 2018) through my adolescence and emerging adulthood (12 to 25 years old) as a gay Chinese Canadian emerging adult. The purpose of this chapter is to examine the way food can be understood as both an influence on one's social identity and physical and psychological wellbeing through culture and sexuality.

Food in Schools

Food as Social Construct

Adolescents often use food to explore and construct their social identities, as well as use food as a vessel to build relationships with their peers. Schools are

DOI: 10.4324/9781003217121-28

an important context for food socialization. The sharing of food in schools can promote the feeling of belongingness to a particular ethnic culture. Previous studies have shown mixed experiences of students' use of food socialization. Nukaga (2008) observed that food was a cultural material that students used to form positive relationships with their peers, often showing pride in their homemade ethnic lunches. In Ludvigsen and Scott's (2009) study where adolescents were ridiculed, a 15-year-old girl mentioned the following experience about an Asian adolescent:

> He used to sit there and cry ... He used to have chicken legs that his mum would have cooked and he would eat like three of them and everyone used to call him "chicken boy" because he would have chicken every day for lunch.
>
> (Ludvigsen & Scott, 2009, p. 428)

As seen by the experiences above, having cultural food for school lunches can act as both a strong, positive connection to adolescents' cultural belonging and opportunities for victimization due to non-normative food choices.

Food as Diet and Physical Appearance

It is well documented that food health is an issue for LGBTQ+ adolescents. Compared to heterosexual adolescents, LGBTQ+ adolescents experience increased likelihood of eating disorders and disordered eating behaviours (e.g., fasting, diet pills, purging, binge eating, food addiction, other unhealthy weight control behaviours, Parker & Harriger, 2020). As this chapter is focused on sexual minority, specifically my experiences as a gay, Chinese Canadian adolescent, LGBTQ+ literature on food will focus on the perspectives of gay adolescents and men. Body dissatisfaction is at a higher percentage for gay adolescents, placing them at risk for unhealthy eating practices and disorders (McClain & Pebbles, 2016). Within the gay community, the focus on culturally defined ideal of body types based on categorical labels (e.g., twinks [thin, lean, stereotypically feminine body], bears [masculine, physically larger, hairy body], Ravenhill & de Visser, 2017) highlights the emphasis gay adolescents place in grooming their bodies to look a certain way. The push and pull of different body ideals places food choices as influential to the self-acceptance of gay identity.

Given that the adolescent developmental period is critical for sexual identity exploration, eating disorders or disordered eating behaviours may disproportionately affect gay youth (Kar et al., 2015). The food choices that gay adolescents make can be influenced by society's outlook on the appropriateness of various foods. For example, their food choices may lean towards restrictive, light food choices (e.g., lean chicken, salads) to model themselves closer to the "twink" stereotype. Therefore, gay adolescents in schools may choose to restrict their food intake during lunch and may skip their school lunch.

Autoethnography as a Gay Chinese Canadian Youth and Emerging Adult

Aligned with the literature surrounding food-sharing as a form of social bonding amongst peers in schools, I experienced mixed responses from my peers due to the differing social environments. During my early adolescent schooling in Hong Kong, from Grades 7 to 9 (2005–2007), it was common and appreciated to share various Asian lunches amongst peers, such as Korean kimbap, Japanese onigiri, or Chinese fried rice. I perceived a sense of belonging to my Chinese culture being in Hong Kong as a Chinese adolescent. However, aligned with research indicating negative food experiences by ethnic minority youth in schools (Ludvigsen & Scott, 2009), when I came to rural Ontario, Canada, for the remainder of my high school education, the reception of having Asian food for lunch was mixed from my peers. For example, I experienced both positive curiosity towards the Chinese fried rice and sautéed vegetables I brought for lunch, but also derogatory comments. For example, I would often hear the comment that I was eating "Chink" food. This made my lunch experiences less enjoyable, and I was more afraid of being victimized during these times. Though I wanted to maintain my pride in sharing my cultural identity with my peers in Canada, I perceived that I was in an unsafe environment due to my non-normative food choices. Bringing Asian snacks, such as seaweed or dried squid, made me feel particularly uncomfortable. I did not want to encounter my peers when having lunch, trying to avoid them whenever possible or trying to bring more normative lunches like sandwiches and pizza.

Eventually, rather than bringing my school lunches to eat at the cafeteria amidst my peers, who were all white, I sought out a group of peers who were Chinese to eat my school lunches, without feeling unsafe or shamed by my peers. This led to me feeling close with my Chinese peers, sharing a sense of cultural belonging and connection amongst each other. My food choices brought me closer and fostered a connection with my Chinese peers, akin to an ingroup–outgroup differentiation where food, instead of bringing all students closer through cultural pluralism and appreciation, made the differences more pronounced and created cultural separations.

However, as I grew older, I was struggling with my sexuality being a gay Chinese Canadian adolescent (details can be read in Leung, 2021). I was being mindful of my food intake, not only due to ethnic-based peer victimization but due to how gay Asian men were predominantly portrayed in media to be lean. One of my other solutions, besides eating with my Chinese peers, was food avoidance. Rather than bringing my Chinese food to school, I felt it was one less issue to worry about while I was at school by simply not bringing my lunch. Instead, I would simply eat one meal a day at night in the privacy of my dormitory room without feeling unsafe. This type of eating habit was both physically and emotionally rewarding. I understood from media portrayal of gay Asian men that having a lean figure was desirable. However, by doing so, I possessed more feminine characteristics and my high school peers in rural Canada would call me "*queer*" or "*faggot*" (Leung, 2021). Though at the time I did not disclose my sexuality, I became frustrated in how I was supposed to look and how to create my body to align with the portrayal of gay Asian men (i.e., twinks) while appreciating my cultural food.

As I began to enter university in an LGBTQ+-welcoming urban city in Canada, I was able to explore my sexuality in a safer environment and publicly self-disclosed my sexuality to my university friends. Though my university friends were not of the same ethnicity, they appreciated and enjoyed eating Asian food and enjoyed Asian culture. Through this cultural connection through ethnic food, I was able to feel closer with my cultural identity with diverse friends. However, though I was able to use ethnic food as a social connection with my friends, I began to gain weight and felt increasingly ashamed in my physical appearance compared to the lean figure portrayed by gay Asian men in the media. As a result, I tended to restrict my food intake whenever I noticed my body gaining weight. This led to years of continuous unhealthy eating practices as I was struggling to balance healthy eating practices and fitting into the stereotypical body type. During my first few years in university, my lean, feminine body type was physically and sexually reinforced, receiving flattering comments from other men. Both media and personal experiences reinforced that a gay Chinese Canadian emerging adult with a lean, feminine physique was considered attractive. Unfortunately, as a result of my unhealthy eating practices, including food avoidance and my one-meal-a-day practice, I had to check into the hospital for digestive complications. I put my body under stress by trying to balance my desire to connect with my culture through its food with trying to lose weight to embody the image of the gay Asian "twink."

The above excerpt of my adolescent and emerging adulthood relationship with cultural food and dieting highlights the complex relationship between my cultural and sexual identity. On one hand, difficulties arise in appreciating and connecting with my cultural identity through healthy and culturally relevant eating practices. On the other hand, difficulties arise in ethnic food consumption and my ability to accept my body image against the stereotypical, idealized body for gay Asians.

Unhealthy Food Practices as a Result of My Intersectional Identities

Though I wanted to have my ethnic school lunches to identify closer with my home culture, particularly in a boarding school away from home, I was shamed and felt like an outcast for my food practices. As I preferred my traditional foods and wanted to maintain my ethnic minority identity and preserve my culture through food practices (Reddy & van Dam, 2020), the message sent by the school and the majority group peers (i.e., white) indicated that this minority culture was not welcomed. Identifying as gay did not help with my food practices. On one hand, to maintain my cultural belonging and identity, ethnic food school lunches provided a social connection whilst being in a Western-dominant environment (i.e., Canada). However, the interaction with my sexual identity and my food practices led me to perceive that I had to conform under social pressure to look similar to the body ideals for gay Asian men pictured in the media via restrictive eating or food avoidance.

I only came to accept myself much later during my emerging adulthood period in part due to the conflict between my Chinese and Canadian identities. My high interest in the cultural food of my Chinese Canadian identity conflicted with my need to be selective about my food choices and restricted my will to eat Chinese cuisine. This led to a continuation of negative self-thought as I was supposed to eat what is socially constructed as "healthy" food: fruits and vegetables, salads rather than food associated with my ethnic culture. Wanting to fit in with how gay Asian men appeared in mass media, I attempted to eat less Asian food, in particular rice, and ate more salads or skipped meals to move towards the lean body figure that is stereotypically seen as attractive for gay Asians. This conflict continued from adolescence through my emerging adulthood.

Ways to Celebrate Ethnic-Minority Food, Identities, and Bodies in the LGBTQ+ Community

Schools are one of the environments where gay adolescents begin to experience restrictive eating or unhealthy eating practices due to the media portrayal of gay individuals. Particularly for LGBTQ+-YOC, media portrayal of body prefer-ences may lead to a possibility for dissociation between cultural belonging and the ability to eat ethnic food, and gay identity. Schools become a place where both cultural and gay identities can be celebrated in a positive manner through food, and social connections (Spencer et al., 2019).

One environment in schools that is an avenue of celebration of diverse food are school gay-straight alliances (GSAs), extracurricular student groups that aim to provide a safe space within schools for LGBTQ+ students and their hetero-sexual peers. GSAs may be the first starting point for LGBTQ+-YOC to feel included in their schools and be allowed to appreciate food that is of their cultural identity and promote healthy eating practices against discussions surrounding body image and media portrayal. However, there have been experiences where LGBTQ+-YOC received a backlash within GSAs due to their racial-ethnic iden-tity and were excluded due to their non-normative lunches, mentioning the food was "weird" and "smelly" (Endo, 2021). Therefore, LGBTQ+-YOC are at a constant conflict with the types of food they eat to fit certain physiques as shown by stereotypical public media and the added layer of being made fun of for non-normative foods in schools.

Overall, schools can be an avenue for future research and programme imple-mentation in two areas: (1) cultural pluralism and (2) positive body image, and how both areas influence students' healthy eating practices. For example, schools with high cultural pluralism endorse cultural diversity approaches through prac-tices that aim at a more holistic understanding of cultural differences. In contrast, ineffective methods of promoting cultural pluralism are through celebrating special events, holidays, and food. Such practices promote cultural pluralism in an exotic manner, separating from the mainstream society rather than an inte-gration of diverse culture within the mainstream society (Civitillo et al., 2017). Evidence in the field of multiculturalism has found that such forms of "lazy" inclusion of multiculturalism can be better programmed by supplementing with critical discussions and elevating the understanding of other cultures through inquiry and questioning. Such questions that teachers can explore through ethnic food can include *"What's missing here?"*, *"What does this tell us about culture?"*, *"Thinking about the ethnic food, where does the food originate from?"*, *"Food may have different meanings in different culture. How is this ethnic food different or similar from our food?"*, and *"How would this make sense with our own body image and who we are?"* (Watkins & Noble, 2019).

As GSAs are extracurricular organizations that house LGBTQ+ students and allies, GSA advisors may be in an ideal position to incorporate discussions with their LGBTQ+ students and students of colour by introducing various ethnic foods and, most importantly, promoting higher-level reflection in how a relationship with food from different cultures can affect their relationship with their own body and body image. As exploring diverse foods is inherently interesting and engaging for students, ethnic food can be incorporated beyond simple exoticism and othering from the mainstream society to fostering critical discussion via ethnic food and its relationship with other identities (e.g., food and body stereotypes).

With respect to healthy eating practices due to media portrayal of gay Asian men's bodies, there is a lack of research investigating programmes that support LGBTQ+-YOC. Rather, there are several broader healthy eating programmes that target body esteem and acceptance, health and nutrition, and media literacy (e.g., *Everybody's Different, Full of Ourselves, Healthy Body Image, and Media Smart*; Larkin & Vernon-Cole, 2015) for students. Though the aforementioned programmes have been implemented in schools, the positive effects (e.g., increased critical media literacy, acceptance of their body, and awareness of health and nutrition) have not been expanded and understood beyond Western populations. It is of interest how healthy eating practices can be understood for LGBTQ+-YOC through an intersectional lens. Taking into account the social pressures to conform and avoid bringing nonnormative cultural food, LGBTQ+-YOC may struggle to understand how their cultural food maps onto Westernized healthy eating programmes.

References

Civitillo, S., Schachner, M., Juang, L., van de Vijver, F. J. R., Handrick, A., & Noack, P. (2017). Towards a better understanding of cultural, diversity approaches at school: A multi-informant and mixed-methods study. *Learning, Culture and Social Interaction, 12*, 1–14. https://doi.org/10.1016/j.lcsi.2016.09.002

Endo, R. (2021). Diversity, equity, and inclusion for some but not all: LGBQ Asian American youth experiences at an urban public high school. *Multicultural Education Review, 13*(1), 1–18. https://doi.org/10.1080/2005615X.2021.1890311

Higgs, S., & Thomas, J. (2016). Social influences on eating. *Current Opinion in Behavioral Sciences, 9*, 1–6. https://doi.org/10.1016/j.cobeha.2015.10.005

Kar, S. K., Choudhury, A., & Singh, A. P. (2015). Understanding normal development of adolescent sexuality: A bumpy ride. *Journal of Human Reproductive Sciences, 8*(2), 70–74. https://doi.org/10.4103/0974-1208.158594

Larkin, A. K., & Vernon-Cole, E. J. (2015). *Nurturing healthy eating and positive body culture at school* [Unpublished graduate thesis]. California State University.

Leung, E. (2021). Thematic analysis of my "coming out" experiences through an intersectional lens: An autoethnographic study. *Frontiers in Psychology*, *12*(654946), 1–15. https://doi.org/10.3389/fpsyg.2021.654946

Ludvigsen, A., & Scott, S. (2009). Real kids don't eat quiche. *Food, Culture & Society*, *12*(4), 417–436. https://doi.org/10.2752/175174409X456728

McClain, Z., & Peebles, R. (2016). Body image and eating disorders among lesbian, gay, bisexual, and transgender youth. *Pediatric Clinics of North America*, *63*(6), 1079–1090. https://doi.org/10.1016/j.pcl.2016.07.008

Nukaga, M. (2008). The underlife of kids' school lunchtime: Negotiating ethnic boundaries and identity in food exchange. *Journal of Contemporary Ethnography*, *37*(3), 342–380. https://doi.org/10.1177/0891241607309770

O'Hara, S. (2018). Autoethnography: The science of writing your lived experience. *HERD: Health Environments Research & Design Journal*, *11*(4), 14–17. https://doi.org/10.1177/1937586718801425

Parker, L. L., & Harriger, J. A. (2020). Eating disorders and disordered eating behaviours in the LGBT population: A review of the literature. *Journal of Eating Disorders*, *8*(51), 1–20. https://doi.org/10.1186/s40337-020-00327-y

Ravenhill, J. P., & de Visser, R. O. (2017). "There are too many gay categories now": Discursive constructions of gay masculinity. *Psychology of Men & Masculinity*, *18*(4), 321–330. https://doi.org/10.1037/men0000057

Reddy, G., & van Dam, R. M. (2020). Food, culture, and identity in multicultural societies: Insights from Singapore. *Appetite*, *149*, 1–12. https://doi.org/10.1016/j.appet.2020.104633

Romito, M., Salk, R. H., Roberts, S. R., Thoma, B. C., Levine, M. D., & Choukas-Bradley, S. (2021). Exploring transgender adolescents' body image concerns and disordered eating: Semi-structured interviews with nine gender minority youth. *Body Image*, *37*, 50–62. https://doi.org/10.1016/j.bodyim.2021.01.008

Spencer, R. A., McIsaac, J. D., Stewart, M., Brushett, S., & Kirk, S. F. L. (2019). Food in focus: Youth exploring food in schools using photovoice. *Journal of Nutrition Education and Behavior*, *51*(8), 1011–1019. https://doi.org/10.1016/j.jneb.2019.05.599

Stets, J. E., & Burke, P. J. (2000). Identity theory and social identity theory. *Social Psychology Quarterly*, *63*(3), 224–237. https://doi.org/10.2307/2695870

Watkins, M., & Noble, G. (2019). Lazy multiculturalism: Cultural essentialism and the persistence of the multicultural day in Australian schools. *Ethnography and Education*, *14*(3), 295–310. https://doi.org/10.1080/17457823.2019.1581821

27 Turning Over a New Leaf

Uncovering Gay Identity Alongside a Vegan Journey

Julia Russell

I was a teenage vegetarian, out and proud. I was a teenage lesbian, repressed and oblivious.

As a vegetarian, I was amongst a small percentage of the population. In the mid-2000's, when I was a newly minted vegetarian in the midst of my teenage years, one British Columbian study found that 6% of the population studied was vegetarian (although they reported that most were not strict adherents to vegetarianism) (Bedford & Barr, 2005). Still, there's safety in numbers. On the other hand, the percentage of Canadian adults of 18 to 59 who identified as homosexual was just 1% in 2004 (Statistics Canada, 2004).

But even before all that it was the 1990s and I was just a girl. In grade two I came home in tears because I thought girls weren't allowed to play hockey, and therefore I wanted to be a boy so I could play too. The next year I was proven wrong, and my parents signed me up to hit the ice in a small, all-girls hockey league. My passion for the sport was enduring and I've played hockey almost every winter since. But then Greco-Roman wrestling came a few years after that initial foray into hockey, and my grandfather told me girls weren't supposed to do that either. Still, I persisted for the next few years, before eventually becoming too self-conscious to pursue the sport further.

The homophobic bullying began around grade six and lasted on and off for half a decade. During those years I had anxious nights filled with shame and fear for what the next day would bring. Around the same time the bullying ended, I became a vegetarian. As far as the bullying went, other people were telling me who I was before I knew who I was myself. It was likely something stereotypical that outed me to others. It's possible it may have been the sports, the tomboy attire, or the short haircut. Whatever it was, I was identified as gay by other kids when I barely knew what the word meant myself. I had no LGBTQ+ mentors in my life. The vitriol with which my peers spit homophobic slurs at me immediately convinced me that being a lesbian was not an option if I wanted safety, love, and acceptance. I avoided clothing I thought looked "lesbian," I grew out my short hair. I changed my aesthetic and others began to react to me differently. I could ignore the strange magnetism, I later realized was attraction, that I occasionally felt towards other girls. I transformed my identity from one that needed protection into a protector. I went vegetarian for the animals and environment.

DOI: 10.4324/9781003217121-29

It may be an oversimplification to say that because LGBTQ+ people have experienced discrimination they are more compassionate, but I believe this has influenced my personal awareness of suffering in the world. Quinn (2021) writes that LGBTQ+ people are more likely to be vegan. I've found no other evidence of this in the academic world but can anecdotally support this claim with experiences from my own life. Perhaps it is compassion as I've mentioned, or perhaps it's related to other trends and fashions within the LGBTQ+ world.

In grade 11, I brought a homemade, vegan, tofu, chocolate cake to share with my biology class after I gave a presentation on vegetarianism. Some people gobbled it up, while others turned their noses up in disgust. I took delight in the experience. I was jazzed by the fact I could fight injustice in the classroom through my mild activism.

My high school had roughly 1,500 students, and a very small number of them were part of a group for LGBTQ+ youth and allies. In contrast to the pride and contented feeling I relished when I proclaimed my (then) vegetarianism, I would hurriedly walk by the classroom when the group was meeting, averting my eyes. Strange feelings of discomfort would envelop me when I had thoughts of this group. I think somehow, I knew I belonged to this group, but I forced myself to point out the external differences that I believed defined the queer, such as clothing choices and hairstyles. I had remedied all that to fit with the acceptable presentation suitable to pass as heterosexual.

Social identity is "part of an individual's self-concept which derives from his knowledge of his membership of a social group (or groups) together with the emotional significance attached to that membership" (Tajfel, 1978, p. 69). What does it mean when one so vehemently denies their identity that they are legitimately oblivious to it, but they are still socially constructed as fitting into that identity, as I was constructed as a lesbian? I was acquainted with only a few vegetarians in my high school days, so I was not more readily able to embrace that identity as a result of any sort of group acceptance. Additionally, the stereotypes I had heard about vegans (vegetarians and/or vegans) were not positive. Still, I was drawn to veganism.

Ruby (2012) describes how among other attributes vegetarians tend to be oriented towards supporting social justice. I still thought I was a strong ally to LGBTQ+ people even if I shirked away from the group meetings, not realizing I was one such person myself. I remember debating with a friend about his religious views that condemned homosexuality and asked him if he would not love his own child if that child was gay. He assured me he would not. I don't recall any debates about vegetarianism. I'm sure I was challenged along the way, but such conversations didn't leave an indelible mark on my psyche.

It has been written that "vegetarians are members of a special type of minority group [...] that (behaviours) are ostensibly beneficial but that others may view as eccentric or even deviant" (Romo & Donovan-Kicken, 2012, p. 406). However, through the benefits of veg*ism to the planet, other lifeforms, and myself, I could justify my being a vegan. Yet ironically, over the years, some people seemed to think I was choosing to risk bodily harm through ill health as a vegan although at times my physical wellbeing was actually jeopardized by homophobes who threatened me with violence. Although these homophobes may have believed my sexuality was immoral, I did not. However, I was not morally compelled to be a lesbian, as I was to become a vegan.

At age 18, I was an adult, and living away from home in Canada's most populous and diverse city, Toronto, and I found it was time to stop living with guilt and embrace my identity, as a vegan. I made new friends who said nothing of my veganism but who hinted that there may be something more to my sexual orientation, beyond heterosexual. I was my own person, demonstrated so I thought by embracing veganism, but I was still constrained. At least now, I happily accompanied the university LGBTQ+ club dancing, in Toronto's LGBTQ+ neighbourhood. I just thought I liked to dance, though something else began to tickle my subconscious.

I chose to be a vegetarian, and later a vegan, at a time when these labels were regarded much more critically than they are today. They marked a person as socially deviant. I am strong in my convictions. But I also wonder, was I trying on a marginalized identity in being vegan before I came out of the closet? Did being vegan allow me to navigate the world, to speak up for myself and who I am without risking too much? To learn how to be myself? I could control being vegan and though I couldn't control peoples' reactions, I was able to see negativity for what it was, whether that was ignorance or simply unfamiliarity. I was also able to see there were positive reactions, curious questions, and for the most part apathy. People simply didn't care what I was doing as long as I wasn't infringing on their own lives in a negative way. Years later, I would find that people's reactions to my being a gay person were much the same. Some things have improved since my teenage years.

As a vegan one must carefully navigate their disclosure of veganism to avoid "alienating" other people in their life (Romo & Donovan-Kicken, 2012, p. 407). Often people may end up framing their vegetarianism as a personal choice to avoid offending another person (Romo & Donovan-Kicken, 2012). The same cannot be done with sexual orientation. Similarly, vegetarians may come to conversations equipped with facts about the benefits of vegetarianism for animal, human, and planetary health (Romo & Donovan-Kicken, 2012). Homosexuality, while adding to the richness and diversity of the human experience, is not inherently more environmentally friendly! The issue of revealing one's veganism can be forced when someone places a dish of meat in front of the vegan who must then explain or excuse their abstention from meat (Romo & Donovan-Kicken, 2012). During the time I misled myself as to my sexuality I had relationships with men. One cannot be a vegetarian in hiding for long, but it is possible to be queer and hidden. Vegetarians can assume that negative reactions from non-vegetarians are possible, and these can include bullying (Romo & Donovan-Kicken, 2012). I experienced homophobic bullying in my youth, so I think comments about veganism never fazed me much. Importantly, although there were negative associations with vegetarianism, they paled in comparison to what I feared others would think of me as a gay person.

When I became a vegetarian, it was only after years of contemplation, beginning at age 11. I was guided by the book, *I'm a Vegetarian* by Ellen Schwartz. This would closely resemble my later experience with coming out as well. Among other approaches I took when trying to decode my sexuality I turned to books on the subject. It was with great trepidation that I signed them out from my university library, but I told myself that I could explain I was simply undertaking research for a class project, if anyone was to ask me about it. No one ever did. In both instances I found strength in the books that enabled me to declare my identity to myself. I stood in front of a mirror and practiced speaking my identity out loud. Did it fit right?

In both cases with my diet and sexual orientation, I began with one identity. First, I was a lacto-ovo vegetarian, first I was a bisexual, then transitioned to another when I was comfortable. I knew I had to transition to veganism. I knew I had to be honest that I was a gay person.

Did I subconsciously substitute one stigmatized identity for another that I could choose for myself? I became vegan at 18 years of age, years before I was fully out as a gay person. I've lived in South America as a vegan and travelled to the Arctic multiple times. I've seen that plant-based food is making inroads, I've seen veggie dogs in Inuvik. I'm not saying veggie dogs are necessarily a good thing, but it shows the spread of influence. At the same time, it seems as if there has been increased acceptance of LGBTQ+ people. But both groups have faced a backlash as well. However, the ranks have swollen, there are now ~8–11% of Canadians who identify as vegetarian (including vegans) (von Massow et al. 2019) while data still indicates that 1% of women identify as lesbian (Statistics Canada, 2019), that doesn't include the full spectrum of LGBTQ+ people whose numbers may be much higher.

Simonsen (2012) likens the coming out process as a LGBTQ+ person to coming out as a vegetarian, although Simonsen notes that one comes with more risk. The processes were similar for me. While in the closet, in both instances I felt ashamed and also fleeting feelings of desperation to be known as my true self. However, I was able to suppress these feelings for years in both instances.

I've been accepted in my own family, first as vegetarian, then a vegan, then as a bisexual, then as a gay person. These things may seem unrelated, but they are intertwined. I come from cultures where meat was a main feature of a meal and making meals for the family was how one showed their love. Therefore, rejecting a meal could be seen as a rejection of the cook, of family, of tradition. If, however, recipes can be tweaked to accommodate vegans, and vegans bring new twists on tradition to the family, then there may be acceptance of veganism as non-threatening. If the family has already accepted and embraced the vegan, it demonstrates that they may be able to move through the same process with other differences as well, such as sexuality. This, in a way, queers the family, of whose members are embedded in different segments of society, thereby potentially influencing wider social change. It also queers the Western notion that family traditions must be passed down from one generation to the next, as embracing new ways of being can also flow upward. It has helped that I have a large family, expectations can be distributed across family members so one person doesn't have to be all things within their family. Granted, my experience cannot be said to be universal.

Nowadays, I am a doctoral candidate studying veganism. However, even before that, veganism was most often what people first learned of my identity followed by my being a gay person. If someone reacted with hostility to my veganism, I would be more cautious about revealing my sexuality. My veganism has long been a shield for me. I realized that I physically depended on it to protect my health, but I've just now come to realize how I've depended on it emotionally as well. I may have often been on the outside because of my vegan ways, but I felt it was better than being excluded for my sexuality.

Looking back, it's quite funny in a sense because veganism has been associated with lesbians by heterosexual males. The authors Alexander and Yescavage mention vegetarian diets in passing as a fashion or identifier of gayness (2012). Maybe there was something queer about veganism all along, and I was not adopting an alternative identity but gradually slipping into my own sexual orientation by first going veg.

References

Alexander, J., & Yescavage, K. (2012). Chapter 3: 'The scholars formerly known as …': Bisexuality, queerness and identity politics. In M. O'Rourke & N. Giffney, (Eds.), *The Ashgate research companion to queer theory* (pp. 49–64). Ashgate Publishing Limited.

Bedford, J. L., & Barr, S. I. (2005). Diets and selected lifestyle practices of self-defined adult vegetarians from a population-based sample suggest they are more 'health conscious'. *International Journal of Behavioral Nutrition and Physical Activity*, *2*(4). https://doi.org/10.1186/1479-5868-2-4

Romo, L. K., & Donovan-Kicken, E. (2012). "Actually, I don't eat meat": A multiple-goals perspective of communication about vegetarianism. *Communication Studies*, *63*(4), 405–420. https://doi.org/10.1080/10510974.2011.623752

Ruby, M. B. (2012). Vegetarianism: A blossoming field of study. *Appetite*, *58*, 141–150. https://doi.org/10.1016/j.appet.2011.09.019

Schwartz, E. (2002). *I'm a vegetarian*. Tundra Books.

Simonsen, R. R. (2012). A queer vegan manifesto. *Journal for Critical Animal Studies*, *10*(3), 51–81.

Statistics Canada. (2004, June 15). The daily: Canadian community health survey. Statistics Canada. https://www150.statcan.gc.ca/n1/daily-quotidien/040615/dq040615b-eng.htm

Statistics Canada. (2019, November 11). Sexual orientation and mental health. Statistics Canada. https://www150.statcan.gc.ca/n1/daily-quotidien/191120/dq191120d-eng.htm

Tajfel, H. (1978). Social identity and intergroup behaviour. *Social Science Information*, *13*(2), 65–93.

Von Massow, M., Weersink, A., & Gallant, M. (2019). Meat consumption is changing but it's not because of vegans. *The Conversation*. https://theconversation.com/meat-consumption-is-changing-but-its-not-because-of-vegans-112332

Part 3

From the Front Lines

Queer Care in Practice

28 The Cerberus Helmet Project

Feast of Wisdom

Lynette A. Peters

Dedication

This art form is dedicated to my beautiful friend, AT. For the joy he continues to bring to our lives and our yearly visits involving feasts. I am thankful for the outcome of camaraderie such feasts provide at the dinner table. We share not only food, but wisdom, acceptance, love, and gratitude when we dine together.

The image in Figure 28.1 is presented to show the early stage of the helmet project, the wet stage of greenware as it dries before underglaze application and bisque firing.

The image in Figure 28.2 is included to show the process of colour application and position in the interior of the kiln.

The image in Figure 28.3 is the completed "Feast of Wisdom." Cone 6, commercial white stoneware with underglazes and poured, black gunmetal glaze (exterior) with lavender and beige-speckled glazes that have been layered and further forced to separate into blues, pinks, and browns using a white fluxing agent (interior). The helmet has been positioned to sit upside down on a pedestal with the extended Rainbow Flag colours. The often unseen or hidden helmet interior is exposed as the food surface.

Inspiration and Art form

In "Rainbow Warrior, My Life in Colour" (2019), Gilbert Baker is presented as a non-conformist who used art as his "weapon" of activism. In 1978, he created the first Rainbow Flag during his service as a US Army medic. Baker and I share similar informal methodologies *of being*: according to his husband Dustin Lance Black, his creativity came in surges and was ethereally connected to his language – and weapon of choice – visual art. Art challenges people to find meaning as prompted by symbols. He mobilized this very well; the Rainbow Flag is a symbol of hope, unity, and inclusion.

Using an "unserviceable" army helmet as a cradle for stoneware clay, this functional piece (raised serving bowl) has renewed meaning while honouring its past identity. Food prepared and served to others can be both a gesture of care, but

DOI: 10.4324/9781003217121-31

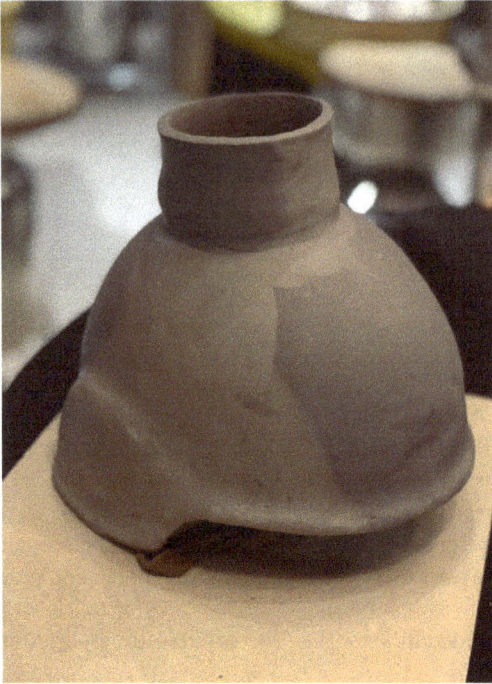

Figure 28.1 Cerberus Helmet Project, "Feast of Wisdom" drying during wet-clay stage. Cone 6, commercial white stoneware. Artist: Lynette Peters. Lynette Peters.

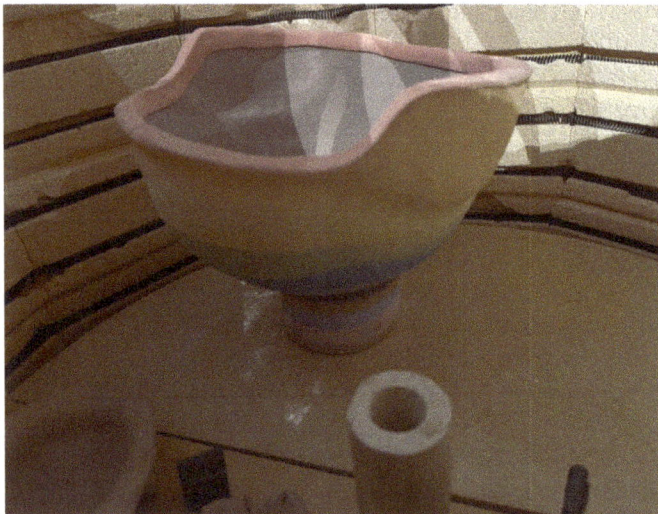

Figure 28.2 Cerberus Helmet Project, "Feast of Wisdom" bone-dry stage with underglaze. Cone 6, commercial white stoneware with underglazes prior to cone 4 bisque firing in a kiln. Artist, Lynette Peters. Lynette Peters.

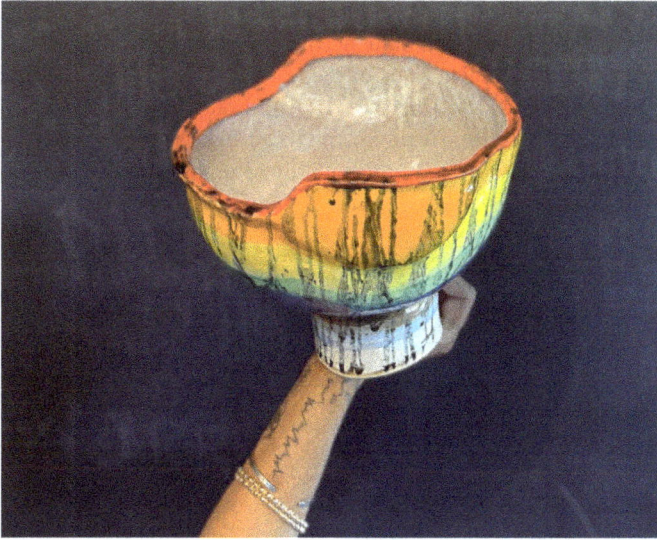

Figure 28.3 Cerberus Helmet Project, "Feast of Wisdom" completed. Artist, Lynette Peters.
        Lynette Peters.

also one of comfort and support and understanding. This Helmet Project is symbolic; it is a medium that reflects substantial institutional harm and profound loss in its design, positioning, and final colour (spatial). It also attempts to include the object's ongoing temporality as one that displays original Rainbow Flag colours and those later included to support gender identities. When no longer viewed as helmet, the spatial position informs future purpose while the colours and dimension invite a canvas for sharing food. Underglaze is used in surface colour layering of greenware before bisque firing. It is beneath the "master" glaze hence it is more intimately connected to the clay body than it is to the surface glaze; ensuring it is less influenced by glaze application. The surface glaze was chosen to coat, to force a unidimensional colour, to heteronormalize – yet – the form is of greater importance to function.

Art can be used as a mode of non-verbal expression for words that cannot be spoken. Visual arts may inspire as the products are tactile symbols representing human meaning through experience. Art has the potential to impact wellbeing from many perspectives (Fancourt & Finn, 2019). Gilbert Baker continues to challenge us to receive his art as a symbolic gift. As a healthcare worker, his artform serves to engage, to unify, and to inspire hope. While art and the processes of art have therapeutic potential for the maker (Pöllänen, 2013), the artform casts special benefit on those beholding it (Mastandrea et al., 2019). Art provides an alternate perspective. Not only did I create this helmet to honour the experiences of those with service histories who identify as LGBTQ+, I intentionally invite curiosity and include this unique population. We have a responsibility to provide for all who commit service on our behalf; however, we cannot properly do so without pushing beyond the stereotypes and interpretations of a monolithic Veteran identity. Service histories are unique and can influence health (Tam-Seto et al., 2019). The Feast of Wisdom Helmet challenges us to reconsider what Veteran identity means. It is one example of the utility of art as a cultivator of cultural competence in the profession of health and care. At the frontlines of healthcare, art may be purposed as a multitool for self-care and understanding human experience. The art-form is then a tactical defensive weapon against inequality.

References

Baker, G., & Black, D. (2019). *Rainbow warrior*. Chicago Review Press.

Fancourt, D., & Finn, S. (2019). *What is the evidence on the role of the arts in improving health and well-being? A scoping review.* Health Evidence Network Synthesis Report, No. 67. World Health Organisation. http://www.euro.who.int/en/publications/abstracts/what-is-the-evidence-on-the-role-of-the-arts-in-improving-health-and-well-being-a-scoping-review-2019

Mastandrea, S., Fagioli, S., & Biasi, V. (2019). Art and psychological well-being: Linking the brain to the aesthetic emotion. *Frontiers in Psychology, 10*, 739.

Pöllänen, S. (2013). The meaning of craft: Craft makers' descriptions of craft as an occupation. *Scandinavian Journal of Occupational Therapy, 20*(3), 217–227.

Tam-Seto, L., Krupa, T., Stuart, H., Lingley-Pottie, P., Aiken, A. B., & Cramm, H. (2019). "Stepping up to the plate": Identifying cultural competencies when providing health care to Canada's military and veteran families. *Journal of Military, Veteran and Family Health, 5*(2), 136–146. https://doi.org/10.3138/jmvfh.2018-0049

29 Fairy Tales

Fables from BC Dietitians

Gordon Ly, Jon Leung, Peter Lam, Gerry Kasten,
Treena Hansen, Shelly Crack, Anna Brisco*, and
Marissa Alexander*

Prologue

Recognizing the relative silence of first-person narratives from queer dietitians within the published literature, the story archivists (AB & GK) sought to compile anecdotes from BC LGBTQ+ dietitians on the interaction(s) between and amongst food and queers. Utilizing a storytelling framework, LGBTQ+ dietitians related their own fables from their lived experiences. Each story is followed by its "moral—" succinct first-person reflections on the deeper lessons or teachings readers could take away from these stories. We are using "morals" in the manner of the fableist Aesop and do not intend to confer any connotations of right or wrong. The focus is on foods and LGBTQ+ persons, incorporating insights obtained from or bounded by the contributors' dietetic practice in British Columbia

Storytellers were purposively recruited via personal networks, leading to six interviews conducted via Zoom between July and September 2021. Each storyteller shared their story, as well as the lessons and morals arising from their story. The sessions were recorded and auto transcribed using built-in Zoom settings. Full transcripts were revised for accuracy, and then due to space constraints, the story archivists abridged each story. To ensure meanings were maintained, the revised fables were verified with the storytellers.

The story archivists conclude this chapter by briefly discussing major themes among the stories. Readers are invited to reflect on and discuss the themes and insights emerging from this collection of contemporary fables that might apply to their lives and dietetic practice.

The Fables and Morals

Gordon's Story

Gordon is a clinical dietitian and dietetic educator, working in Vancouver.

* Contact Authors/Story Archivists

DOI: 10.4324/9781003217121-32

Gordon grew up within an immigrant/refugee family from Southeast Asia in a small town in BC, knowing he was different from other boys well before he understood he was gay. He also felt quite different from his highly religious, conservative family; in a family of loud partiers, he was quiet and shy.

Reflecting on how his career as a dietitian, his passions, and many of his hobbies all relate to food, Gordon traced it back to early positive experiences in the kitchen. Despite the kitchen being a highly gendered space, his mom and grandma welcomed him in and supported his skills and interests. This recognition and support contrasted with other areas of life, where he often felt criticized or looked down on.

> Food was the one thing that made me feel like I belonged. I was good in the kitchen, and everyone in my family loves food.

For Gordon, food was the key that unlocked his sense of belonging; cooking was not just a skillset but also something that brought him safety and security.

> Food is so meaningful for me. I realized it's probably because cooking was my escape and my safe place to be authentic. It's also the great unifier because everyone has to eat, and everyone has some sort of connection to food. So, the fact that I had some skill or knowledge about food ... that helped build my confidence and helped me to accept myself. It signalled to me that I, too, can be good at something and be accepted.

Gordon is grateful that he had found a way to channel his passion for food, understanding how differently his life would have turned out without this safe place to explore himself.

> I honestly feel so blessed because once I discovered cooking, I feel like my life really took off. As soon as I put energy into these things – sciences, dietetics, nutrition, food, and cooking – my life became exponentially better. I left the city to pursue higher education ... and now I'm really thriving. How unfortunate it would have been if I didn't find that safety ... I don't even know where I would be – maybe not alive.

Moral

> Every person deserves something in their life to feel comfortable and safe in, whether that be a community, a hobby or idea. If we deny that to people, they can't be their authentic selves. There's no safe place for them to take space and that is tragic.

Peter's Story

Peter is a dietitian with a consulting practice, working in BC's Lower Mainland.

Peter's story begins some years ago, when he and his partner Haakon met a younger couple while walking in Vancouver's gay village. They invited the couple for dinner, and over the years, those young men told other young men, and now they regularly host gatherings for 40-something people: "it's like the … shampoo commercial – s/he tells two friends and so on and so on." The gatherings are a mix of some dietitians and others from various vocations. Peter questions whether the young dietitians yet feel safe to be out during their training and early career: "We haven't quite gotten to that level of indifference yet, where the nutrition and dietetics department would feel indifferent about a young man who is queer, who's gay." These gatherings are not only about sharing food and learning more about the food itself: Getting together also helps the participants learn about entertaining and socializing:

> it has, I think, provided some life lessons to this … "potluck of people." They have evolved and grown up to, you know, see examples of how to entertain, how to welcome others unconditionally. And I think in a really kind of informal way, there was a bit of a mentoring process that was going on through the years.

The gatherings have evolved to a "multigenerational" family. The younger members may or may not be thinking of Peter and Haakon as "gay parents," as the first members did:

> And, you know, it has been over 20 years … there's a bit more of an age gap now between us and some of the younger ones, they may want to talk to somebody that's a little closer to their age. Right? So it doesn't feel like talking to their gay parents, or gay grandparents …

They are forming mentor/mentee relationships with some of the people who are closer to their own ages:

> we've now been able to step away a little more and just observe and see how things are going. And now … you're mentoring the mentors, right? Some of the older ones will come and say, You know what … we're talking about this [and we] don't quite know how to manage it or handle it … Now, how can we best sort of guide them? So, you know, it's kind of fun.

Hence, the group has become very personally important to all of the people who attend, perhaps more than their own families, particularly if they aren't out to their families, as yet:

> Many of them actually view the special occasion mealtime with this group, [as an] even more important an event, than they would celebrate with their own families. Right, particularly the ones that are, you know, not quite out of the closet yet.

And so, Peter and Haakon continue to host these get togethers, building community, fun and enjoyment, and providing safe space for folks to get together:

> It really doesn't matter what setting or what group or a population of people you are interacting with … All it takes is a bit of willingness. Right? And, a sprinkle of that generous spirit to just get things started. Everybody appreciates a safe space. Everybody appreciates a place where they feel appreciated.

Moral

> Don't underestimate the power of food. The power of a meal, no matter how simple or fancy it might be. The power of the "potluck of people" … This is a forum for people to help each other get better and if you bring that kind of spirit to it, I think it just flourishes all on its own, without very much effort.

Treena's Story Is called "Love, Recipe, and Alzheimer's"

Treena worked as a clinical dietitian and educator in Vancouver, BC and Tillsonburg, O.N. She now lives in Calgary, AB.

This story begins with two people. Treena's dad who grew up in Standard, AB, a Danish community, and her mom growing up in Yorkton, SK. Her parents met in Calgary eventually marrying and adopting five kids. Treena's mom was taught by her Danish grandmother to cook many Danish dishes. Treena grew up as a "pink sheep" in a large family. One particularly fond memory is of coming home for lunch, to a stack of Danish doughnuts called Æbleskiver. She recalls:

> I would eat as many as I could not taking the time to think of the labour that went into making the delectable Danish doughnuts. Once I finished eating, off I went, back to school to play.

Treena's mother was recently diagnosed with Alzheimer's disease, and subsequently admitted to long-term care in Qualicum Beach, BC. Treena's mom's memory had now settled in the past when she lived in Calgary. Treena would talk about the times growing up in Calgary. One day while going through her belongings, she found an Æbleskiver pan along with the recipe for the sweet treats (Figure 29.1).

So, she made them (recipe provided, see Figure 29.2) and went on Facetime to visit with her mother as her brother was with her. And when she showed her mother the Æbleskiver, "Her eyes just lit up!" and she went on to make comments and ask questions about Treena's experiences making them:

> They are nice and round … and have a good amount of sugar coating," "Did you use a knitting needle to turn them?" I was like, "No, mom. Unfortunately, I don't knit." [Laughs] So I said I used a skewer to flip them over.

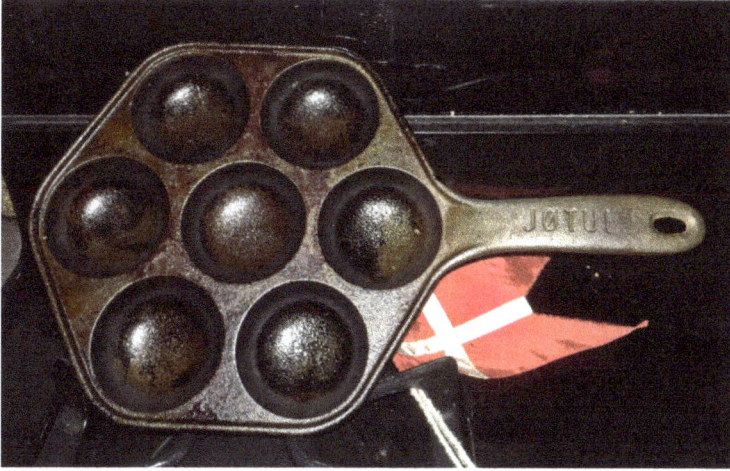

Figure 29.1 Æbleskiver pan. Treena Hansen.

Treena found this very heart-warming, because making Æbleskiver was such a clear memory that her mother could enjoy. They were also able to talk about making these treats, and that really made her mother smile.

> I didn't realize how much work went into making Æbleskiver when all of the five kids come home from school, and you had like 50 or 60 of these in these massive mounds, and we just ate them down like they were nothing and, and off we went back to school.

It was a chance for Treena to let her mother know how much she appreciated the work she did for her family. Her mother, "was very taken by my attempt at Æbleskiver. And she … had gone back in time and she commented, 'Oh, they must be so proud of you as a dietitian in Vancouver'."

And so, Treena encourages people who have a loved one living with Alzheimer's to try to find new ways to communicate and bring joy to them such as making a recipe because the memories of those foods will bring them a lot of happiness:

> That was probably the best memory of mom … living with Alzheimer's. It brought great happiness to her and a joyful memory to remember her by. It was just a beautiful moment in time.

Treena finished by dedicating this story to her parents, Lois and Carl Hansen.

Moral

> Be fearless! Alzheimer's rips away memories from your loved ones. Take the time to think of what could put a smile on your loved one's face. Food is one means to communicate love. Take out a family favourite recipe and try it.

Don't be afraid … you're bringing joy to them, and you're bringing a happy memory to yourself. Food is more than food groups. Food is culture, food is language, food is memories, food is love, and food is delicious!

Danish Doughnuts (Æbleskiver)
Ingredients: 2 cups flour ½ teaspoon salt 1 teaspoon sugar 2 cups buttermilk (or 2 cups milk, soy milk or other milk alternative and 2 tablespoons lemon juice or vinegar) 2 eggs, separated 1 teaspoon baking soda Melted butter Jelly or applesauce
Directions: 1. Mix flour, salt and sugar. 2. Beat together buttermilk and egg yolks, and add the flour mixture. 3. Add soda and fold in stiffly beaten egg whites 4. Heat the pan and put melted butter in each hole in the pan. 5. Pour batter into holes, but do not quite fill them 6. Place over low heat and turn quickly when half done 7. Serve very hot with jelly or applesauce.
Note: Danish doughnuts are baked on top of the stove in a special pan with a hole for each doughnut. Æbleskiver pans may be purchased at most gourmet cookware shops.
From Jensen McDonald, J. (1984) *Delectably Danish: Recipes and Reflections.* Penfield Press.

Figure 29.2 Æbleskiver recipe. Treena Hansen.

Jon's Story

Jon Leung is an Asian Canadian clinical dietitian, working in Vancouver, BC

Jon's story begins with the positive reaction of his friends in the dietetic programme when he came out to them; they were supportive and kind, which helped

Jon feel more comfortable coming out to more people. However, as an intern and new grad, the following incidents left Jon feeling unsure that he could be fully himself in the profession.

One afternoon, Jon's boyfriend came to pick him up from his internship placement. In his words:

> Just by chance, one of my preceptors happened to see us as I was showing him around the hospital. The next day, [my preceptor and I] were chatting and I shared, "That was my partner." She responded, "Oh, that's nice. That's interesting that you brought him because it might be perceived as unprofessional."

While the preceptor was non-judgemental in their tone, Jon was surprised and wondered if she would have made similar remarks to a straight intern.

At the end of year, interns were encouraged to bring family and friends to a graduation celebration. At this time his family did not know about his boyfriend, so Jon wrestled over who to bring. He attended with his boyfriend, eliciting the following reactions:

> I think people didn't really know what to make of us. One of the dietitians came up to me and said, "Oh is that your brother?" That was kind of awkward … One of the other [dietitians] came up to me and asked, "Oh, is this your" pause "special friend?"

While Jon was grateful that he didn't experience overt homophobia during his internship, both these incidents signalled he should tread carefully around sharing his personal life in order to be seen as "professional."

A few years later, at a social gathering of mostly LGBTQ+ dietitians from across Canada, Jon experienced a surprising racist microaggression when a dietitian touched his hair and exclaimed that it looked, "so oriental," highlighting the intersections of Jon's experience as a gay East Asian man within dietetics. Jon was stunned that his boundaries were crossed by another dietitian: a potential colleague who he expected would have awareness and cultural competency.

These incidents of unintentional othering contrast strongly with Jon's current situation, where he feels supported in his workplace, and values his gay dietitian mentors and friends.

> I think I've been quite fortunate to be able to work [here] … it's super welcoming and a safe space … Even just where the building is situated in the gay village, you have to walk past all the pride flags to get there … [With] the staff here, you kind of know … you're not the only one … we can talk quite openly about our relationships and things like that, so that's been quite nice.

Moral

> I think it's easy for me to speak to this now, but you know, had I been some-body without these supports, somebody more marginalized, more vulnerable … I suspect it would affect somebody [very deeply] … I think there is a lot of power in those kind of interactions … Working with others, the language you choose … it holds power, whether you realize it or not and … regardless of the intent or the tone behind it … I think there can be unintentional offences that can happen. And [dietitians need] to be mindful about that.

Marissa's Story

Marissa Alexander is a Regional Dietitian who works with Indigenous communities across Northern BC.

Marissa shared how, throughout their life, they did not feel like they were enough. They perceived a lack of fit between their nuanced experience and the mutually exclusive options they felt were available. The pressure to "choose a box" made Marissa feel like they couldn't accept or share aspects of themselves unless they were 100% certain. When combined with prevalent identity stereo-types, they didn't initially see the diversity within any identity marker or see them-selves as part of those communities.

In working past these limiting boxes, Marissa pointed to the central role of gathering around food.

> I always felt a little bit like I didn't belong, until I started just sort of speaking to people who I also realize didn't necessarily belong … and a lot of those conversations happen at, you know, at dinner or at drinks, or when you're out with those people that you feel really safe with … What I learned through all of those experiences and exploring that with everybody is that there really is no right way to be queer, or to be biracial, or to express your intelligence. All those things are just so unique to the individual.

Marissa's deepening self-understanding through food experiences connects to the privileges and responsibilities dietitians have:

> We know that when people share about food, we learn so much more about them … As dietitians, we have so much power and privilege, that we get to talk to people every day and learn about them and their food and where they come from in their culture. Because of that, I think it's really important that we're actively working against all of those binaries, especially when … it comes to healthy eating, or what healthy food looks like … Just like there is no right way to be queer, there's no right way to eat.

Their experiences being accepted while working with Indigenous peoples have deeply influenced their story. In contrast to the binary pressures of mainstream culture, they shared that, "… being able to work in spaces where Indigenous peoples' ways of knowing are highlighted, expected, and honoured really makes me … and a lot of people feel safer. It is a very accepting place to be."

Despite the challenges of questioning a binary world, Marissa's story concluded on a positive note:

> I hope that there's some sort of pansexual biracial aspiring dietitians out there who can see their experiences reflected in my journey. And I hope that the dietetics profession continues to work towards making space for people who don't fit into those boxes and are very much in-between.

Moral

> The more time you spend trying to be true to who you are, the more you can support other people … Whether that's somebody that you are caring for as a dietitian or just a loved one or family member, people you just experienced in your life … the more authentic you are to yourself, just the more you bring to this world and to the relationships you have.

Shelly's Story

Shelly is a community dietitian, working in a small town in rural BC.

Shelly tells the story of growing up in rural Ontario, and not learning about things like residential school, racism, colonization, or queer culture. While at university, her worldview opened through literature, dialogue about social issues, and exposure to diverse cultures. While seeing her first female lover off at the airport, she happened upon a book about India's ashrams, which led to a gap year.

> it was a really life-changing moment to find that book, and … within four months get on a plane and spend a year in India with that book as my travel guide.

She returned to University of British Columbia (UBC) for her second year, and then took another gap year and travelled in South America. On returning to UBC, she found that the dietetics programme had moved from the faculty of science to agriculture:

> I was so thrilled to be in agriculture. I just was like, "these are my people" and I loved how nutrition fit into the broader conversation about food systems.

Shelly became a registered dietitian, applied for a job, moved north, and met her wife in a small community. Over the next 10 years Shelly and Traci raised two children and set down roots, establishing careers, family life, and small-town living.

> I applied for one job out of university and one job only and that is this job that I'm in right now. I came ... here in my internship year ... and I just locked in. I just knew I wanted to create a home. I met my wife here, had two children, created a home and we are raising our children here, in a community that does not offer anonymity. In a small community all aspects of yourself are exposed to everyone you work and live with. It is what made me want to stay here and deepen my connection with the people and land of this community. The fact that this community asks you to be authentic; that you can't be one way at work and another way at home – in a smaller town where everyone knows everyone, I felt called to live a more accountable and authentic life.

Not to say that it's always been easy: Shelly describes many moments of humility, discomfort, and navigating challenging relationships with friends and colleagues.

> You have to face these issues with the people you live with. Maybe in a larger city you can avoid conflict, but here you keep seeing your community again and again and that forces you to push through conflict and possibly deepen your connections. It never felt like an option to hide who I was or our family structure, because there was nowhere to hide.

Shelly reflects how being queer has affected her practice as a registered dietitian. Shelly feels that she brings a special awareness to her practice that might not otherwise be there:

> over my career I have had the gift of stories, stories from queer folks, elders, survivors of residential school, people who have experienced trauma. I have spent 16 years listening to stories of resilience, stories of strength, and stories about people's relationship to their bodies and food. These stories are gifts to me because these stories inspire me to stand in strength and my own power. And when I use the word power, I am referring to my most authentic self. Coming from a place of white privilege has made me blind to so many injustices and these stories help remove the filters over my eyes. Living as an openly gay women and touching into the LGBTQ+ injustices throughout time brings me closer to the community members who have lived similar injustices. At the end of the day, I have such gratitude for all the stories this career has gifted me with, and I send a big thank you to all those storytellers.

Moral

> I feel gratitude to live in a place rich with culture, resilience and a deep connection to food and the land. Living alongside people who know where they belong, know their ancestral roots and traditions makes it more available to live my most authentic self. And I think that coming here and being infused with ... that authenticity of a culture ... that's just been here for, generation

after generation … I think that it opened me up to the possibility that I could be anything that I wanted to be.

Epilogue

The story archivists, with input from the storytellers, identified the following themes from the fables and associated morals.

The first theme is that food is never just food – it facilitates mentoring, learning, and the creation of safe spaces. Food is a pathway to relationship, where gathering around a meal can contribute to building chosen family: deep, intimate, and honest relationships that hold space for complexity. Food is a safe space for many queers, but this, too, is complex, as food preparation is a highly gendered activity. Food can also provide important connections to families of origin.

Further themes explored belonging and safety. In early practice, people don't feel very comfortable being out, in part due to the heteronormativity of the profession. For example, in some of these stories, "professionalism" is weaponized and used against LBGTQ+ people, so as to avoid being explicit about prejudice and assumptions. As students and early in their careers, LGBTQ+ dietitians don't necessarily want to be tokenized as queer – the objective seems to be for people to be indifferent to whether one is gay, hetero, queer, pansexual, or …? As people practice for longer and feel community support, they stop trying to hide queer aspects of their lives, and intentionally or unintentionally provide mentorship to younger queers. Practising dietitians and dietetics students should develop cultural humility and language awareness to facilitate more equitable relationships with LGBTQ+ colleagues, students, and clients.

Queer dietitians exhort others to be fearless and be true to who you are, whether trying new recipes, living out and proud, or exploring the complexity of life and practice. Dietetics positions practitioners within systems of power and privilege, and we need to be cognizant of that and work towards equitable relations with clients. Critical reflection and embodied authenticity are necessary first steps towards power-conscious dietetic practice.

Throughout their stories, the participating BC queer dietitians provided thoughtful and reflective examples of excellence of practice in all fields of dietetics. As the archivists and storytellers read and re-read each other's stories, recognizing shared experiences, we built networks of solidarity across generations and geographies. Also, although the option was offered, none of the storytellers chose to publish under a pseudonym, revealing a shared sense of strength in vulnerability. Always remember that when people share stories about their relationship with food, it is precious and should be treated as a gift.

30 Still Dreaming After All These Years that Dietetics Be (Made) Relevant

Jacqui Gingras and Lucy Aphramor

Inconceivable

What Is a Queer Imaginary?

It will feel like all you have/known is shattering/but it is only/a tongue/a soft tongue/ tearing you to pieces

J: I don't know for sure. I guess that is a starting place, the "for sure." A queer imaginary holds nothing as "for sure." It is a theory, a way of seeing and being in the world that invites unruliness and direct confrontation of that which has harmed; that which has reinforced a heteronormativity and white supremacy, which has harmed. This theory was introduced to me in my encounters with Butler (1997, 1999, 2004, 2005), primarily. Reading Butler unravelled me and my thinking. She got my mind whirling and gave language to the injustices I was seeing and experiencing around me. Maybe some would argue that Butler's writing is nothing more than a solipsism – a position that insists that the self is sure to exist, self-aggrandizing, intellectualisms – but I read her differently. She moved me, compelled me to consider that perhaps what I was holding so tightly as truth was not "for sure." That the world as I had come to know it (through my positivist dietetic training) was not a sure thing and that certainty being fed to me and others (Rochefort, Senchuk, Brady, & Gingras, 2016) was worthy of, actually demanded, a second look. And from there a queer imaginary took hold in me and I ventured towards other post-structural texts. I learned a language of disruption and that language mingled ravenously with my hunger for social justice, multiple voices, curiosity, and rampant questioning. Yes, a queer imaginary permits the questions, "What if this were true? What then?"

After grappling with queer texts, I felt an obligation to disrupt the (dietetic) education process for those who were coming through it after me. It was crucial for me and many others to turn our critical gaze to the anti-queer educational process, the horizontal violence, and the other harms that had been permitted in our names (Gingras, Brady, & Aphramor, 2014). It became a time of urgent, breakneck politicizing and unruliness in dietetics. Sparks were flying between and among us, but it did not come without risk.

DOI: 10.4324/9781003217121-33

L: *The hugely influential womanist educator bell hooks says she came to theory to save herself – "because she was hurting"* (hooks, 1991). *It sounds like that's what you're saying too, that you wanted some way of making sense of your feeling response to injustice and this is what Butler offered. It was the same for me in work and life. So we're talking praxis, right? Praxis (which means iteratively building theory from action and taking action informed by this theory) is about reworlding for justice, and this is for all of us. But there's a WEIRD (Western, educated, industrialized, rich, and democratic,* Henrich, Heine & Norenzayan, 2010) *leaning to anti-intellectualism in dietetics that loves decontextualized and compartmentalized theory that aligns with essentialism and capitalism, like behaviour change, dieting, intuitive eating. At the same time, it snubs deep theory. This keeps people/ us stuck imagining the liberal is transformational. In mainstream dietetics that's tackling fat stigma while promoting dieting; in critical spaces, it's refusing the o words (that is, obesity, overweight) but perpetuating white supremacy.*

Anti-intellectualism represses theory/praxis/queering in dietetics via ridicule, through an exceptionalism that locates responsibility for theory in certain academics and leaders, in plain old silence, by disciplinary policing, and so on. It also severs theory from real bodies, real places, and real consequences by treating it like a party game. I can't recall which educator said that white students approached theory like intellectual masturbation, BIPOC students knew their lives were at stake. To be reckless with theory is to be reckless with response-ability.

The term, theory, sounds very head-based, but the theory of a queer imaginary doesn't consider the head or even the self as a stand-alone unit. So when I talk about queer learning I'm talking about learning that involves process, opening, and witnessing, that can find words but need not start with them, that might never be set into a sentence. It's the theory and learning we make possible when we let go of what stops us from worlding differently.

So, theory is for life and queering is an anti-colonial politic. It's a way of relating to the world, not an attribute that's synonymous with identity. Queer covers the story that formal (Western) logic can't describe or contain. Heterosexual nutritionists can write very queer; queer nutritionists can write very straight.

Queer knowing leads us astray. It insists that we need to get lost to find our way (Hemphill and Hemphill, 2021). *It exposes the liberal humanist/imperialist project of coloniality, and hence dietetics, as irredeemable. I'm not saying dietitians have nothing to offer, I'm saying we need an ontological reconfiguring – rupture, not repair.*

Sharman (2022) opens her book on LGBTQ+ healthcare by asking "what if queer and trans people loved going to the doctor?" That's wild, right? That's queering. It about changing conditions in service of liberation not paternalistic benevolence for practitioner feel-good.

Where does queer take you in real time? It would be interesting to know how you queer from within the university, as well as beyond.

J: Your question caught me off guard. How do I queer the institutional from within the university? The practices of freedom are so tightly bound to who I am, it is difficult to answer quickly because, as you have already said, a queer imaginary is a process, not only an identity. I should first admit that although this is a Queering Nutrition and Dietetics book, I am not a faculty member in nutrition anymore. I moved from nutrition to sociology, which is not typical for folks in the ironclad, discipline-bound institutional space called university. Nonetheless, it was a strategy for my own survival and some prescient leaders helped make it happen. One reason it had to happen was because I was insolently queer in my daily practices and beingness to stay.

And that would be another story for another day. For right now, I am in sociology, and I am surrounded by equity-minded folks who have created the conditions for queerness to flourish; again, not the queerness that concerns itself only with upending heteronormative practices, but with every single injustice that we carry in our bones, and we witness with our whole selves, and we witness around us. This is a most beautiful, vital academic home.

What does my queering look like in the university? Many things, because the university is a place where many injustices reside and are reconstituted in daily routines and actions.

I adapted a textbook on the sociology of education in so-called Canada to focus on how the state colonized Indigenous people through residential schooling, land dispossession, and the Sixties Scoop. This version of the textbook is open access and available for everyone (https://pressbooks.library .ryerson.ca/socedind/). It is under continual revision. I wrote a grant that would enable the hiring of Indigenous students who comprised the advisory council for the text and then conducted an inquiry on how students in the class received and acted upon the attempt to decolonize. Some of them reminded me that this course was the first time they had heard about residential schools.

I continually talk back to the administration regarding how they misrepresent themselves to students. I write to the president asking why he has not instituted a tuition waiver during a pandemic. I ask the administration to remove a statue that reflects our adherence to a person who created the curriculum of the genocidal residential schools.

Also, I queer the way educators might reframe academic misconduct and integrity by offering students online, open-book, collaborative exams. What might it mean for us as academics to promote ways for students to work together instead of punishing them with charges of academic misconduct? How might educators reorient themselves to the radical idea that taking time to create relational means of evaluation and assessment will not only strengthen their relationships with students but leave them better prepared for their collaborative work outside the university.

And I wonder how I might use my position as a tenured professor with white, cis privilege to disrupt business as usual? I have been here for 16 years, and I have learned some things about how this place works and I actively seek to unsettle those policies and practices that tend to dehumanize. I am thinking lately of Ahmed's (2021) latest work on *Complaint* where she reveals that "To become a complainer is to become the location of a problem." I have noticed that to be even more true the longer I find myself in the academy. Reading Ahmed's queer phenomenology of complaint has given me a language for the labour and resistance I have experienced as a complainer;

one that seeks to queer the institution in the name of justice. This language of recognition along with the solidarity and connection with colleagues and comrades keep me afloat.

I was caught up recently in reading an Ahmed post from her Feminist KillJoy blog (2018) where she talks about complaint as scratches into the wood panelling of those colonial spaces. Ahmed describes those enduring marks made by feminists as carrying their own message *"we were here, we did not get used to it."* I want to leave similar marks that can be read long after I am gone. I hope I did that in dietetics with the writing we left. We were here and we did not get used to it.

And there are so many ways I can do queer process differently, better. I am still learning. For instance, I find it hard to "be strategic" and wait for "the right time" to act. I tend to want to act now and face the consequences of my impatience later. I have this burning pit of urgency in my gut that says, "We have been waiting long enough." This is a place where I can be more discerning for the greater good, for the long conversation.

L: *The Black Lives Matter uprisings in 2020 compelled me to ask and to keep on asking "what am I missing." I was trying to recognize – and then change – my own commitment to whiteness. I turned to scholarship that values indigenizing, intersectionality, animism, to new practices, and performance/poetry.*

I came to realize that I'd wrapped previous work around coloniality. A key error is that I hadn't grasped the fact that evidence-based medicine, aka colonial medicine, aka Eurocentric, biased medicine, is a vector for scientific imperialism. So in the book Body Respect (2014) *for example, my co-author Lindo Bacon and I present evidence-based medicine conventionally, as the judicious use of the best available evidence. We argue that public health practice corrupts the neutral, valuable, methodology of evidence-based medicine because of conscious and unconscious bias. Our metanarrative is that the proper, rigorous use of colonial medicine would root out fat stigma, neoliberalism, and other infestations of oppression and move us further towards health equity.*

But of course, colonial medicine isn't neutral, evidence-based medicine isn't an objective methodology – it's an intentionally anti-Black ideology that presumes the only possible, real, way to collate evidence, "be healthy," relate to plants, or conduct science, is the white way. Our education inculcates us with ideas and values that programme us to scoff at ritual and ceremony as healing modalities, to be contemptuous of Indigenous concepts like cosmovisions, ancestor worship, and plant medicine. The ideology of evidence-based medicine legitimates these feelings and opinions for us. On the occasions where dietetics acknowledges healing interventions from beyond Western science, it teaches us to regard these as useful because evidence-based medicine has said so, as if Western science is the final arbiter of Truth.

It was hard coming to know this.

Hard to step outside of the delusion of white supremacy (helped by staying away from spaces shaped by orthodoxy or comfort); hard to own the sheer magnitude of my ineptness; hard to allow for the implications of everything else I must be missing; hard to reckon with forces that will/ed silence. And an utter relief, liberatory

These Are the Anti-Queer Tactics

J: A community that creates a handful of experts to curate the approved script is one that starves the queerness of the meanderers from morsels that nourish them. I see an example of anti-queer tactics in the copyrighting of health at every size (HAES). This is an action that quells growth, movement, and dissent. And it is entirely problematic (Gingras & Cooper, 2013). Are you aware of being starved? I remember a time that I questioned one of my instructors as to the legitimacy of eco-centred ways of knowing. It was there for the taking, for the gentle embrace I could have made with it, but I was far too far gone in the stranglehold of egocentricism. I could see this was marginal knowing within dietetics and I could smell the blood of that shadowy epistemology. I went for the kill and only returned humbled years later. Responding queerly means learning to say "sorry" to those I have harmed, bowled over, and trashed along the Right Path. My becoming has placed me in front of decent teachers, and I have not always been receptive (Gingras, 2004). I found myself learning to say sorry.

L: What does response-ability entail? Some combination of apology, reckoning, repair. For me it includes apologizing for cementing coloniality and for misrepresenting HAES as liberatory; changing the narrative so that evidence-based medicine is understood as a technology of whiteness in need of dismantling, not a foundationally sound project in need of tweaking.

By learning together queerly we're saying "this is where my thinking is at the moment. I'll probably change my truth on this sometime and I might also totally be wrong." That's not an abdication of our duty of rigour or care or repair.

If we understand ourselves as mouthpieces of white domination now, why didn't/wouldn't/couldn't we know differently before?

The tactics of the anti-queer are to batter us into shape by forces of belonging that want us to stay on the straight and narrow; forces we barely register as long as they are the wind behind us, plain sailing. They're the power of cultural hegemony deciding what ideologies will be unremarkable, desirable, superior. The best way to expose them is to disagree and notice what happens.

Which is to say that the collective decides what narratives to establish, which knowledge matters, what personhood entails, whose feelings to care about, when to impose silence, the voices to emulate, acceptable terms and cosmologies, who and what histories to erase. Naming the role of the collective here isn't a ruse to exonerate me and my co-author Lindo Bacon from authorial accountability in the Body Respect example. I'm not rationalizing away our culpability but highlighting the fact that the decision-making collective plays a significant role in amplifying or repressing any potential impact of individual actions. Scholars have differential impact according to the privileges we are granted, our iteratively situated social standing. Power-as-community determines what Truth(s) matter(s).

Communities create leaders and agendas. I'm haunted by poet David Whyte's observation that the only thing wrong with (UK neoliberal politician) Margaret Thatcher is that no-one stopped her.

While queering holds plurality it welcomes singularity and queries. For the record, my story of Body Respect is one of failure, the disruptive and generative queer art of failure that Judith Haberstam (2011) explores. If these thought-strands enter a hostile culture they'll get killed off – dysbiosis. They could land in another culture that permits their reproduction, allows them to mutate and merge with other life-affirming fragments of story. We'll see.

Dietetics as a culture nourishes some ways of knowing superbly, and this creates a medium that is poisonous to growing learning through failure, dissent, creativity, uncertainty, plurality, animism, Blackness, fatness, queerness. Deep knowing means rejecting consistency, universality, respectability – being unsortable:

I thought I'd be sorted by fifty

of course I wasn't at all, not by a long shot
mainly because I was still alive
to things becoming always more
exuberant and confusing and the pleasure of reckoning seduced me
so I found myself being out of step with the crimping etiquette of straightness and whiteness
that said settle
that said be consistent
Don't revel. That's it.
don't risk it, be careful yeah? stay clever what if you unravel, what if
I am so out of sync with protocol I might tell even occasional lovers everything
all of it
my late arriving my precious self-obsession I am so done pretending
so utterly off-beat with what's expected from respectability that I only insisted on storying trauma, sold tickets to strangers, wrote all about embarrassment, outright aired my ignorance and my glory staged this whole freakin' show of things I didn't know until I did shed so much shame and shushness that transjoy found me, flung euphoric arms around me, swung me high high.

References

Ahmed, S. (2018). *Refusal, resignation, and complaint.* Feminist Killjoys.

Ahmed, S. (2021). *Complaint!* Duke University Press.

Bacon, L., & Aphramor, L. (2014) *Body respect.* Benbella.

Butler, J. (1997). *The psychic life of power: Theories in subjection.* Stanford University Press.

Butler, J. (1999). *Gender trouble: Feminism and the subversion of identity.* Routledge.

Butler, J. (2004). *Undoing gender.* Routledge.

Butler, J. (2005). *Giving an account of oneself.* Fordham University Press.

Gingras, J., & Cooper, C. (2013). Down the rabbit hole: A critique of the ® in HAES®. *Journal of Critical Dietetics, 1*(3), 2–5.

Gingras, J., Brady, J., & Aphramor, L. (2014). Harm has been done: Ethical transgressions in becoming and being a dietitian. *Journal of Critical Dietetics, 2*(1), 52–62.

Gingras, J. R. (2004). Like cold water or a kiss: Reflections on transformative teachings. In G. Smith, M. L. deZwart, & L. Peterat (Eds.), *Home economics now: Transformative practice, ecology, and everyday life, a tribute to the scholarship of Eleanor Vaines* (pp. 67–75). Pacific Educational Press.

Halberstam, J. (2011). *The queer art of failure*. Duke University Press.

Hemphill, P., & Hemphill, E. (Hosts) (2021, May 3). Hope, questioning, and getting lost with Bayo Akomolafe. (No. 52) [Audio podcast]. https://www.findingourwaypodcast.com/individual-episodes/s2e3

Henrich, J., Heine, S., & Norenzayan, A. (2010). The weirdest people in the world? *Behavioral Brain Science*, 33(2–3):61–83.

hooks, b. (1991). Theory as liberatory practice. http://www.uwyo.edu/aded5050/5050unit12/theory%20as%20liberatory%20prac.pdf

Rochefort, J., Senchuk, A., Brady, J., & Gingras, J. (2016). Spoon fed: Learning about "obesity" in dietetics. In J. Ellison, D. McPhail, & W. Mitchinson (Eds.), *Obesity in Canada: Critical perspectives* (pp. 148–174). University of Toronto Press.

Sharman, Z. (2022). *Care we dream of, the: Liberatory & transformative approaches to LGBTQ+ health*. Arsenal Pulp Press.

31 Being Trans in Dietetics

A Step in the Movement towards Trans and Queer Liberation through Collaborative Conversation

Kathryn Fraser, Nat Quathamer, and Marin Whebby

The experiences of lesbian, gay, bi, trans, queer, and other sexual- or gender-minority identities), (LGBTQ+) individuals, and in particular trans people, have rarely been heard within the world of nutrition and dietetics, either as students, interns, or dietitians. The impetus for this chapter was to provide space for three queer and trans people who have lived through dietetic pedagogy to have a conversation about their personal experiences and reflections about the education received and its underlying dominant discourses. Despite going to three separate institutions, these experiences were largely similar, showing the systemic nature of these issues within dietetics. The information in this chapter is specific to our experiences and does not speak for all of the trans and queer people who have experienced dietetics, in particular, the perspectives of queer and trans folks who are Black, Indigenous, or people of colour (QTBIPOC).

Although this is sharing that has been done voluntarily by the authors it is crucial to note that these conversations were emotionally and physically draining for the participants. This is not an invitation for dietitians and healthcare professionals to rely on queer and trans people to speak about their trauma for the purpose of their learning. It is, however, an invitation for cisgender and heterosexual people (cishets) to do their own learnings on LGBTQIA+ health care and begin critical conversations around sexuality and gender in dietetics.

During analysis and interpretation of the resulting transcript, three main themes were developed: the representation of health, food, and bodies in dietetic pedagogy, and subsequently, how those representations impacted the authors' queerness and transness. These themes represent the interpretation of the education and training provided, whether that knowledge was explicit, such as overt dietetic theory and professional standards, or implicit, in terms of tacit knowledge and the unspoken rules of a professional performance (Burwood, 2007).

Health

In our dietetic education, health, and knowledge were presented as rigidly binary and fixed. As a medical profession in our society, there was only one valid form of wellness, a form steeped in colonial, fatphobic, ableist, white supremacist, and

DOI: 10.4324/9781003217121-34

cisheterosexist ideas of morality and worth. Within dietetics this was presented as explicit and implicit rules of how to correctly achieve health, which is eating to discipline the body into something more normative – such as being thin, cis, and white-passing. The binary foundation of knowledge presented in our dietetic educations left no room to consider or be anything else within dietetic culture and reinforced cisheteronormativity by enshrining two static, opposite, and separate sexes: "*So health was very binary and dietetics was very binary. I felt like there wasn't room to explore beyond the 'one path to go on'.*" There was no space for us to talk about or experience transness and queerness. It has been left up to us as trans and queer people to carry the emotional weight of opening up this dialogue and advocating for ourselves, resulting in exhaustion, anxiety, and the risk of potential harm.

For us as students, this view of health became embodied in a mandatory "health" performance – an externalization of health that replicated the appearance of "health" but did not serve us or our wellbeing as people: "*I feel like it wasn't an option. You're a health professional, it was mandatory, and there was only one way to achieve health.*" We were taught that there was one right way of achieving health, and little else was presented to us as an option; unsurprisingly, performing health according to these standards made us sicker. Our disordered eating behaviours fit right into the framework we were learning, and for each of us, our mental health worsened. However, we all experienced the sense that we were doing such a good job at being the "good" dietetic student and even believed at the time that we were being "healthy." Disordered eating was a coping mechanism and a way to successfully assimilate into the dietetic profession.

As we got better at embodying the harmful image of health so often cherished within dietetics, we got further away from ourselves. For some of us, it was a way of continually selling the fantasy of cisheteronormativity to ourselves even though we felt different within the social system of dietetics: "*I think for me, it was a way to continue selling myself cisnormative discourses. I just needed to be a 'Good girl' and comply with all the associated gender roles around health, food, and bodies, and everything would be okay.*" Possibilities for exploring transness and queerness were stifled by the static, oppressive foundation of dietetics, as was our sense of selfhood. How could we begin to conceptualize a different way to exist when difference was absent? No one had to tell us that transness was wrong, we just knew because it was never talked about in our education, therefore, it couldn't be right or healthy. There was always a fear of being discovered as doing health and cisness wrong, even as we could not hold back the fact that our health was deteriorating – because "failing" at dietetics implicated you as the problem, not as the result of an unjust system. This resulted in the suppression of our authentic selves and kept us in the closet longer, causing an intense amount of shame.

Food

The dominant representation of food in dietetics for us was that it was simply a vehicle through which you obtained health and morality – a means to an end. Conceptions of food were rooted in the discourses around health, offering a physical model to display the right, and wrong, way to achieve health. As students, food became performance riddled with anxiety and shame. The crunch of crisp vegetables as the soundscape for learning was welcomed by students and educators but the rustle of a chip bag was a deafening offence. For us, food was an opportunity to demonstrate that you were literally devouring the tomes of dietetics; embodying what it meant to be considered the right kind of dedicated student; showing you belonged; and providing a sense of self for the consumer.

> *It felt like every time you ate, it was an opportunity to prove yourself, improve your health. It wasn't an opportunity for exploration, it wasn't an opportunity for new flavours, it wasn't an opportunity for pleasure. It wasn't an opportunity to learn that you didn't like something – it was an opportunity to show that you were right.*

The undercurrent of this message was that of deprivation. Food was framed in the negative, an opportunity to avoid the "wrong" things and behaviours. Moving towards pleasure or joy from food was rarely discussed with us by dietetic educators, except when it stemmed from the use of food as a means to achieve optimal health, disease prevention, and outward appearance.

The lack of discussion around pleasure or joy and the focus on puritanical ideals bled into our daily lives and habits, making our exploration of queerness and transness even more difficult in a cisheteronormative society. Notably, achieving the dietetic standard of "healthy" eating was intimately bound to one's ability to be a good person and a good citizen, that society already deems impossible for queer and trans people (Serrano, 2016). Furthermore, the presentation of food as a moral dichotomy of "good" or "bad" made exploring outside the binary in other aspects of life, such as with gender and sexuality, feel unsafe. In addition, the resulting obsession with food was time-consuming and energy-sapping and was a way to numb our desires or needs around sexuality and gender.

> *It's easy for rhetoric around healthy eating to obfuscate queerness and transness, because what's good and right is so tied up in being a cishet person, and being good in dietetics is specific for being a woman or specific for being a man. And so, in order to be good at healthy eating, you have to be good at being a woman or a man, and there's no room for failure, or blurring the boundaries."*

Bodies

Within the confines of dietetic education and training, there were two physical options presented to us in any category: for example, man or woman, normal shape or abnormal shape (i.e., too fat or too thin), and healthy or unhealthy. What it meant to have a healthy body was also wrapped up in oppressive ideals of what it means to be a good and productive member of society. Though brief instances of counter-narratives were presented to us, specifically about fat bodies, these were small points in time against an overwhelming message of bodies that are acceptable according to specific standards, and bodies that are fundamentally disobedient. This binary was particularly absolute regarding sex and gender:

> *It's very binary. There were two options, and those were cishet options of ideal bodies wrapped up in fatphobia and colonial ideas of what is to be pursued, what is desirable. Those two ever present silhouettes of a buff, but not too buff, man and slender hourglass woman. There are two bodies.*

Thus, much like the presentation of food, bodies were stripped of their important social context and humanity. They were framed as both method and project in obtaining idealized health and happiness according to biomedical standards based on two idolized forms of bodies.

For much of our schooling, there was no representation of queer and trans people or their experiences within dietetic education, unless it was explicitly sought out. In addition to these messages about bodies that permeate the dietetic curriculum, much of the performance of a dietitian-to-be was wrapped up in flawlessly demonstrating this knowledge with one's body, such as presenting the correct body shape and ability, one that was in accordance with rigid standards of looking "professional" and achieving cisfemininity. It felt as though there was no space for transfemininity or anything outside the binary. There was little joy in having a body within this framework; instead, there was always a new goal or something to pursue in order to have a "healthy" body. Each of us put a lot of energy, time, and effort into trying to fit our bodies into these standards of health and gender in dietetics.

Steeped within the binary knowledge and culture of Canadian dietetic education, we felt a lack of connection to our bodies. We experienced our bodies from an external vantage point, even going so far as to feel dissociated from ourselves. This manifested in a feeling that our bodies and experiences didn't belong to us, and instead were a performance meant to secure us belonging, connection, and acceptance into dietetics:

> *I didn't really feel like I belonged to myself anymore. It felt like masking. I remember exactly what I wore because I spent so much time planning it, and that was specifically to impress them. And I had so much makeup on. I remember looking in the mirror that morning [of my internship interview] and I didn't even recognize myself, I had a weird out of body experience. I didn't want them to see that I was crumbling inside.*

Having a body viewed as "unacceptable" gave us a significant level of fear and anxiety, whether that was a way of dressing, a certain body shape, or even having piercings. We felt unable to move toward what would bring us actual health, joy, and wellbeing. Even as some of us made secretive strides forward into exploring what it meant to be queer or trans, dietetics held us back and prevented us from fully developing into our transness and queerness due to the all-encompassing fear of being rejected.

These are particularly troubling issues given the ostensibly "apolitical" nature of the dietetics profession (Gingras, 2009), which purports itself in being evidence-based, objective, and neutral. For each of us, social concerns were framed as a niche topic for dietitians, and fundamentally only as barriers to "helping" people achieve the correct body. This absence of human social context ignores that bodies are already politicized and does not critically question the underlying assumptions made about what makes a correct and healthy body. The rigid and exclusive framework of health in dietetics also remains silent and unquestioned until seen or experienced by those who are impacted by its assumptions and are othered as "wrong." Many of the messages that we received as students were implicit and framed in the negative. We were not often explicitly told which body was the most correct body, we simply intuited which bodies were more acceptable based on what was described as less desirable, which bodies were represented, and the absence of other bodies. Therefore, students had to intuit the right way to be in the world, both as a person and as a dietetic student. It could be so subtle that we would blame ourselves for being the wrong type of person when we inevitably "failed" and didn't fit the right mould:

> *They just describe everything that's wrong and you intuit the right thing. And of course because they don't get "political" and they don't explicitly say what the right thing is, it means that they're not doing anything wrong so you can't even question it, because they're not taking an active stance against anyone, but they're not taking an active stance for anything that's remotely inclusive either. When you're in it, it's so subtle that it digs you apart and makes you feel like you're the inherently wrong one.*

This resulted in a lot of shame, guilt, and anxiety for each of us trying to navigate dietetic knowledge and education, as being different, including being trans or queer, and it felt like deviance.

Final Considerations

For all three of us, the ultimate result of these experiences was disenfranchisement, disillusionment, and resentment towards dietetics, as well as the need to step away from the knowledge and culture of the dietetic profession. Either temporarily to have breathing space before re-entering the profession at a later time, or permanently for the sake of self-preservation: "*I had to step away from academia, in general. I had to take a critical look at the knowledge that I had gained. A big thing for me was seeing the breaks, it allowed me to weasel my way through into exploration beyond binary thinking.*" Though we may have received encouragement to stay within the profession, this was not a tenable course of action given the significant costs to our mental health and wellbeing that resulted from remaining in that environment:

> *Being in dietetics was killing me. It's one of the things that kept me in the closet and prevented me from developing a sense of my own transness and my own trans-femininity. I couldn't find any sort of liberation within dietetics. And so, I left, and have never regretted that decision once.*

This was not an easy decision, given the extensive mental, emotional, social, and financial investment that we each made in the dietetic profession. It was more than walking away from a degree, it was walking away from who we were in those moments and choosing to prioritize our wellbeing by living a more authentic life regardless of the likely consequences to our social circles and professional paths as people who had "failed" to complete dietetic education in the linear, intensive fashion expected for many "successful" students. Outside of the all-encompassing nature of dietetic education, we have each been able to gradually process our experiences and emotions, as well as explore new forms of knowledge from less binary and rigid perspectives on human experience and health. Importantly, this space has allowed us to critically examine our experiences and develop into our queerness and transness. By stepping away, we have all become happier, healthier people, and feel a deep sense of gratitude for the queerness and transness that lit the way.

This reflection upon our experiences also made us consider how to promote queer and trans liberation in nutrition and dietetics, not only for the benefit of future, current, and past LGBTQIA+ students, but also for the field overall and all those it serves. Queerness and transness offer dietetics the opportunity to blossom beyond the binary, creating new visions of health, food, and bodies that are kinder and more compassionate. In order to make dietetics a safer space for LGBTQIA+, we suggest starting with the foundation of dietetics, breaking down the rigidity around food, bodies, and health in an intersectional manner. This may look like disrupting current assumptions around gender, sexuality, race, and ability within the profession, and the oppressive standards that follow, such as unpaid internships and requirements of elitist "professional" attire. Specifically, explicitly representing and including important social context into the dietetic curriculum, such as the experiences and voices of LGBTQIA+ people with their consent and compensation, is critical to disrupting this rigidity. In addition, this should entail creating space for personhood outside of dietetics and integrating pleasure as an essential part of the human experience. In this, different ways of knowing, being, and finding joy through food and bodies would not only be valued but would actively be seen as foundational to the minimum practice standards of dietetics.

References

Burwood, S. (2007). Imitation, indwelling and the embodied self. *Educational Philosophy and Theory, 39*(2), 118–134.

Gingras, J. (2009). The educational (im)possibility for dietetics: A poststructural discourse analysis. *Learning Inquiry, 3*(3), 177–191.

Serano, J. (2016). *Whipping girl: A transsexual woman on sexism and the scapegoating of femininity.* Seal Press.

32 Light of a New Day

Fabien Lutz-Barabé

I was diagnosed with squamous cell carcinoma (tongue cancer) in 2016. The radiation treatment that followed the surgery caused me to lose weight. I went from 180 lbs to my current 128 lbs because of the difficulty in eating and swallowing.

Getting back to my art was uninspiring as I went through a severe depression. The only thing that brought me back was returning to my love of cartooning. This digital drawing is entitled *Light of a New Day* (Figure 32.1). It represents a hopeful outlook on the future. I chose to use light and shadow to best reflect my optimism I feel when looking through a window at the rays of sunlight on a new day.

I still struggle with my diet and what I can and cannot eat. In the last month, I have gone to 90% vegetarian. A lot of these types of foods are easier to consume, and it has helped in many ways as I feel more energetic, physically and mentally.

DOI: 10.4324/9781003217121-35

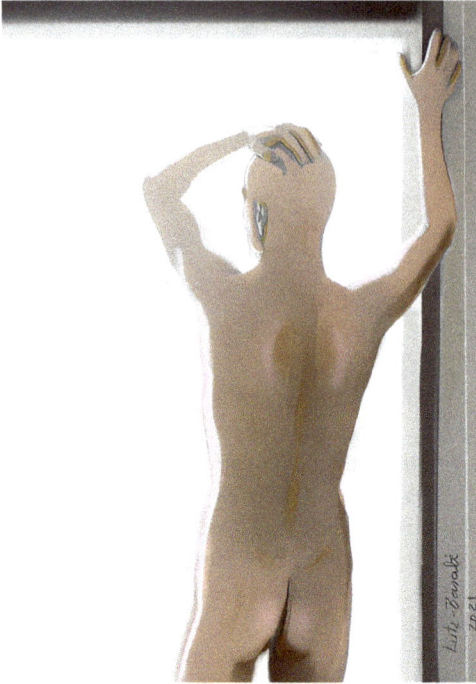

Figure 32.1 Light of a New Day. Fabien Lutz-Barabé.

33 How Recovering from an Eating Disorder Made Me Queer

Kelsey Moran

The Eating Disorder Part

When I was in middle school, back when I thought I was a cishet (cisgender and heterosexual) girl, I remember not wanting to eat much at lunch. I remember feeling too self-conscious about how I looked, instead waiting until I got home to eat. I remember getting home from school and grabbing snacks for myself while I watched TV, and then grabbing more snacks, and more snacks. I remember feeling ashamed when I realized how much I had eaten and deciding to hide the evidence so that no one would know. I remember friends expressing concern about how little I was eating at school, and I remember feeling angry that they were drawing attention to what I was eating, fuelling an increasingly desperate need to hide my eating habits from the world. I remember feeling self-conscious about my body changing as I entered high school and the relief of getting out of my head and shifting into autopilot when I got home and opened the fridge. I remember going through college and deciding to count calories to help myself manage what I was eating, feeling proud of myself for going to bed hungry every night and for fitting into clothes that I hadn't fit into in years. I remember feeling devastated when I stopped counting calories and started gaining back the weight that I had lost. I remember feeling like I had failed.

Looking back at myself during those 11 years from the perspective of someone who (finally) has a positive relationship with food and their body, in addition to a doctorate in clinical psychology, I mostly just feel sad. I feel sad that I spent so much of my life fixated on food, my weight, calories, clothing sizes, and hate. I feel sad that I didn't have the skills I do now that help me filter out all of the garbage narratives society has about "good" and "bad" foods, about beauty, about the worth of bodies. I feel sad that I worked so hard to hide my binge eating disorder (BED) and that I ignored the concerns from my friends, delaying my ability to get the help I needed for years. I feel sad that I let the mean and thoughtless comments that people made about me contribute to the mean and thoughtless ways I talked to myself. I feel sad that I didn't have a higher opinion of myself, that I didn't look at myself with the compassion that I deserved. I feel sad that because I was singularly focused on the way I looked and what I ate, it took me years to get

DOI: 10.4324/9781003217121-36

to know other parts of myself, parts of myself and my identity that are way more important and interesting than a number on a scale.

But I also feel proud, and relieved, and grateful. I'm absolutely grateful for the work that I did and the support I had from my family and friends, but honestly I'm mostly grateful for the therapists who helped me change my life.

The Therapy Part

In my first semester of graduate school, I heard from a number of professors that if we hadn't been in therapy before, we should consider trying it now. Given that I was learning to become a therapist, I figured that it made sense and I scheduled my first appointment. I told myself that I didn't have anything in particular to talk about, so throughout the six appointments that I had with that therapist over winter break we mostly just chatted about my sense of self. She was primarily an Internal Family Systems therapist, meaning that she helps people understand themselves by looking at the different "parts" of the self and how they interact with each other to function as an internal system (IFS Institute, n.d.). We tried to identify some of the parts of myself that might be getting bullied by some of the more dominant parts of myself, specifically the part of myself that felt ashamed. We wrapped up our work together once I moved back up to graduate school for the spring semester, and I remember thinking about shame more intentionally and thoughtfully than I had before. It felt wildly overwhelming but important to really look at how shame was preventing me from acknowledging my eating disorder even within myself, let alone being able to talk about it with someone else. Even though it was brief, that first experience in therapy helped me feel a little more comfortable feeling vulnerable with a therapist, allowing me to find a new therapist later that year who was closer to graduate school and who specialized in eating disorders.

I ended up working with this therapist for about three years, and in that time I learned more about myself than I believe I ever would have on my own. She was brilliant, compassionate, insightful, and kind of a hard ass, but in the best and most caring of ways. I remember feeling pretty defensive at first, not wanting to be any more vulnerable than I already felt talking about something I had never talked about with anyone before, but over time we built up our relationship and I really started trusting her. And not just trusting her to hold the secrets I was sharing, but trusting her to understand me, to challenge me, and to care about me. I remember the first time I was able to sit in her office without holding a pillow in front of me to hide my stomach and how she helped me celebrate that moment. I remember her helping me visualize my BED, guiding me through an exercise to help me understand how big and uncontrollable it still felt at that point. It was hard work, and it was scary to look my eating disorder in the eyes after running from it for so long but doing that work alongside this therapist made that feel a little easier. There were a few times where things got worse before they were able to get better, but she was there to help talk me through my first panic attack and to help me feel less hopeless about ever feeling free from my eating disorder. She helped me figure out how to talk about what I was going through with my family and friends, gently nudging me to be more open about my experience with the people I trusted.

Eventually I got to a point where I didn't feel like food, my weight, and my appearance were taking up the majority of the space in my head, where I could just eat something without it feeling like I was going into battle with myself. I stopped binge eating in secret, I stopped counting calories, I stopped hating the size of my body, all of it. It certainly didn't happen overnight, and I'm still a human with insecurities who lives in a society with a toxic perspective on bodies, diet culture, and florescent lighting in changing rooms so it's not all rainbows and sunshine, but overall, I really do feel good. I get that that might not sound like a big deal to some people, but if you've struggled with an eating disorder and especially if you're still in the midst of it, you get how big a deal it is to be free of that perspective. I haven't looked at a scale in years, so I don't know how much I weigh these days, but I know that I weigh more than I've ever weighed before. And every time I realize that and really think about how much happier I am with myself and my awesome, fat body now than when I was at my thinnest as an adult, I feel like I'm on top of the fucking world. As I'm typing this right now my foot is tapping, and my leg is bouncing, and my thigh is jiggling, and I just feel so happy. I owe so much of my current happiness to that therapist who believed in me and stuck with me through the biggest growth period of my life.

Years later, I still wholeheartedly believe that she saved my life. And not just because of the work we did with my eating disorder but also because of the work we did with my sexuality for the final year of our work together.

The First Queer Part

As I got to the point in my eating disorder work where I started to feel more stable and actually shifted into recovery, something I previously didn't think would ever be possible, I noticed that I had way more brain space than I had before. I was halfway through my graduate programme and had always been able to manage the student part of my life well enough, but this was the first time in my adult life that I felt like I had a little latitude to maybe understand myself better as a human, beyond the monopoly of shame that had been front and centre for so long. I started noticing some patterns in my interests, specifically around LGBTQ+ (lesbian, gay, bisexual, trans, queer/questioning, and all other people who exist under the rainbow) topics. Among other clues, I realized one day that I had watched this one particular coming out video on YouTube, without exaggeration, over 100 times. I remember thinking about that one night as I started up the same video again, and the metaphorical lightbulb over my head started flickering on as I realized that I was maybe trying to work through something by watching and rewatching this video.

The way that I understand all of this for myself is that my eating disorder was like a balloon in my brain. It started small enough, totally deflated, and then every critical comment or shameful moment around food and my body was another breath of air to fill that balloon. It got so full that it pushed everything else about myself that had previously taken up space or had the potential to one day take up space off to the side, wedged so deeply into the nooks and crannies in my brain that they couldn't be found. That balloon got so full that it almost burst, and it was taking all of my attention and energy to try to keep it from bursting. My eating disorder brain was running the show, and it barged ahead for almost a decade until I went to therapy and started trying to poke some holes in it. Little by little, my therapist and I were able to deflate it until it finally looked small again, or at least as small as it's capable of being in the society we live in. And little by little, there was space in my brain again. The parts of myself that had been driven away into hiding started to come out (pun intended), and eventually I realized that they were there, and I could start interacting with them, getting to know them.

As it turns out, a lot of those emerging parts were pretty queer. I started thinking about past relationships and moments with a new perspective, realizing with more and more clarity that I was perhaps not as straight as I once thought. I sat with this by myself for a few months before hitting a point where I needed to process it with someone else. As much as I trusted my family and friends to be supportive, my therapist was the only person I wanted to talk to about it. At this point in our relationship we had established a solid foundation, and I felt completely comfortable with her, but it was still terrifying to say it out loud. It took me a few sessions to feel brave enough to bring it up with her, but I finally told her that I thought I might be bisexual. She paused a moment, blinked at me a few times, and finally responded with "Kelsey, how the fuck did I not see that?!" Which admittedly caught me a little off guard, but I absolutely loved her reaction. The immediate reassurance that me coming out to her did not in any way change our dynamic was such an unbelievable relief. We had a fairly candid way of talking with each other as well as a very similar sense of humour and laughing with her about how "I didn't know before now; I don't know how the fuck you were supposed to know!" was just the best. We spent the rest of the session talking through that moment and processing my understanding of my sexuality with a great deal of care and respect, but that moment of levity and reassurance is what gave me the confidence to eventually start coming out to the other most important people in my life.

This therapist helped me through so many challenges and transitions in my life throughout our time working together. For my last year of graduate school, I had to move halfway across the country for an internship, bringing our time together to an end. I hated that I had to say goodbye to her. I still think about her and how grateful I am to her for helping me get to a point where I was lucky enough and able to build the life that I have today. The skills she helped me develop to understand and take care of myself have been reinforced by other great therapists since then, but she's the one who did the heavy lifting and made it possible.

The Second Queer Part

More recently I've been going through a similar process, but this time instead of the resolution of an eating disorder creating space for sexuality exploration, it's a pandemic creating space for gender exploration. In hindsight it shouldn't have taken a pandemic to jumpstart my non-binary awakening, but here we are. Years earlier, I wrote my dissertation on gender identity and the language used to describe it, and that same amazing therapist very gently asked me if there was any reason in particular that I chose to research trans identities. My answer at the time was that I was just trying to be a good ally, but I can now look back and understand that there was part of myself that resonated with the concept of living outside of a gender binary.

My growing understanding of myself has certainly been meaningful and heal- ing for me personally, and I hope it helps me become a better therapist for my clients. When I think of my LGBTQ+ clients, especially those who have difficult relationships with food and their bodies, I feel deeply connected to and in awe of the bravery that it takes to share their experiences with me. I've thankfully had the training and support to keep my own experiences in the back of my head rather than taking up space in the session that belongs to my clients, but their stories resonate with me more than they know. I remember how important it was for me to know that my therapist believed in me, and I hope that they know how much I believe in them. I want to be clear that this story is my own and does not in any way describe a universal experience for all people in the LGBTQ+ community and/or who have experienced difficult relationships with food and their bodies. I'm sharing this with the hope that fellow therapists will have a better understand- ing of what their clients may be experiencing and that clients who are struggling with the same things that I struggled with may feel a little less alone. Thank you for taking the time to share in this with me.

Reference

IFS Institute. (n.d.). *The internal family systems model outline*. Retrieved September 14, 2021, from https://ifs-institute.com/resources/articles/internal-family-systems-model-outline

34 Nutrition in Chemsex

Jason Simpson-Theobald

Chemsex is the term used to describe the taking of certain recreational drugs either preceding or during sexual intercourse between men who have sex with men (MSM) (Bourne et al., 2014). This is sometimes referred to as "Party and Play" or "PnP." The chemsex drugs include gamma hydroxybutyrate (GHB), its precursor gamma-butyrolactone (GBL), crystal methamphetamine, and mephedrone. Mephedrone is a synthetic cathenone; more recently chemsex definitions have expanded to include other chemicals within this class (Stuart, 2019).

The drugs increase sexual desire and stamina, resulting in sessions which can last for extended periods (Bourne et al., 2014), with some parties going on for several days (Macfarlane, 2016). The drugs are often taken in combination to maximize the desirable effects and to modify the onset and duration of the "high;" mephedrone users begin to feel subjective effects after about 15 minutes from administration, peaking at around 45 minutes (Papaseit et al., 2016). Crystal methamphetamine may have a slower onset time, depending on route of administration, but its half-life is around 11 hours (Kish, 2008).

The prevalence of chemsex is difficult to accurately assess as it involves illegal drugs, and those using them are from a marginalized community. Prevalence data in the literature varies due to the heterogeneity of study designs (Tomkins et al., 2019). Lifetime chemsex drug use in the United Kingdom and Republic of Ireland in MSM ranges from 10.1% (Blomquist et al., 2020) to 18% (Frankis et al., 2018)

Direct Drug Effects

Chemsex drugs all have anorectic properties to varying degrees. Kirkpatrick and colleagues (2012) compared the effects of 20 mg and 40 mg of methamphetamine with 3,4-methylenedioxymethamphetamine (MDMA/ecstasy) and a placebo. They reported a statistically significant reduction in all macronutrients (in grams) and total caloric intake for both doses of methamphetamine compared to the placebo. Both doses of methamphetamine had a statistically significant reduction in the number of eating occasions compared to placebo despite free access to food (10.1, 5.7, and 5.5 for placebo, 20 mg and 40 mg methamphetamine, respectively). This demonstrates a direct drug effect rather than any associated impact of the context of "real world" drug taking as the study was undertaken

DOI: 10.4324/9781003217121-37

under laboratory conditions. To this author's knowledge there are no comparable studies for mephedrone or GHB/GBL. There is evidence to suggest that GHB has appetite-suppressing effects, although this is limited (Kapoor et al., 2013), but 81% of mephedrone users reported "no appetite for food" as an acute drug effect (Winstock et al., 2011). Studies cite the appetite-reducing properties of crystal methamphetamine as the main reason for use (García-Gómez et al., 2009; Neale et al., 2009). These studies were in the context of eating disorders, but given this is a direct drug effect, the results are likely transferable. Some studies indicate a possible compensatory mechanism, with 14% of participants taking GHB reporting an increased appetite after cessation of drug use (Barker et al., 2007) and 33% of mephedrone users reporting an increased appetite as a withdrawal effect (Winstock et al., 2011). It should be noted that this figure is notably lower than those reporting the appetite-suppressant effects whilst taking the drug, which may suggest that the overall effect of the drug would reduce the subject's oral intake.

One of the most commonly reported effects of taking these drugs is the increase in libido; the reported frequency of this depends on the design of the study but can be up to 66% for mephedrone (Winstock et al., 2011), 100% in GHB/GBL (Palamer & Halkitis, 2006) and 48% in methamphetamine (Reback et al., 2003). This can impact nutritional status in two ways: increased energy expenditure and prioritization of sex over other activities such as eating.

Sexual intercourse has an increased energy expenditure. The energy required to undertake certain activities is measured using metabolic equivalent time (MET) by using oxygen consumption as a proxy marker; a MET of 1 is the amount of oxygen used sitting at rest (Jetté et al., 1990) and increments proportionally. "Passive sex" has a MET of 1.3, whereas "active vigorous sex" has a MET of 2.8 (Ainsworth et al., 2011). When this occurs over many hours, up to several days, there is likely to be a meaningful impact on energy balance, particularly if this occurs on a regular basis. It should be noted that the literature does not provide sufficient detail as to how long participants are likely to be actively engaged in sexual activities as opposed to how long the session lasts overall. Some qualitative studies suggest that there are periods of inactivity due to excessive drug consumption or due to using geosocial dating applications or so-called "hook-up apps," to find others to join the party (Milhet et al., 2019)

Due to the drugs, participants have a greatly increased sexual desire and during the parties participants are largely focused on having sex with little regard to other aspects of daily life. Qualitative interviews provide insights. In the study by Milhet and colleagues (2019), one participant describes the effect it has on him: "You always want it … nothing satisfies you. You can fuck for hours and hours … and you always want more" (p, 16). In the Reback and colleagues (2003) study, one participant is quoted as saying "I have total focus on just having sex. Nothing else matters." (p, 779), another says "I can't be bothered to stop and have a sandwich" (p. 780). This shows that the entire focus of the session revolves around sex, with other aspects of daily life, including eating, being neglected, compounding the impact of increased energy expenditure and the anorectic properties of the drugs on the participants' nutritional status.

Practical Impacts of Chemsex

Participation in chemsex also has the potential to impact the participants' nutritional intake in more wide-ranging ways, including before the event has even started. Some men who intend to have receptive anal intercourse prefer to undertake rectal douching prior to sex to ensure they are "clean;" data are limited as to the proportion of people who do this, but one small study reports 66% (n = 16) of their participants undertake a rectal douche prior to intercourse (Schilder et al., 2010). Anecdotally, some chemsex participants, particularly those intending to have prolonged sessions, may have a reduced intake on the day of the session or may not eat at all. They cite aiming to minimize the chance of them having to open their bowels during the session once they have undertaken a rectal douche so that they can remain "clean." This may be particularly important for those who undertake activities such as fisting or more "extreme" anal play. Harm-reduction advice targeted at those intending to participate in chemsex, suggests eating a good meal before the session begins so that the participant has sufficient energy for the party (NUAA, 2020; Terrence Higgins Trust, 2018); in reality however, some participants skip meals prior to the party starting. This further extends the period of poor or no oral intake.

Chemsex is not defined by the location in which it occurs, but often occurs in private residences, saunas/bathhouses, or other commercial sex-on-premises venues (Bourne et al., 2014). This means that access to food, or facilities to prepare it are likely lacking, further compounding the anorectic properties of the drugs themselves. The lack of nutritional intake has also been cited as a reason for non-adherence to HIV medications that have food requirements (Reback et al., 2003), but it is beyond the scope of this chapter to explore this further.

A further concern is for those who have insulin-dependent diabetes mellitus (IDDM); prolonged reduced oral intake alongside increased energy expenditure is likely to lead to erratic capillary blood glucose (CBG) levels and may require dose adjustment of insulin. Those who use crystal methamphetamine have lower CBG levels than controls, although these remain normoglycaemic (Zhang et al., 2017; Lv et al., 2016); data are not available for GHB/GBL and mephedrone. Regular CBG monitoring should be encouraged, particularly as some of the effects of the drugs are similar to those experienced during a hypoglycaemic episode (Barker et al., 2007; Winstock et al., 2011; Diabetes UK, 2021). It should be acknowledged that checking CBG levels whilst under the influence of drugs is likely to be significantly more difficult as the drugs affect the central nervous system and can cause blurred vision, tremors, poor concentration, and reduced motor function amongst others (Schifano et al., 2011; Rusyniak, 2014). The checking of the CBG level is a multistage process including thinking to check them, having the dexterity to do the test alongside the mental capacity to interpret and act on the results; all of which are likely to be more difficult when under the influence of drugs. Healthcare professionals should be encouraged to discuss this risk with their patients.

Conclusion

Participating in chemsex has the possibility of impacting on a person's nutritional status. The extent of the impact is likely to be influenced by a number of factors; frequency of attendance at chemsex parties is likely to be the biggest factor, if this is a weekly occurrence, a significant part of the week is likely to involve reduced or negligible oral intake, whereas if this occurs infrequently, the participant will likely compensate for the reduction in intake in between sessions. The quantity of drugs used will also likely have an impact; prolonged sessions with multiple doses of drugs are more likely to be clinically meaningful than when single doses are taken. The participants' baseline nutritional status will also affect the magnitude of the nutritional implications; those who are underweight or who have a poor diet may be more impacted as they have a limited nutritional reserve.

The Art of Dietetic Practice: Recommendations

People who partake in chemsex should be encouraged to take ready-to-consume foods with them to the parties to facilitate nutritional intake as food is unlikely to be available. People may also take with them over-the-counter nutritional supplements or meal replacements. However, it should be acknowledged that some of these supplements contain polyvalent cations and can have significant drug nutrient interactions with the integrase inhibitor class of anti-retroviral medications for HIV (Rock et al., 2020) and may not be a suitable recommendation for those taking this class of drug.

Traditional "food first" nutritional support strategies such as food fortification should be encouraged between drug use in those whose weight is either below-recommended guidelines or is decreasing unintentionally to facilitate nutritional adequacy averaged over the week, acknowledging that the person is likely to be in negative energy balance on days drugs are used.

Those who have IDDM should be encouraged to regularly check their CBG and adjust their insulin accordingly. It should be encouraged that they use waterproof dressings or gloves following the checking of their CBG to minimize any risk of blood-borne virus transmission due to blood exposure (Simpson-Theobald, 2019). It would also be recommended that people with IDDM should have appropriate treatment for hypoglycaemia with them and some form of medical identification such as a necklace/bracelet so that others at the party are more likely to suspect a hypoglycaemic episode rather than a drug overdose; although the practicality of this within a chemsex party setting could be debated.

All healthcare professionals should discuss chemsex drug use, and recreational drug use more generally, with their patients using non-judgemental language to establish the patterns and frequency of use and how their drug use impacts them. Clinicians and services should be mindful of the nuances of how chemsex fits within the MSM community to ensure appropriate language is used and that they recognize the complexity of chemsex drug use beyond a physical addiction to drugs.

This author recommends:

- Using the patients'/clients' preferred pronouns and terms to refer to their sexual identity.
- Acknowledging that MSM do not necessarily identify as gay or bisexual.
- Ensuring that assumptions based on demographics are not made. As shown in Barker et al. (2007) those using chemsex drugs come from diverse cultural and socioeconomic backgrounds.
- Using non-judgemental terms such as recreational drugs as opposed to illicit or illegal.
- Using terms more associated with chemsex such as "partying" and "slamming" rather than more generic drug use terms, although these will vary by country/region.
- Acknowledging that even those who inject drugs do not always identify as intravenous drug users.
- Being mindful that even regular chemsex participants who experience problematic drug use may not identify as being a drug addict. Chemsex users may take the drugs for reasons such as trying to manage internalized homophobia; it is beyond the scope of this chapter to explore this further but the article by Stuart (2019) expands on this.
- Being mindful that mainstream harm-reduction services may not adequately be able to address the causes for chemsex use (Stuart, 2019), a holistic assessment of the role that chemsex plays in the individual's life may more adequately address the needs of this group rather than a more traditional medical model of treatment, although some aspects, such as needle exchanges may be helpful.

References

Ainsworth, B. E., Haskell, W. L., Herrmann, S. D., Meckes, N., Bassett Jr, D. R., Tudor-Locke, C.,Greer, J. L., Vezina, J., Whitt-Glover, M. C., & Leon, A. S. (2011). 2011 Compendium of physical activities: A second update of codes and MET values. *Medicine & Science in Sports & Exercise, 43*, 1575–1581.

Barker, J. C., Harris, S. L., & Dyer, J. E. (2007). Experiences of gamma hydroxybutyrate (GHB) ingestion: A focus group study. *Journal of Psychoactive Drugs, 39*, 115–129.

Blomquist, P. B., Mohammed, H., Mikhail, A., Weatherburn, P., Reid, D., Wayal, S., Hughes, G., & Mercer, C. H. (2020). Characteristics and sexual health service use of MSM engaging in chemsex: Results from a large online survey in England. *Sexually Transmitted Infections, 96*, 590–595. https://doi.org/10.1136/sextrans-2019-054345

Bourne, A., Reid, D., Hickson, F., Torres Rueda, S., & Weatherburn, P. (2014). *The Chemsex study: drug use in sexual settings among gay and bisexual men in Lambeth, Southwark and Lewisham.* Sigma Research, London School of Hygiene & Tropical Medicine. http://www.sigmaresearch.org.uk/chemsex

Diabetes UK. (2021). What is a hypo? Retrieved August, 2021, from https://www.diabetes.org.uk/guide-to-diabetes/complications/hypos#symptoms-hypo

Frankis, J., Flowers, P., McDaid, L., & Bourne, A. (2018). Low levels of chemsex amongst men who have sex with men, but high levels of risk amongst men who engage in chemsex: Analysis of a cross-sectional online survey across four countries *Sex Health*, *15*, 144–150.

García-Gómez, M. D. C., González, J. O., del Barrio, A. G., & García, N. A. (2009). Rhabdomyolysis and drug abuse in a patient with bulimia nervosa. *International Journal of Eating Disorders*, *42*, 93–95. https://doi.org/10.1002/eat.20583

Jetté, M., Sidney, K., & Blümchen, G. (1990). Metabolic equivalents (METS) in exercise testing, exercise prescription, and evaluation of functional capacity. *Clinical Cardiology*, *13*, 555–565.

Kapoor, P., Deshmukh, R., & Kukreja, I. (2013). GHB acid: A rage or reprieve. *Journal of Advanced Pharmaceutical Technology & Research*, *4*, 137–178. https://doi.org/10.4103/2231-4040.121410

Kirkpatrick, M. G., Gunderson, E. W., Perez, A. Y., Haney, M., Foltin, R. W., & Hart, C. L. (2012). A direct comparison of the behavioural and physiological effects of methamphetamine and 3,4-methylenedioxymethamphetamine (MDMA) in humans. *Psychopharmacology (Berl)*, *219*, 109–22. https://doi.org/10.1007/s00213-011-2383-4

Kish, S. J. (2008). Pharmacologic mechanisms of crystal meth *Canadian Medical Association Journal*, *178*, 1679–1682. https://doi.org/10.1503/cmaj.071675

Lv, D., Zhang, M., Jin, X., Zhao, J., Han, B., Su, H., Zhang, J., Zhang, X., Ren, W. and He, J. (2016). The body mass index, blood pressure, and fasting blood glucose in patients with methamphetamine dependence. *Medicine*, *95*, 1–4. https://doi.org/10.1097/MD.0000000000003152

Macfarlane, A. (2016). Sex, drugs and self-control: Why chemsex is fast becoming a public health concern. *Journal of Family Planning and Reproductive Health Care*, *42*, 291–294. https://doi.org/10.1136/jfprhc-2016-101576

Milhet, M., Shah, J., Madesclaire, T., & Gaissad, L. (2019). Chemsex experiences: Narratives of pleasure. *Drugs and Alcohol Today*, *19*, 11–22. https://doi.org/10.1108/DAT-09-2018-0043

Neale, A., Abraham, S., & Russell, J. (2009). "Ice" use and eating disorders: A report of three cases. *International Journal of Eating Disorders*, *42*, 188–191.

NUAA. (2020). Chemsex. *User's News Issue #94 Gender & Sexually Diverse Edition*. https://indd.adobe.com/view/3fdc7fdd-3fc3-4446-bac7-3a8549a1ec59

Palamar, J. J., & Halkitis, P. N. (2006). A qualitative analysis of GHB use among gay men: Reasons for use despite potential adverse outcomes. *International Journal of Drug Policy*, *17*, 23–28.

Papaseit, E., Pérez-Mañá, C., Mateus, J.-A., Pujadas, M., Fonseca, F., Torrens, M., Olesti, E., de la Torre, R., & Farré, M. (2016). Human pharmacology of mephedrone in comparison with MDMA. *Neuropsychopharmacology*, *41*, 2704–2713. https://doi.org/10.1038/npp.2016.75

Reback, C. J., Larkins, S., & Shoptaw, S. (2003). Methamphetamine abuse as a barrier to HIV medication adherence among gay and bisexual men. *AIDS Care*, *15*, 775–785.

Rock, A. E., DeMarais, P. L., Vergara-Rodriguez, P. T., & Max, B. E. (2020). HIV-1 virologic rebound due to coadministration of divalent cations and Bictegravir. *Journal of Infectious Diseases & Therapy*, *9*, 691–696. https://doi.org/10.1007/s40121-020-00307-4

Rusyniak, D. E. (2014). Neurological manifestations of chronic methamphetamine abuse. *Psychiatric Clinics of North America*, *36*, 261–275. https://doi.org/10.1016/j.psc.2013.02.005

Schifano, F., Albanese, A., Fergus, S., Stair, J. L., Deluca, P., Corazza, O., Davey, Z., Corkery, J., Siemann, H., Scherbaum, N. and Farre, M. (2011). Mephedrone (methylmethcathinone; meow meow'): Chemical, pharmacological and clinical issues. *Psychopharmacology*, *214*, 593–602.

Schilder, A. J., Ochard, T. R., Buchner, C. S., Strathdee, S. A., & Hogg, R. S. (2010). Insert discourse: Rectal douching among young HIV-positive and HIV-negative men who have sex with men in Vancouver, Canada. *Sexuality & Culture*, *14*, 327–343. https://doi.org/10.1007/s12119-010-9077-7

Simpson-Theobald, J. (2019). Sex, drugs and…nutrition? *HIV Nursing*, *19*, 61–64.

Stuart, D. (2019). Chemsex: Origins of the word, a history of the phenomenon and a respect to the culture. *Drugs and Alcohol Today*, *19*, 3–10. https://doi.org/10.1108/DAT-10-2018-0058

Terrence Higgins Trust. (2018). Taking drugs, prepare and repair, before. Retrieved August, 2020, from https://www.fridaymonday.org.uk/taking-drugs/prepare-and-repair/before/

Tomkins, A., George, R., & Kilner, M. (2019). Sexualised drug taking among men who have sex with men: A systematic review. *Perspectives in Public Health*, *139*, 23–33. https://doi.org/10.1177/1757913918778872

Winstock, A., Mitcheson, L., Ramsey, J., Davies, S., Puchnarewicz, M., & Marsden, J. (2011). Mephedrone: Use, subjective effects and health risks. *Addiction*, *106*, 1991–1996. https://doi.org/10.1111/j.1360-0443.2011.03502.x.

Zhang, M., Lv, D., Zhou, W., Ji, L., Zhou, B., Chen, H., Gu, Y., Zhao, J. and He, J. (2017). The levels of triglyceride and total cholesterol in methamphetamine dependence. *Medicine*, *96*, 1–4.

35 Ace(ing) ED

Mikey Anderson

The comic is a six-panel digital comic about the author's experience as a queer, non-binary, white, able-bodied, mental health clinician living at the intersections of the asexuality spectrum and a history of an eating disorder (ED). From the top of the page is the title Ace(ing) ED in bubble letters. The comic shows how their experience with asexuality, dating, body image, and eating are all intertwined. The thought bubbles in the comic represent the ongoing flashbacks the author has from their history of ED. These flashbacks are harsh reminders of the effect the ED had on the author's body and mind (Figure 35.1).

Panel one is Mikey on a scale that says "12000" and a thought bubble that says, "7 years ago," with another scale that says "97" with an arrow with "All day" above it pointing to panel two.

Panel two is a self-portrait of the author with times, food, and the ace symbol swirling around their head.

Panel three is the author's exposed stomach with hands around them with a thought bubble that says "No, not there … I want to, but I just can't." With an arrow pointing at dating app symbols with the text "self worth" with an arrow pointing to panel four.

Panel four is the author grabbing their arm with a realistic heart drawn on their chest. On their arm it says "At one point my hand went around my whole arm," with a thought bubble on their face that says, "Maybe you have autism??"

Panel 5 is a self-portrait of the author with their legs crossed with their hand over their lap with their fingernails chipping off. Around the panel are fibre bars with three thought bubbles that say, "Memories of my nails chipping off," "Therapist always ate fiber bars in therapy," and "Was this a test??"

Panel 6 is a self-portrait of the author's chest with long hair on their shoulders. The panel has a heart drawn in the middle with food drawn inside of it with the letter "ED" in the heart.

The comic disrupts the bias perpetuated by many academic writings that pathologize queer folx bodies. Instead, the comic opens a space for queer folx to feel comfortable with sharing their experiences in the therapeutic space and beyond. The comic draws upon queer theory by how it subverts the traditional comic panel frame by flowing organically from panel to panel with arrows to direct the reader. By queering the comic's layout, the way disordered eating has

DOI: 10.4324/9781003217121-38

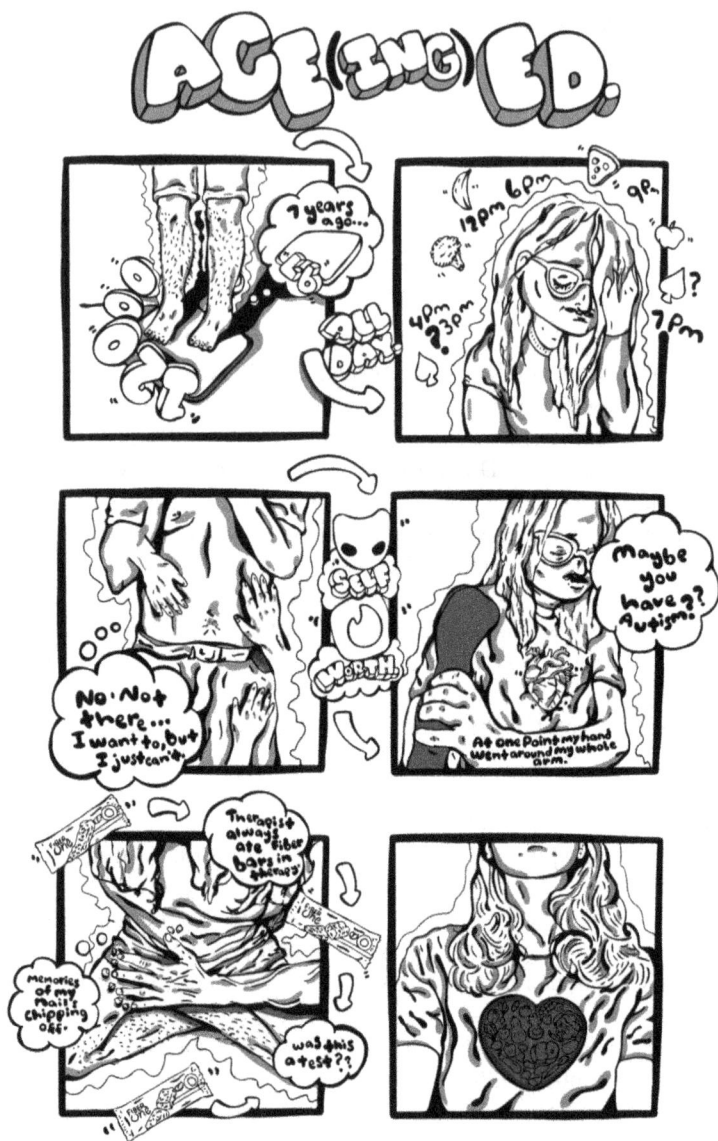

Figure 35.1 Ace(ing) ED. Mikey Anderson.

impacted their life, the symptoms they experienced, and ongoing struggles to accept their body are revealed. This form of comic-making displays their internal and external experience living on the asexual spectrum and their past with ED.

Though the comic shows the painful side-effects of living with an ED, it ends with hope: a continuing process of working toward queer body self-love. The author aims to shed light on how therapists face their own mental health concerns as a result of living in a heteronormative society, just like many of the queer clients we work with. The author's intention by creating this comic is to deepen clinicians' understanding of how disordered eating impacts the queer community and challenges stereotypes around EDs.

36 "Going from Invisible to Visible"

Challenging the "Normal" Ranges, Cut-Offs, and Labels Used to Describe the Sizes and Shapes of Transgender and Gender-Diverse Bodies

Whitney Linsenmeyer and Melik D.H. Coffey

Measuring a patient's body size and shape is a perfunctory component of a registered dietitian's nutrition assessment. With those values, we then provide labels such as underweight, normal, overweight, or obese, and often recommendations on how to achieve a "normal" body weight (Centers for Disease Control and Prevention, 2021). The stakes are high for these labels in many cases; they may be used as criteria to justify certain mental health diagnoses, surgical interventions, or insurance claims.

"Overweight" and "obesity" have become household terms, with attention from leading organizations such as the World Health Organization (WHO, 2021), United States Department of Health and Human Services (United States Department of Health and Human Services, n.d.), and the Centers for Disease Control and Prevention (CDC, 2021). At the same time, weight bias and obesity stigma are now recognized for their wide-ranging detrimental effects including physical harm, psychological damage, and inadequate medical care (Rubino et al., 2020).

Pushback to the focus on body size and hypocaloric diets to achieve a "normal" body weight has also catalyzed the emergence of non-dieting approaches such as mindful eating, intuitive eating, and health at every size (HAES) (Fuentes Artiles et al., 2019; Ulian et al., 2018). These approaches, while not yet mainstream in the medical community, aim to de-centre the emphasis on body size and instead focus on the whole picture of a person's health. Emerging evidence supports these approaches and do have some beneficial effects, yet the totality of resulting health outcomes is mixed (Fuentes Artiles et al., 2019; Ulian et al., 2018).

Considerations for the Transgender and Gender-Diverse Community

Labels for body size and shape have unique implications for the transgender and gender diverse (TGGD) community given their intersection with gender identity

DOI: 10.4324/9781003217121-39

and expression. The World Professional Association for Transgender Health (WPATH) (Coleman, et al., 2012) defines gender identity as a person's intrinsic sense of being male (a boy or man), female (a girl or woman), or an alternative gender (i.e., boygirl, girlboy, transgender, genderqueer, eunuch) (Bockting, 1999; Stoller, 1964). Gender role or expression is defined as the characteristics in personality, appearance, and behaviour that in a given culture and historical period are designated as masculine or feminine (Ruble et al., 2006).

TGGD individuals may seek a different body size that is a more authentic expression of their gender identity. Though not limited to these trends, transfeminine individuals may desire a smaller body size, and this "drive for thinness" may contribute to increased body dissatisfaction (Witcomb et al., 2015). Transmasculine individuals may seek a larger body size that may or may not be distinguished by muscularity (Kamody et al., 2020; Linsenmeyer, Drallmeier, & Thomure, 2020; Murray et al., 2016).

Relatedly, a growing body of research emphasizes the increased risk of eating disorders and disordered eating among the TGGD population. In contrast to 2.8% of the general adolescent population, an estimated 4.3% of transmasculine youth and 4.2% of transfeminine youth reported a lifetime eating disorder diagnosis (Becerra-Culqui et al., 2018; Coelho et al., 2019; Swanson et al., 2011). The theorized rationale for this health disparity is closely intertwined with gender identity and expression; TGGD individuals may utilize disordered eating or exercise behaviours to attain or accentuate body features that are consistent with one's gender identity, to delay pubertal development of secondary sex characteristics that are not consistent with gender identity, or to mask the presence of body features with additional adiposity (Avila et al., 2019; Becerra-Culqui et al., 2018; Coelho et al., 2019; Diemer et al., 2015; Donaldson et al., 2018; Guss et al., 2017; Linsenmeyer et al., 2021; Watson et al., 2017).

This interrelationship is compounded by the known effects on body size and shape that are associated with masculinizing or feminizing hormone therapy (HT). While both are associated with weight gain, masculinizing HT typically results in increases in lean body mass and decreases in fat mass, while feminizing HT has the reverse effect (Coleman et al., 2012; Klaver et al., 2016). HT also affects body shape in that masculinizing HT tends to promote fat deposition in the central abdominal region while feminizing HT tends to do so in the hips and buttocks (Klaver et al., 2018). Therefore, body size and shape are not only interwoven with gender expression but are expected to undergo significant changes starting as early as three months after initiating HT (Coleman et al., 2012).

Narratives of a Transgender Man and Cisgender Ally

In this section, we illustrate the limitations and cisnormativity of nutrition assessment methods related to body size and shape. We will share our personal narratives as a 35-year-old African American, transgender male (Melik) and as a white, cisgender dietitian and ally to the transgender community (Whitney). We then close with a discussion on how dietitians can confront their own biases, foster more nuanced conversations with their TGGD patients regarding their goals for body size and shape, and ultimately provide better nutrition care for the TGGD community.

Melik's Narrative: *Going from Invisible to Visible*

I started on T [testosterone] about eight years ago. At the time, I wanted to get to a certain size. It was all about having more of a presence and filling out my space. As you transition, you feel more strength. You feel empowered. You feel stronger. You feel more solid. You're not going to blow over. You're more rugged, solid, stocky. You feel yourself becoming more visibly who you've always been.

It's the process of going from invisible to visible. It's almost like bringing yourself to life.

My size fit my own perception of masculinity. It was like I needed to have some type of machismo or presence. If I'm in a room with other guys, they will see me as, "Oh that guy – he's a stocky guy – he's built like his grandfather."

I'm here now.

I'm visible.

I'm taking up space.

I have a voice.

It was also about wanting a size so that I could feel more masc. If I was questioning, "Can you see my chest? Can you not see my chest?" I wanted people to see me and think, "That's a big dude. That's normal." Your ideal body image might come from the men in your life or stereotypes – which might not always be the healthiest. For me, it was my six-foot-five-inch big-and-tall grandfather. Or, the construction worker. Or, the Hollister model. It's whoever is in your mind that you look at and think that he is an undeniable, irrefutable man.

When I started taking hormones, I just wanted my size. I was consumed by wanting to start testosterone. Then, wanting my beard to grow. Then, wanting to have surgery. Now that I've had top surgery, I don't need that size anymore. I'm thinking to myself: Where do I want to go? How do I want my body to change? What do I want it to look like? How do I want to feel in my body? Do I want to be this heavy? Am I content being this heavy? Is it the healthiest thing for me to be this heavy? Now I just want to be healthy; I want to be the healthy guy who can touch his toes, put his socks on, and take walks around his neighbourhood.

Plus, now that I'm comfortable in my body, I can also be more physical. I can get back to swimming, which I avoided for a long time, or I can go lift weights. I can go to the gym, and I don't feel uncomfortable going to the men's locker room. Now it feels good to me. Versus focusing on if I'm blending in or not.

I really like my life now.

I get to be a husband.

I get to live my life as I am.

I want to preserve that!

It's also about recognizing that these things – my size or my physical abilities – they don't define my masculinity. If I'm in this space, and this is authentically who I am, then I am that person. I've always been the guy who holds the door for you, and that's not going to change. Ever since I was a little person, four or five years old, I've been the one saying, "I got the door!" Those things are organically me; they're who I am. If these external things change, I'm still me. I feel safe in my own body now.

I have a sense of wholeness.

I can just be me.

Whitney's Narrative: Confronting Bias and Learning to Be a Better Ally

I consider myself to be a "classically trained" dietitian in that energy balance, hypocaloric diets, and motivational interviewing took centre stage in my education about weight management. The focus was on how patients could make small behaviour changes that would set them on a path of slow yet sustained weight loss until they reached a "normal" body mass index (BMI). Mindful and intuitive eating were considered fringe topics during my education, and the term HAES was brought to my attention only years after graduating.

Although I understood obesity to be a multifactorial disease, my understanding of my role as a dietitian was to support a patient in changing their behaviours to lose weight. I never considered that an obese patient would not want to lose weight – that their size held a particular meaning for them or that they would genuinely desire a larger body size.

I had been practising as a dietitian for about a decade when I met Melik and had the privilege to learn his story. Although my line of research was coming into focus as nutrition care for the transgender population, up until then I had only worked with overweight or obese transgender patients who were seeking to lose weight. This served to confirm my subconscious assumption about the universal desire to "achieve" a "normal" BMI.

My bias was brought into the light when I listened to Melik talk about his experience of coming out as transgender, medically transitioning, and celebrating his larger body size. His language such as "going from invisible to visible," "having a presence," and "filling out my space" have never left my mind. His larger body size is a physical manifestation of his masculinity ("more power, more strength").

Although clinicians would label Melik's body as obese, his size is also an expression of his most authentic self. I do not seek to minimize the known health outcomes associated with high levels of adiposity, but I do recognize that labelling Melik's body and automatically recommending weight loss could also be damaging to his health. As a cisgender person, I can't earnestly fathom the amount of courage it takes for someone to come out as transgender to friends and family, to go through the emotional labour of redefining their lives, to medically transition if they desire to do so, and ultimately to live as their most authentic self. To undermine that courage with a one-word label simply isn't worth the potential damage.

My new perspective, thanks to Melik and others, is to be an ally first and a clinician second. I have the privilege of working with transgender individuals and honouring their authentic selves, which includes their body size and shape. Weight management can take a back seat to making sure my patients are supported, listened to, and respected.

How Dietitians Can Do Better

It can be rather counterintuitive for dietitians to set aside the labels for body weight. We tend to treat our assessment of body weight like a vital sign ("Mr Jones is a 55-year-old male with a BMI of 39.0, obese class II"). It can even feel incomplete to chart on a patient without leading with an assessment of their weight status.

But of course, dietitians can do better. We can start by confronting our own biases about BMI and weight loss. Do we assume that all overweight or obese patients are not content with their body size? Do we blindly launch into motivational interviewing for weight loss? Do we label our patients' body size without also considering what their size may mean to them? Confronting our own biases does take effort, but it is the first step to truly supporting our patients. For those that identify as allies to the TGGD community, we can't fully advocate for our patients until we are honest with our own limitations.

Next, dietitians can foster more nuanced conversations with TGGD patients regarding their goals for body size and shape. Especially when working with patients who are initiating HT and will soon be experiencing changes in body size and shape, we can help our patients explore their feelings about these changes, what body size and shape means to them and their gender expression, and how nutrition and physical activity can play supporting roles.

Ultimately, dietitians as allies can commit to humility and lifelong learning. We can accept that our own understanding of the transgender experience will be inherently limited but can always be expanding. We can be allies first and clinicians second.

Melik's Closing Thoughts

As I take time reflect on this experience and my ability to share the trans voice in spaces where it may not have been previously included, I am filled with gratitude. I am grateful for clinicians like Whitney who have made it a priority to challenge the "norms." It is extremely important for the medical community to understand how body size and shape are interconnected with gender expression and gender identity.

It is also important to remember that when TGGD individuals seek services within the healthcare system, there are often numerous barriers in place that can impact the quality of care. Therefore, it is essential to not only educate ourselves on issues surrounding transgender healthcare, but also check in on our own biases that may influence our ability to see each patient as a unique individual.

Lastly, we need more opportunities like this, where the medical community creates space for the TGGD community to share our experiences. Clinicians can commit to not just listening, but genuinely hearing each patient's unique perspective.

References

Avila, J. T., Golden, N. H., & Aye, T. (2019). Eating disorder screening in transgender youth. *Journal of Adolescent Health, 65,* 815–817.

Becerra-Culqui, T.A., Liu, Y., Nash, R., Cromwell, L., Flanders, W.D., Getahun, D., Giammattei, S.V., Hunkeler, E.M., Lash, T.L., Millman, A., & Quinn, V.P. (2018). Mental health of transgender and gender nonconforming youth compared with their peers. *Pediatrics, 141*(5), e20173845.

Bockting, W. O. (1999). From construction to context: Gender through the eyes of the transgendered. *Siecus Report, 28*(1), 3–7.

Center for Disease Control and Prevention. (2021, June 7). *Defining adult overweight & obesity.* https://www.cdc.gov/obesity/adult/defining.html

Coelho, J. S., Suen, J., Clark, B. A., Marshall, S. K., Geller, J., & Lam, P. Y. (2019). Eating disorder diagnoses and symptom presentation in transgender youth: A scoping review. *Current Psychiatry Reports, 21*(107), 1–10.

Coleman, E., Bockting, W., Botzer, M., Cohen-Kettenis, P., DeCuypere, G., Feldman, J., ... & Zucker, K. (2012). Standards of care for the health of transsexual, transgender, and gender-nonconforming people, 7th version. *International Journal of Transgenderism, 13*(4), 165–232.

Diemer, E. W., Grant, J. D., Munn-Chernoff, M. A., Patterson, D. A., & Duncan, A. E. (2015). Gender identity, sexual orientation, and eating-related pathology in a national sample of college students. *Journal of Adolescent Health, 57,* 144–147.

Donaldson, A. A., Hall, A., Neukirch, J., Kasper, V., Simones, S., Gagnon, S., ... & Forcier, M. (2018). Multidisciplinary care considerations for gender nonconforming adolescents with eating disorders: A case series. *International Journal of Eating Disorders, 51,* 475–479.

Fuentes Artiles, R., Staub, K., Aldakak, L., Eppenberger, P., Rühli, F., & Bender, N. (2019). Mindful eating and common diet programs lower body weight similarly: Systematic review and meta-analysis. *Obesity Reviews, 11,* 1619–1627.

Guss, C. E., Williams, D. N., Reisner, S. L., Austin, S. B., & Katz-Wise, S. L.. (2017). Disordered weight management behaviors, nonprescription steroid use, and weight perception in transgender youth. *Journal of Adolescent Health, 60,* 17–22.

Kamody, R. C., Yonkers, K., Pluhar, E. I., & Olezeski, C. L. . (2020). Disordered eating among trans-masculine youth: Considerations through a developmental lens. *LGBT Health, 7,* 170–173.

Klaver, M., De Blok, C. J. M., Wiepjes, C. M., Nota, N. M., Dekker, M. J., de Mutsert, R., ... & Den Heijer, M. (2018). Changes in regional body fat, lean body mass and body shape in trans persons using cross-sex hormonal therapy: Results from a multicenter prospective study. *European Journal of Endocrinology, 178*(2), 163–171.

Klaver, M., Dekker, M. J. H. J., de Mutsert, R., Twisk, J. W. R., & den Heijer, M. (2016). Cross-sex hormone therapy in transgender persons affects total body weight, body fat and lean body mass: A meta-analysis. *Andrologia, 49*(5), 1–11.

Linsenmeyer, W., Drallmeier, T., & Thomure, M. (2020). Towards gender-affirming nutrition assessment: A case series of adult transgender men with distinct nutrition considerations. *Nutrition Journal, 19,* 74.

Linsenmeyer, W. R., Katz, I. M., Reed, J. L., Giedinghagen, A. M., Lewis, C. B., & Garwood, S. K.. (2021). Disordered eating, food insecurity, and weight status among transgender and gender nonbinary youth and young adults: A cross-sectional study using a nutrition screening protocol. *LGBT Health, 8*(5), 359–366.

Murray, S. B., Griffiths, S., & Mond, J. M. (2016). Evolving eating disorder psychopathology: Conceptualizing muscularity-oriented disordered eating. *British Journal of Psychiatry, 208*, 414–415.

Rubino, F., Puhl, R. M., Cummings, D. E., Eckel, R. H., Ryan, D. H., Mechanick, J. I., ... & Dixon, J. B. (2020). Joint international consensus statement for ending stigma of obesity. *Nature Medicine, 26*, 485–497.

Ruble, D. N., Martin, C. L., & Berenbaum, S. A. (2006). Gender development. In N. Eisenberg, W. Damon, & R. M. Lerner (Eds.), *Handbook of child psychology* (6th ed., pp. 858–932). Hoboken, NJ: John Wiley.

Stoller, R. J. (1964). A contribution to the study of gender identity. *International Journal of Psychoanalysis, 45*, 220–226.

Swanson, S. A., Crow, S. J., Le Grange, D., Swendsen, J., & Merikangas, K. R. (2011). Prevalence and correlates of eating disorders in adolescents: Results from the national comorbidity survey replication adolescent supplement. *Archives of General Psychiatry, 68*(7), 714–423.

Ulian, M. D., Aburad, L., da Silva Oliveira, M. S., Poppe, A. C. M., Sabatini, F., Perez, I., ... & Baeza Scagliusi, F. (2018). Effects of health at every size interventions on health-related outcomes of people with overweight and obesity: A systematic review. *Obesity Reviews, 19*(12), 1659–1666.

United States Department of Health and Human Services: Office of Disease Prevention and Health Promotion. (n.d.). *Overweight and obesity.* Healthy People 2030. https://health.gov/healthypeople/objectives-and-data/browse-objectives/overweight-and-obesity."

Watson, R. J., Veale, J. F., & Saewyc, E. M. (2017). Disordered eating behaviors among transgender youth: Probability and profiles from risk and protective factors. *International Journal of Eating Disorders, 50*(5), 515–522.

Witcomb, G. L., Bouman, W. P., Brewin, N., Richards, C., Fernandez-Aranda, F., & Arcelus, J. (2015). Body image dissatisfaction and eating-related psychopathology in trans individuals: A matched control study. *European Eating Disorders Review, 23*(4), 287–293.

World Health Organization. (2021). *Obesity.* https://www.who.int/health-topics/obesity#tab=tab_1

37 A Case Study Exploring Relations between Creativity, Queering and Undoing Coloniality in Dietetic Theory

Lucy Aphramor

Things Fall Apart

I am writing from Shropshire which is on the England/Wales border. It's a squally, copper-leafed autumn afternoon. My intent in writing is that we support each other in learning and healing and develop leaders among us who are courageous and accountable.

Writing poetry and creating hands-on art has been a way of me revealing my history as a survivor to myself bit by bit. It enabled me to titrate the risk of sharing, to pace the overwhelm of shame. This allowed me radically new ways of being in the world and significantly altered my dietetic practice.

I'm a poet but I have also made textile pieces. It feels too grand to label this as sculpture or textile art, but I guess these are the closest approximations.

The first textile piece I made is a huge red quilt (Figure 37.1). Hand-sewn, it took me several years to finish. Creating it became a feature of my leisure time as I'd tack and sew when I met friends. I carried red fibres in my clothes the way cat owners carry cat hairs. I'd build up a pile of hexagons over a few weeks, sew them together into long segments, and every so often I'd have a session stitching these sections into the quilt at home. I wasn't working to a pattern or plan or end date. In that sense, I knew what I was doing in the moment, but I didn't know what I was doing it for.

I gave it the title The Red Quilt but if I think of it now, it's The Scream.

My friend, sculptor Kathryn Caswell (2007), wrote about it for an exhibition:

> There is one, certain thing that can be said about The Red Quilt. It cannot be ignored. The vast expanse of vibrant colour is instantly arresting; its presence is irrefutable; its impact is rich and powerful.
>
> … The offence to all the senses is powerfully delivered directly from eye to mind by the jarring disruption of colour and texture of the central entrance. Here, in brutal contrast to the elegance of the making, the whole is marred by the outrageous disruption of aggressive burrs in indelible black and spiky silver and snatches graphic imagery from childhood … In the dissonance of colour, texture and form, there can be no underestimation of the woundings

DOI: 10.4324/9781003217121-40

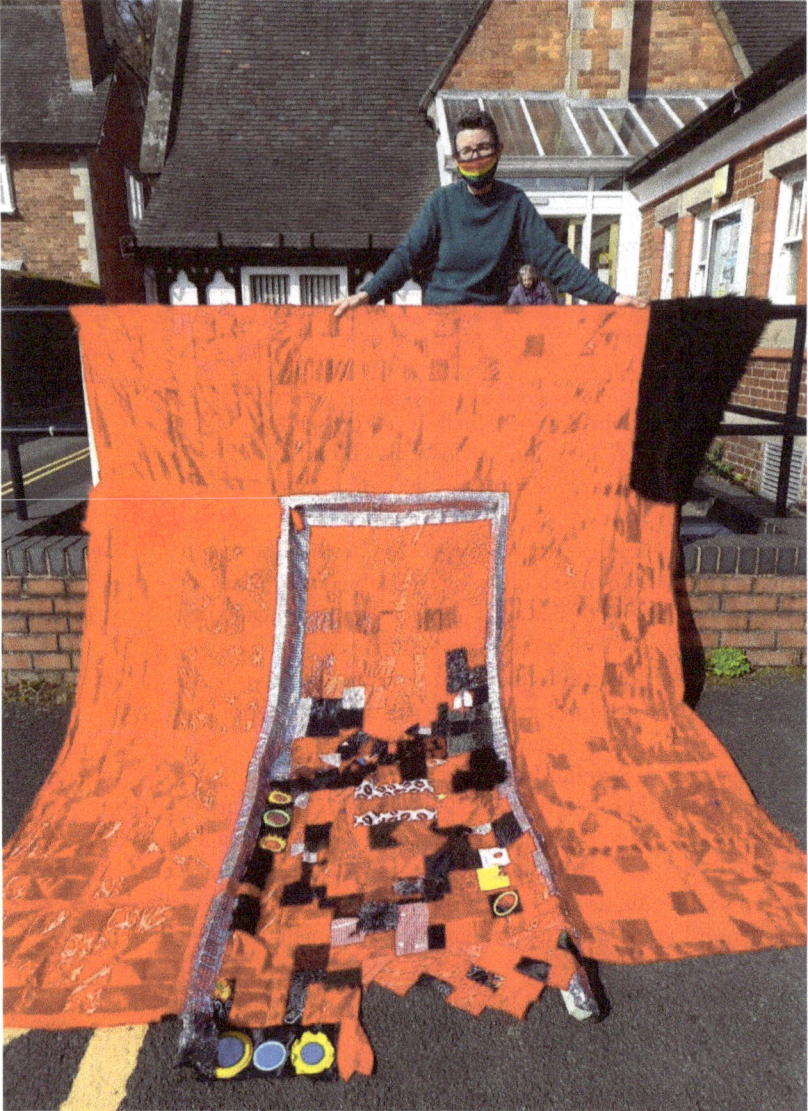

Figure 37.1 The Red Quilt. Lucy Aphramor.

that remain as explicit scars, eventually grown around and stitched across but not healed over. There is an overwhelming disarray of coarse black and spits of silver and slick lipsticked slit of adult mouthprints. Most poignant are the innocent patches of summer gingham, reminiscent of school dresses. Mirrors disconcertingly involve the viewer with the turmoil.

… This vast, double-sided hanging is mesmeric. Its visual hold is consuming rather than meditative. It is a simple move for the viewer to turn her back on the quilt: it is not easy to dislodge the image from the back of the mind. It is a banner of strength and empathy, an assertion of the right to autonomous life for survivors of childhood abuse.

There were lots of reasons why it was impossible for me to talk about this at the time. The Scream said it all.

Many dietetic programmes refuse applicants with a history of eating disorders. The sort of applicant who is more likely to have experienced abuse. The sort of applicant who might make a quilt like this.

As a middle-class teenager it was easy for me to escape being diagnosed with first one eating disorder, and later another, because no one really wanted to know or could grasp knowing. It was enough to tell teachers and concerned others that "I had to be thin for running." I was still telling myself this when I applied to university. Where the form asked about any current or previous eating disorder I ticked "no" and so my application made it through.

There were two posts available at my first dietetic job interview, one in the community and one in eating disorders. The psychologist explicitly stated that anyone with history of mental health problems was barred from working in eating disorder services. That was probably illegal, certainly discriminatory.

I was appointed to the community post. Several years later the same psychologist invited me to share my innovative scholarship with the eating disorders team he managed. He mentioned my work in his book on compassion in eating disorders.

Next year I'm co-delivering a panel talk at an eating disorders conference with "The Mad 5." We'll be using a Mad Studies framing to explore mad- and fat-affirming liberatory practice in eating disorder work (and) for collective liberation. We explained that challenging ableism, saneism, healthism, and colonialism is integral to this agenda. That as a panel, we enter this work through a shared experience of Madness.

Professional ableism goads us to bury our story and suffocates creativity.

> *who are your colleagues? What standard biases let one Mad dyke suffice? I am not your idea of what psychiatric looks like which freaks you slightly you feel deceived, nervous, aggrieved cheated of easy recourse to stereotype you suspect I owe you something yours by right detail explanation reassurance. (Aphramor, 2018)*

Self-disclosure is costly. The price alters with the market value of our professional (gendered, raced, sized etc.) capital. How can those of us most protected by our proximity to white supremacy use our privilege to expose and disrupt Saneism?

The second piece I made (Figure 37.2) tells a story that questions and queers dietitians' investment in colonial tropes of Progress and Modernity. Where the Quilt/Scream conveys dissolution and disarray, the fragments in *Truth Is Not*

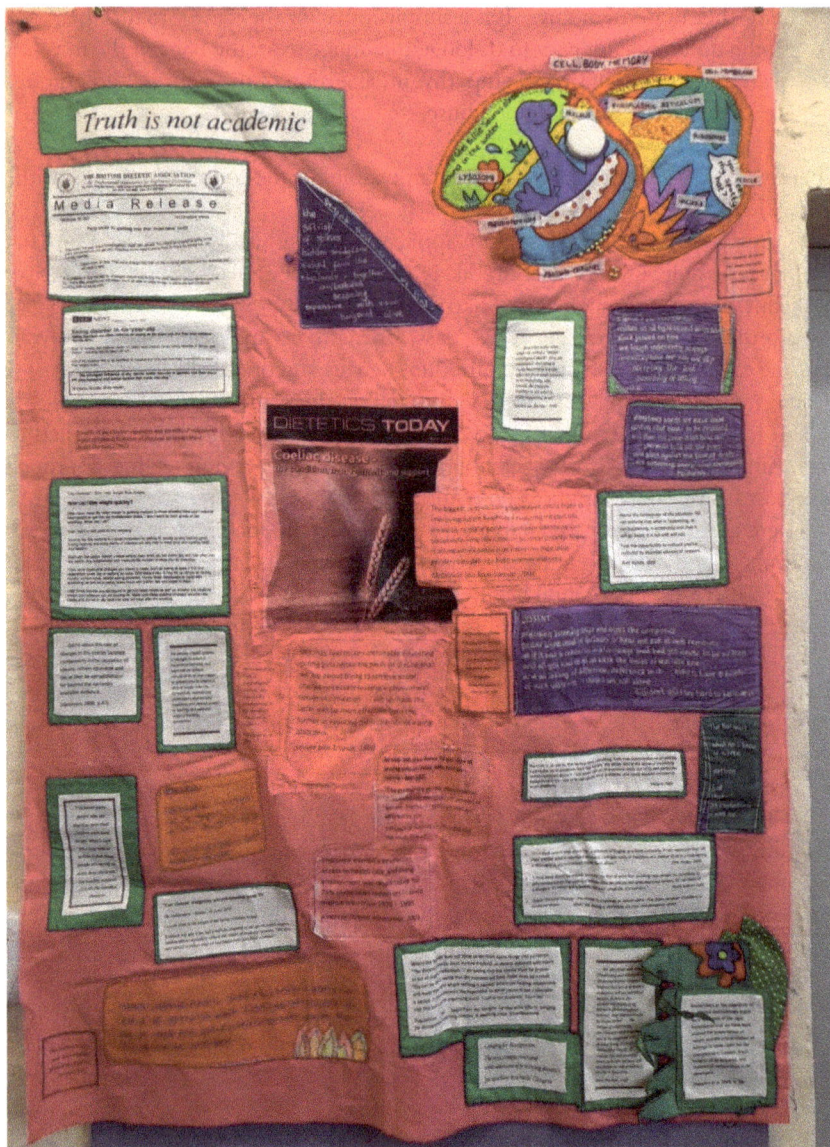

Figure 37.2 Truth Is Not Academic. Lucy Aphramor.

Academic interlock to form a disjointed narrative. It has a coherence that musses coherence.

The pieces are photocopied text, silk paintings, and babies' cloth books. Topics covered include tips for alterative behaviours to bingeing; gender and childhood sexual abuse; anti-queerness; self-harm; the association between eating disorders and young women's experiences of violence; misogyny in dietetic imagery; domestic violence; data on patriarchy and public health; dietitian Jacqui Gingras's book *Longing for Recognition* (2009); comments from a range of womanist and feminist philosophers and pedagogists on the need for new language and methods. Most of these themes are absent from mainstream dietetic texts.

Jangling these concerns together suggests there is a way of making sense of them through interconnections and foregrounds context. The effect is to steer the viewer to organize their responses, knowledge, thoughts, and feelings into something usefully disturbing. There is a projection of hope, the belief that growth – as the forest not the megapolis – is possible.

I made it to take to a seminar, Beyond Nutritionism, at Ryerson University in 2009. I had no idea how I would bring it into the discussion, if at all. And when I did, Cath Morley – dietitian, film maker, and textile artist – jumped up to unfurl her textile poster. This workshop led to the founding of the World Critical Dietetics movement. Borrowing the ecofeminist phrase, we spent the time "hearing each other into speech."

The Quilt/Scream and poster made my unknowings tangible and discussable. They helped me acknowledge the unworded terror, chaos, and confusion that backboned my life.

More recently I made another huge piece. I've only shown it to one person so far. The Tear. Like the Quilt/Scream, it's been made from survival mode. It's overwhelming, disturbing. Even for the person I showed it to who knows me well, who knows that I'm no longer debilitated by daily struggling with the chaos and pain it captures, it was still overwhelming, disturbing. Like the Quilt/Scream, the perturbation registers viscerally. It disturbs me to look at it, like a whole-body dysphoria that lingers. I keep it rolled up and out of sight, the monstrosity in the closet. It's a tangible reminder that there's more deep learning, more unravelling, more freedom available. There is no sorted. Ha.

Making each of these pieces enabled a letting go into deep learning. Not learning as additional facts: I "just" stop blocking what I already know in some way. I am honest with myself. As a result, something changes around shame, acceptance, joy, spaciousness. I am rearranged. Living my life gets easier (notwithstanding immediate consequences of upheaval) and my thinking can shift, my identity too.

Creativity helps me to know "Cognitively, erotically, viscerally, verbally, poetically, indeterminately, certainly, narily, spiritually, in the tears we shed, in the pain that screams us, in our injury and pleasures in our heartache and broken sleep in our bones." (Dark & Aphramor, 2021)

It's more often poetry, particularly spoken-word poetry, that I've turned to at the push-pull of no longer being able to ignore the feeling that there is something (dangerous) lurking, demanding acknowledgement. The feminist novelist Virginia Woolf says, "If you do not tell the truth about yourself you cannot tell it about other people" (Woolf, 1947). Poetry has let me tell the truth about myself to myself, and then to others, which has profoundly changed what I know.

There's something particular that happens when the saying involves the physicality and energetic exchange of performance. Repeating the hard, painful, taboo thing to an audience metabolizes it into something that lives, integrated, generatively insinuated, in my bodymind. It frees me up to be with people and place differently, to know the next awkward or explosive thing and to know differently. Once, warming up for a show I fell bodily into the memory I was recounting, connecting with it emotionally for the first time. As one reviewer says, on stage it looks like I could genuinely break down at any minute (Turnbull, 2017). Performing has let me know I can tap terror and not get trapped there. It's an incredibly liberating experience.

The audacity of the Performing Self scares me: they are bold, shameless, impatient, sorted, ready to tackle the flack. And then there's me. Not so bold. Being politically committed to challenging white supremacy and breaking silences doesn't annul trepidation.

The first time I said "cunt" on stage was a big deal. Theatre (like ceremony) means we get to present differently than we feel. Each respected, connected telling makes telling less costly. We sink deeper into the darkness of our mind.

I want you
to fuck
me
up the arse
hard
so it hurts
as real learning
must
thrusting us
into a knowing
beyond anything yet wordable
I want to hover over wholeness
my body a concoction rendered receptive by the yearning that precedes
the reworlding I dare to imagine is possible

I let myself know and say disruptive and uncomfortable things through poetry, things I'm not ready for and then live into them. Creativity makes the unthinkable thinkable and allows us to say the unsayable. This happens through the entanglement of a personal (healing) process, identity shifts, bodily receptivity, and scholarly readjustment. This disregard of binary borders is also a queering. Like Queerness, Creativity leaves behind the discrete, autonomous, Rational self of coloniality, separate from the environment and in dominion over Nature and presumes an enmeshed world. This is a world whose cosmologies exceed those of white supremacy's binary paradigm.

In this way, the not-knowing and coming-to-know and confusions of Creativity and Queerness have significantly altered my own learning and/as healing and what I can offer, receive, and create around healing and/as learning. As Rachel Naomi Remen (2021) says, "At the deepest level, the creative process and the healing process arise from a single source. When you are an artist, you are a healer; a wordless trust of the same mystery is the foundation of your work and its integrity."

Rapture and Rupture

They realize at last that change does not mean reform, that change does not mean improvement.

(Fanon, 2007)

The nebulous promptings of Creativity jostled me to a place of rupture where I recognized the onto-epistemological flaws in my own arguments endorsing an approach to dietetics called health at every size (Aphramor, 20, 2021).

Creativity helped me incorporate trauma and reconcile with my failings and foolishness so I could move into and out of relationship in ways that broke with silencing.

I became less conflict avoidant. In this and other ways Creativity has helped me stray further and further from whiteness. I get now that stitching The Scream was a practice. It was a practice I committed to over several years because I knew it was important even though I didn't know what I was doing (making) at the time. The same calling draws me to land-based practices where I don't know what I'm doing but I know it is important to do it.

Creativity schools us in uncertainty, indeterminancy, confusion, queerness, and humility. It urges us to go off-grid into wild imaginings, into sensuosity, ineptitude, spirituality, and the erotic. It screws with colonial borders and launches us into a bewildering pluriverse of possibilities. This pluriverse doesn't cage knowing to whiteness's binary but flamboyantly and strategically exceeds the limits of our colonial-schooled imagination. It lives and shape-shifts beyond my faculties for comprehension or perception. It reorganizes food work beyond the choice of Diet or Non-Diet or Well Now in the other worldings (Harrison, 2021) of Aboriginal Food Ways, Via Campesina, Nalgona Positivity Pride, Gordibuena, the Zapatista, and galaxies of other cosmologies.

Diving into the Wreck

White supremacy is continually disseminating spores that embed in the world and adapt to local circumstances to nurture anti-Black, anti-fat, anti-queer orientations currently streaming as Rationality, Progress, Modernity, Certainty, Perfectionism, and the ideology of evidence-based practice.

Creativity and Queering challenge whiteness as they are intimately and reciprocally intrarelated with Blackness, Indigeneity, and animism. Each of these orientations reject dietetics' colonial constructs of "self" and "'health," of humans as other-than Nature, of linear time. Creative practice made me receptive to these truths, to the other worldings that Black scholars write into being (Akomolaf, 2020; Harrison, 2021).

Creativity and Queerness are anti-colonial and also (re)indigenizing. They know that the logic of evidence-based practice is the logic of whiteness, one that presumes Western science is the only credible science. The logic that fetishizes Randomized Controlled Trials as the pinnacle of useful data is a logic of clean lines, clear divisions, extracted variables, an inert context, Universal truth, linear time. In other words, of Rationality, Linearity, Modernity, Progress and as such it is inherently anti-Black and anti-Queer, and anti-Creativity.

We are schooled to perpetuate the myth of evidence-based practice as the judicious use of the best available data for the greater good. When it is the obedient use of whatever white supremacy considers relevant as data for the good of white supremacy.

An education that has us believe evidence-based practice is neutral may have so thoroughly imbued us with anti-Blackness that words like animism and cosmology and deities provoke disdain. Anti-Blackness may be so rooted in us that a dietetics that respects the personhood of lettuces feels laughable, the need for land-based knowledge preposterous. We may believe that any transformative potential of dietetics hinges on what our white bodies can register and measure, on what we understand and value. But we'd be wrong.

For sure, animism, and cosmology and deities are troubling words for a dietitian to use respectfully because they break the contract with white supremacy. The problem is not that they suggest tree-hugging, sex magic, singing plants and singing to plants, entities, voodoo, food as medicine, ancestral reverence, and other manifestations of Blackness and Queerness. The problem is that white supremacy has taught us to feel and think ourselves superior to Blackness and Queerness, to feel and think Blackness through words like superstition, esoteric and "barbarism" that render it disposable. As a result, we feel entitled, obliged even, to dismiss Black knowledges out of hand, justifying derision via an assemblage of body signals that confirm our infallibility and righteousness to ourselves.

The novelist and scholar James Baldwin declared that "The American Dream is at the expense of the American Negro" (1965). Our allegiance to evidence-based practice is an allegiance to whiteness made at the expense of liberation and of our Indigenous colleagues, our Black colleagues, and our colleagues who are People of Colour.

Respect to Indigenous dietitians for their wisdom and endurance. Respect to those who share and develop the teachings of Blackness. Respect for the human and non-human Beings who hold knowledges that coloniality still trains us to erase.

Liberation, and the scientific attitude, require us to make best use of what we know collectively to survive and strategize. I hope I have demonstrated the vital role of recognizing white supremacy as we build knowledge for freedom. I hope I have also impressed on (white) readers the need to train ourselves to value Blackness and to engage in this work from an ethic of care and repair.

I hope I have left you with a sense of how creativity and queerness helped me survive and start to flourish, and how they are implicated in liberatory knowledge creation. I hope there is enough to corroborate my claim that dietetic norms make us oblivious to the ways we nurture white supremacy. And enough to prompt you/us to counter this by noticing and undoing whiteness so that things fall apart.

References

Akomolafe, B. (2020, January 22). On slowing down in urgent times. *For the Wild Podcast.*

Aphramor, L. (2018, August 14–26). Enough. Solo theatre show. Venue 42. Edinburgh Fringe. Director Tian Glasgow.

Aphramor, L. (2021, June 30). Hey! are you one of 401k people misled by our HAES theory? *Medium.* https://lucy-aphramor.medium.com/hey-are-you-one-the-401k -readers-misled-by-our-haes-theory-14bc3b02276e

Baldwin, J. (1965). In *the famous Baldwin-Buckley debate still matters today* by Gabrielle Bellot. https://www.theatlantic.com/entertainment/archive/2019/12/james-baldwin -william-f-buckley-debate/602695/

Caswell, K. (2007, April). In "it could have been so beautiful - Coventry circa 2007" mixed media exhibition. St Mary's Guildhall, Coventry.

Dark, K., & Aphramor, L. (2021). Fat politics as a constituent of intersecting intimacies. *Fat Studies Journal.* In Press.

Fanon, F. (2007). *The Wretched of the Earth*, p. 79, Grove/Atlantic, Inc.

Gingras, J. (2009). *Longing for recognition: The joys, complexities, and contradictions of practicing dietetics.* Raw Nerve/UK.

Harrison, D. L. (2021). *Belly of the beast: The politics of anti-fatness as anti-blackness.* North Atlantic Books.

Remen, R. N. (not given). In creativity and spirituality. Retrieved December 5, 2021, from https://www.sanctuaryspiritualcare.com/creativity-and-spirituality

Turnbull, J. (2017, September 6). The naked dietitian: A true radical. *DisabilityArts* Online. https://disabilityarts.online/magazine/opinion/naked-dietitian-true-radical/

Woolf, V. (1947). *The moment and other essays.* Retrieved October 30, 2021, from https:// gutenberg.net.au/ebooks15/1500221h.html

Index

Note: Page numbers in *italics* indicate figures and **bold** indicate tables in the text